DBT

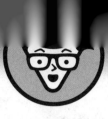

DBT

by Gillian Galen, PsyD, and
Blaise Aguirre, MD

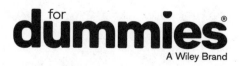

DBT For Dummies®

Published by: **John Wiley & Sons, Inc.**, 111 River Street, Hoboken, NJ 07030-5774, www.wiley.com

Copyright © 2021 by John Wiley & Sons, Inc., Hoboken, New Jersey

Published simultaneously in Canada

For general information on our other products and services, please contact our Customer Care Department within the U.S. at 877-762-2974, outside the U.S. at 317-572-3993, or fax 317-572-4002. For technical support, please visit https://hub.wiley.com/community/support/dummies.

Wiley publishes in a variety of print and electronic formats and by print-on-demand. Some material included with standard print versions of this book may not be included in e-books or in print-on-demand. If this book refers to media such as a CD or DVD that is not included in the version you purchased, you may download this material at http://booksupport.wiley.com. For more information about Wiley products, visit www.wiley.com.

Library of Congress Control Number: 2021935362

ISBN 978-1-119-73012-5 (pbk); ISBN 978-1-119-72567-1 (ebk); ISBN 978-1-119-73016-3 (ebk)

Manufactured in the United States of America

SKY10027237_052021

Contents at a Glance

Table of Contents

Introduction

In our professional experience, at no other time have we seen more of a demand for compassionate, effective, and comprehensive mental health care than we did in the strange year of 2020. The mental health toll caused by the isolating impact of the COVID-19 pandemic, the financial uncertainties of the economy, the divisive polarization of social justice causes, and the doubt and suspicions magnified by political extremes has impacted those without mental health issues, significantly impacted those with mental health issues, and even affected mental health practitioners. We are, after all, human beings whose brains respond to stress, strong emotions, and lack of connection.

We all need to take care of ourselves, and we don't have time to spend years contemplating our lives. The changes you make today will reverberate throughout the rest of your life. Now is the time to start behaving in ways that are consistent with your values and your aspirations. Of course, you need the help of others — even the most powerful of quarterbacks cannot win without a supportive team — but you can also take charge of some of your own self-care. You don't need the blessing of others to start changing your behaviors, by eating healthier food, exercising more regularly, getting to bed on time, reducing your alcohol intake, and practicing some meditation every day. And then, when you're a healthier person, you bring a more skillful version of yourself to your life and to the relationships that you care about.

We have told our patients, friends, families, and colleagues that DBT — dialectical behavior therapy — is not just for our patients but is also a life enhancer for everyone. When we practice DBT, we are better able to take care of ourselves and our relationships, we are more compassionate, and we make less judgmental assumptions. We don't say these things simply because we authored this book, but because we have seen the benefits of DBT in our personal and professional lives.

About This Book

DBT For Dummies is a book for our time. The world in 2020 — when we wrote this book — was full of the most unexpected of challenges. There was a global pandemic, a contentious election, and demonstrations that highlighted significant divisions within our communities. These are experiences that demand the most of us, and yet can also bring out our weaknesses and struggles.

For those who already fight against underlying mental health conditions, the need to be able to regulate, connect effectively, tolerate difficult moments without sinking deeper into despair, and pay attention to the present moment, each other, and ourselves makes the need for the skills in this book timely and essential. These are skills that, if learned, used, and practiced on a regular basis, will get us not only through this moment but through all future moments, whether or not they are filled with uncertainty.

Almost everything you need to know about DBT is in this book, whether you're new to the therapy or an expert practitioner looking for new ideas. We want to be very clear that this book is no substitute for expert therapy. Reading it will inform you and give you some good ideas as to what to do, but it takes a therapist skilled in DBT to help you if you're struggling.

Along our own journey with DBT, we've had many patients tell us that they did DBT before and that although we use many similar terms and practices, what we did was different. Many of our protocols will be identical to those of other DBT therapists. However, because DBT is not only protocol-based but also principle-driven, there is also an art to DBT, and that is the way in which it is delivered. Many of the ideas in this book come directly out of our own clinical practice, and different therapists may apply the therapy differently.

As with all *For Dummies* guides, you won't have to read this book from start to finish as you would so many other books. If the only thing you're interested in is how to practice emotion regulation, how to use mindfulness to improve your relationships, or how to apply DBT to a specific mental disorder, the information is here, easily found, and ready to be read and comprehended in minutes.

A quick note: Sidebars (shaded boxes of text) dig into the details of a given topic, but they aren't crucial to understanding it. Feel free to read them or skip them. You can pass over the text accompanied by the Technical Stuff icon, too. The text marked with this icon gives some interesting but non-essential information about some of the more technical procedures in DBT.

One last thing: Within this book, you may note that some web addresses break across two lines of text. If you're reading this book in print and want to visit one of these web pages, simply key in the web address exactly as it appears in the text, pretending as though the line break doesn't exist. If you're reading this as an e-book, you've got it easy — just click the web address to go directly to the web page.

Foolish Assumptions

Dear reader, we make a few assumptions about you. No, you're no dummy; however, you're reading this book because you want a clearer, less jargon-filled understanding of dialectical behavior therapy. You may have some basic knowledge about the therapy, and you may have heard that it's useful to treat certain conditions, but this book will offer a much clearer picture of this fascinating therapy.

We also recognize that no book is a substitute for expert therapy, and we assume that anyone who is in need of help will seek it out, even if they use this book as a guide for understanding. Finally, we assume that readers who are suffering might do so in ways that make it hard to learn new approaches. We value you tremendously and support you in your efforts to improve, despite the obstacles that life may have thrown at you.

Icons Used in This Book

We include some handy icons that you may notice in the margins of this book. They point you to certain types of information, so be sure you know which is which.

We include some text that tips you off into certain directions — this icon makes sure you notice. These aren't substitutes for practicing the skills as they are intended, but they are reminders that might make it easier to remember a skill.

Although we'd like you to remember everything we say, we have seen time and again just how easy things are to forget. We will repeat things, because we know that repetition is a great way to learn, and if you tend to forget, if you see this icon, be sure to ingrain this information in your brain.

Just as we want you to remember everything we say in this book, and that we'd love for you to *do* everything we recommend, it's possible (okay, highly likely) that you'll only do half (okay, a quarter) of what we suggest. But to truly stay away from pitfalls that can create significant obstacles to your healing, you should heed any warnings that you see associated with this icon.

Just like any expert, we do have nuggets of knowledge that only some of our most persistent patients and DBT junkies could love. But we know that you may want to know more and delve deeper into subjects like neural pathways and brain chemicals. If these excite you rather than putting you to sleep, we welcome you to dive in with us. However, if you prefer, you can skip the information associated with this icon. This is *the only* icon that points you to information that you can skip if you prefer to.

Beyond the Book

In addition to the material in the print or e-book you're reading now, this product comes with some access-anywhere goodies on the web. Check out the free Cheat Sheet for interesting information on what to expect from DBT, the components of DBT, and useful skills you'll discover. To get this Cheat Sheet, simply go to www.dummies.com and search for "*DBT For Dummies* Cheat Sheet" in the Search box.

Where to Go from Here

At this point. . .browse! Check out the detailed table of contents and go straight to those chapters that grab your interest. This isn't a novel that you need to read from start to finish. It's more like when our children open up the fridge and take the things they want. If you're totally new to DBT, though, we do recommend starting with Chapter 1.

As you understand more and more about DBT, and maybe even teach your therapist a thing or two, keep coming back to this book and discover more information, which will increasingly be accompanied by "aha" moments, and do let us know. We thank you for including us on your journey.

1

The Nuts and Bolts of DBT

Discover how DBT (dialectical behavior therapy) was developed.

Understand the components of a comprehensive DBT treatment.

Recognize the elements of a contemplative mindfulness practice as a core part of DBT, and figure out how to accept multiple points of view.

Interweave behaviorism into mindfulness practices to develop a complete therapy.

Chapter **1**

Entering the World of DBT

E ntering the world of DBT (dialectical behavior therapy) is entering into a world that focuses on the philosophical process of dialectics, while also attending to the psychological process of behaviorism and change. Imagine entering into a therapy that tells you that everything is composed of opposites, that these opposites are all true, that everything changes except for change itself, and that the way out of suffering is to start by accepting that all of these things are true. This chapter introduces the basics.

Looking at the Main Pillars of DBT

REMEMBER

DBT stands on three big philosophical and scientific pillars. These pillars are specific assumptions that hold the treatment together:

>> **All things are interconnected.** Everything and everyone is interconnected and interdependent. We are all part of the greater tapestry of all things, a community of beings that supports and sustains us. We are also connected to our family, friends, and community. We need others; others need us.

>> **Change is constant and inevitable.** This is not a new idea. The pre-Socratic philosopher Heraclitus said, "The only constant in life is change." Life is full of suffering, but because change happens, change being the only thing of which you can be certain, your suffering will change as well.

>> **Opposites can be integrated to form a closer approximation of the truth.** This is at the core of dialectics. A dialectical synthesis combines the thesis (an idea) and the antithesis (its opposite). In coming up with the synthesis of the two ideas, the process never introduces a new concept not found in either the thesis or the antithesis. Strictly speaking, the synthesis incorporates one concept from the thesis and one from the antithesis.

Check out Chapter 2 for more about DBT's main pillars.

Getting an Overview of DBT's Treatment Modes and Functions

DBT was originally developed by Dr. Marsha Linehan for the treatment of people who struggled with self-destructive and suicidal behavior, and it subsequently became the gold-standard treatment for the condition known as borderline personality disorder (BPD), which we review comprehensively in Chapter 20. The treatment appeals to many therapists and patients, not only because it is very helpful, but because it integrates four essential elements in a comprehensive treatment by addressing the biological, environmental, spiritual, and behavioral elements of a person's struggle. It's also unique in its focus on balancing the need for a person to change while being completely accepted for who they are in the present moment.

As you find out in Chapter 2, DBT delivers the treatment through four modes, and these four modes address the five functions of a comprehensive treatment.

The four modes of therapy

There are four modes of therapy, which are detailed completely in Chapter 14:

>> **Individual therapy:** In this mode, a trained therapist works with you to apply newly learned skills to your personal life challenges.

>> **Group skills training:** In this mode, together with a group of other patients, you're taught new behavioral skills, you complete homework assignments, and you role-play new ways of interacting with others.

>> **Phone skills coaching:** In this mode, you can call your therapist between sessions to receive guidance on coping with difficult situations as they arise.

>> **Therapist consultation team meetings:** In this mode, your individual therapist meets with other therapists who are also providing DBT treatment. These meetings help therapists navigate difficult and complex issues related to providing therapy, and give them new ideas for what to do when they are stuck. Chapter 17 goes into more detail on the consultation team.

The five functions of treatment

As you see in the previous section, DBT is a comprehensive treatment program. In this way, DBT is a collection of treatments, rather than a single treatment method conducted by a single therapist and a single patient. Any program, whichever you choose to do, should address five key functions of treatment (which are fully reviewed in Part 4):

>> **Increasing your motivation to change:** Changing self-destructive and maladaptive behaviors can be very difficult, and it can be easy to become disheartened. Your individual therapist will work with you to make sure you stay on track and reduce any behaviors that are inconsistent with a life worth living. Within individual and group therapy, your therapist will ask you to track your behaviors and use skills coaching in order to achieve this goal.

>> **Enhancing your capabilities:** DBT assumes that people who struggle either lack or need to improve several important life skills, including skills that help you regulate emotions, pay attention to the experience of the present moment, effectively navigate interpersonal situations, and finally, be able to tolerate distress.

>> **Generalizing what you've learned in therapy to the rest of your life:** If the skills you've learned in group and individual therapy sessions don't transfer to your daily life, then it's going to be difficult to say that the therapy was successful for dealing with your problems.

>> **Structuring your environment in order to reinforce your gains:** An important function is to make sure that you don't slip back into maladaptive or problematic behaviors or, if you do, to make sure that the impact isn't enduring. Structuring the treatment in a manner that promotes progress toward your goal is a way to do this. Typically, your individual therapist will make sure that all of the elements of effective treatment are in place for you. At times, they may intervene for you if you aren't yet skilled enough to do so for yourself, with the understanding that such intervention is temporary until you have acquired the skills to manage.

>> **Increasing your therapist's motivation and competence:** Although helping people who come to therapy with multiple problems can be very rewarding for both patient and therapist, the behaviors that people present with can be very taxing for the therapist, and so the therapist needs help to stay in the game of DBT. This is where the DBT consultation team that you read about in the previous section comes in.

Focusing on the DBT Theoretical Framework

The practice of DBT relies on three central theories:

>> **The biosocial theory:** Dr. Linehan's biosocial theory essentially states that people who struggle in regulating their emotions do so because of an enduring interaction between that person's biological makeup — one that makes them more emotionally sensitive, more emotionally reactive, and slower to return to their emotional baseline — and what she termed the invalidating environment.

An *invalidating environment* is one where a child's emotional experiences aren't recognized as valid or tolerated by significant people in the child's life. When this happens, and a child's emotional experiences aren't validated until the child has escalated emotionally and with high intensity, the child effectively learns that they have to escalate to be heard. When they get punished for expressing high emotions, the child might take their difficulties underground and try to regulate by using maladaptive behaviors such as self-injury. This, in turn, leads to even greater emotionality, as the child experiences shame and guilt. Flip to Chapter 2 for more about the biosocial theory.

>> **Behavioral theory:** The behavioral theory seeks to explain human behavior by analyzing the antecedents of the behavior. *Antecedents* are the events, situations, circumstances, emotions, and thoughts that preceded the

behavior — in other words, the events that were happening before the behavior occurred — and the *consequences* of the behavior are the actions or responses that follow the behavior. It's in understanding the elements that are causing behaviors to manifest — and then further understanding what keeps the behaviors going — that the behavioral theory is applied in order to reduce maladaptive behaviors and increase adaptive responses.

An important element to this theory is that maladaptive behaviors are maintained because a person lacks the skills for more adaptive functioning due to problems in processing emotions and thoughts, which is why there is such an emphasis on teaching helpful emotion regulation skills. We discuss regulating your emotions in Chapter 10.

>> **The philosophy of dialectics:** Essentially, *dialectical theory* states that reality is the tapestry of interconnected and interwoven forces, many of which are opposing one another. It is the continuing synthesis of opposing forces, ideas, or concepts that defines dialectics. Chapter 15 has more information on dialectics.

Checking Out the DBT Stages of Treatment

DBT consists of five stages of treatment, one of which is pretreatment:

>> **Pretreatment:** This is the period of time when the person is making a direct commitment to themselves and their therapist to do DBT therapy. In this stage of pretreatment, the patient also creates a hierarchical list of problem behaviors that interfere with their living the life they want to live.

>> **Stage 1:** In this stage, the main goal is to reduce the most severe behaviors that greatly impact a person's life. These include life-threatening behaviors such as suicide and self-injury, therapy-interfering behaviors such as being late to therapy or not completing homework assignments, and quality-of-life-interfering behaviors such as substance misuse and hurtful relationships. Finally, they want to increase behavioral skills that are done in the skills-group format.

>> **Stage 2:** In this stage, the person focuses on emotional experiencing and attending to the trauma in their life, trauma that has often led to misery and desperation.

>> **Stage 3:** In this stage, residual problems such as boredom, emptiness, grieving, and life goals are addressed.

>> **Stage 4:** In this final stage, the person works on deepening their self-awareness and their sense of incompleteness, becoming more spiritually fulfilled, and recognizing that most of happiness lies within the self.

Surveying DBT Skills

DBT assumes that many of the problems that people experience occur because they don't have, or can't effectively use, the skills to manage emotionally charged situations. More specifically, the failure to use effective behavior when it's needed is often a result of not knowing skillful behavior or, if known, how to use it. Consistent with this idea of skills deficit, the use of DBT skills during standard treatment — in group, individual therapy, and coaching — has been found to lead to a reduction in suicidal behavior, non-suicidal self-injury, and depression, and to improve emotion regulation and relationship problems. In Part 3, we thoroughly review these skills:

>> **Mindfulness:** In part derived from Zen and mystical meditative practices, DBT teaches people the importance of how to be mindful. It involves reflecting on two considerations: "What do I do in order to practice mindfulness?" and "How do I practice these mindfulness skills?"

>> **Interpersonal effectiveness:** DBT teaches more effective ways for people to get what they need and what they want, how to reduce interpersonal conflict, how to repair relationships, and how to say "no" to unreasonable requests. The focus is on helping a person build self-respect, improve their self-advocacy, and recognize their needs as valid.

>> **Distress tolerance:** Whereas many approaches to mental health treatment focus on changing stressful situations, DBT focuses on teaching people skills that allow them to tolerate these situations, which are often fraught with emotional pain or distress. Within the skills, there is also a recognition of the importance of distinguishing between accepting reality as it is and approving of this reality.

>> **Emotion regulation:** Central to many of the problems in which DBT is effective is the finding that people who struggle with regulating their emotions lack the ability to do so effectively. The focus of this skills module is to get people to know what emotion they are experiencing, what the vulnerability factors are to dysregulated emotions, what the functions of emotions are, and then how to deal with the emotions when they are disproportionate to the situation.

Walking through the Mechanics of DBT

As mentioned earlier in this chapter, a comprehensive DBT treatment goes beyond individual therapy and includes group skills training, phone coaching, and a consultation team for the therapists. The group sessions are typically held once per week and run for two-and-a-half hours. In the group, the four skills modules that are mentioned in the preceding section — mindfulness, interpersonal effectiveness, distress tolerance, and emotion regulation — are taught. (These are extensively reviewed in Part 3 of this book.)

REMEMBER

It typically takes six months to get through all the components of all the modules, and many people who do a course of DBT repeat it. As a result, it takes about a year in total. It can take longer if there are co-occurring disorders such as post-traumatic stress disorder.

In the skills-group session, the first part is dedicated to reviewing the previous week's assigned homework, while the second part is used for learning, teaching, and practicing new skills. In individual therapy, the skills learned in the group are reviewed within the context of the person's individual treatment needs and goals. One way to think about this is that the skills groups put the skills into the person, while the individual therapy extracts them in the context of the person's life.

Treating Specific Conditions with DBT

Most studies on the efficacy of DBT have been completed in people who struggle with borderline personality disorder; however, DBT has been studied in many other conditions (which are more fully reviewed in Part 5). DBT has been shown to have a degree of effectiveness, either on its own or in combination with other behavioral therapies, for conditions such as the following:

>> Post-traumatic stress disorder (PTSD)

>> Substance use disorder (SUD)

>> Binge eating disorder (BED)

It has also been used in diverse populations:

>> Adolescents (see Chapter 13)

>> Prison populations

>> People with developmental disabilities

>> Family members of people with borderline personality disorder

>> Students who would benefit from a social-emotional learning curriculum in schools

Chapter **2**

Understanding Dialectical Behavior Therapy

Dialectical behavior theory (DBT) was initially developed by Marsha M. Linehan, Ph.D., a psychologist at the University of Washington, to help adult women with a condition known as borderline personality disorder (BPD). BPD is characterized by intense swings in emotions, difficulties with intimate and close relationships, self-destructive behavior, and at times suicidal behavior. For many people with BPD, the possibility of death by suicide makes it one of the most difficult of mental health conditions to treat. In fact, before DBT, BPD was considered a uniquely difficult psychiatric condition to treat; neither medications nor psychotherapy seemed to provide any kind of immediate relief.

However, because people who were suicidal were not "just" suicidal but also had many other problems, having a therapy that dealt with *all* of a person's problems was essential to having a comprehensive, supportive, and successful treatment. Further, the treatment needed to be useful to both patient and therapist, because many therapists would often find themselves terrified of treating suicidal patients, and so they also needed support.

Enter DBT. In this chapter, you discover the basics of this therapy, including the biosocial theory, treatment functions and goals, modes of treatment, and the dialectical process.

Beginning with the Biosocial Theory

REMEMBER

Dr. Linehan recognized that certain conditions and disorders such as BPD were characterized primarily by *emotion dysregulation* — in other words, difficulty in regulating (through recognizing and then skillfully either tolerating or effectively dealing with the impact of powerful and at times painful) emotions. She stated that these difficulties emerged from the transaction between an individual's biological and genetic makeup and specific environmental factors (a concept known as the *biosocial theory*). She noted that people with conditions like BPD had three prominent characteristics:

>> They tended to be very emotionally sensitive, which means that they tended to react very quickly and with more intensity than the average person to events that led to emotional experiences.

>> When emotions flared up, they had difficulty controlling them, and this in turn led to behavior that was dictated by their mood state; as a result, when a person with BPD was in a good mood, they could get almost anything done, and when they were in a bad mood, they had a difficult time meeting the expectations of the moment. This type of behavior based on mood is termed *mood-dependent behavior.*

>> When the person experienced these intense and heightened emotions, it took them longer than the average person to get back down to their emotional baseline.

The following sections discuss dysregulation and environmental factors in more detail.

Types of dysregulation

Over time, people who were emotionally sensitive and who didn't have the skills to manage difficult situations and relationships in their lives would develop enduring difficulties in regulating five areas of daily experience. The term used by therapists for an inability to regulate is *dysregulation*, and so people with conditions like BPD had the following five areas of dysregulation, a conceptualization originally described by Dr. Linehan in 1993:

>> **Emotion dysregulation:** *Emotion dysregulation* is the inability to flexibly respond to and manage one's feelings in the context of emotional responses that are highly reactive. Typically, these are brief episodes, lasting a few hours, but they feel overwhelming. Although a person with BPD might have difficulty regulating all emotions, irritability and anger are specified in the *Diagnostic and Statistical Manual of Mental Disorders* (DSM), which is the manual that mental health experts use to classify psychiatric conditions.

>> **Interpersonal dysregulation:** *Interpersonal dysregulation* is characterized by a fear, whether real or imagined, that the person with BPD will be abandoned by those closest to them. In this context, the person with BPD will then become desperate to prevent the abandonment from occurring and will then behave in ways to stop it from happening. These ways will often appear to be extreme to the person on the receiving end of the behavior, and at times can be the reason why that person no longer wants to have anything to do with the person with BPD.

Another hallmark of this is that people with BPD tend to develop intense relationships with others, and these are characterized by extremes of, at times, idealizing the other person and then, at other times, devaluing the other person. These fluctuations can happen very quickly and leave the other person feeling bewildered.

>> **Self-dysregulation.** *Self-dysregulation* is characterized by having an unstable sense of self and the experience of feeling empty inside. People with BPD can have a very difficult time defining themselves in terms of who they are as people, what their values are, and what their long-term goals and life direction are. At times they look to others and others' behavior, and try to copy it in order to fit in, but they often recognize that when they simply behave differently, it does not always feel authentic. Another aspect of self-dysregulation is the experience of emptiness, which is an intense feeling of disconnectedness, aloneness, and feeling misunderstood.

>> **Cognitive dysregulation:** *Cognitive dysregulation* is characterized by relatively brief episodes of paranoid thinking, and this is particularly true during periods of stress. This means that when the person with BPD has high stress levels, they can begin to imagine that others are intentionally out to get them, even when there is no evidence that this is true. People with BPD can also experience *dissociation,* which is the feeling or thought that they are not real or that the rest of the world is not real.

>> **Behavioral dysregulation:** *Behavioral dysregulation* in people with BPD is characterized by extreme, sometimes impulsive, and at times dangerous behaviors. These behaviors are often used as a way to deal with intense and unbearable emotions, and can include self-injurious behaviors, such as cutting and suicide attempts. Other such behaviors include eating behaviors, such as binge eating, substance use as a way to fit in or self-medicate, dangerous sexual behaviors as a way to feel connected, and dangerous driving or excessive spending as ways to feel a rush of positive emotions.

The invalidating environment

The environmental factor that Dr. Linehan proposed was most significant in the development of BPD in a person who had the emotional makeup in the previous section was what she termed the *invalidating environment*. The invalidating environment has certain characteristics, as you find out in the following sections.

Intolerance of emotional expression

The invalidating environment is *intolerant* of another person's expression of private emotional experiences and, in particular, emotions that aren't supported by observable events. For instance, if a person believes that they are unlovable and becomes extremely sad because of this, it's typical for others to tell them that it isn't true and that their statement that they aren't lovable isn't supported by the facts. A person feeling unlovable isn't something that another person can observe, and so simply telling the person who is struggling with such thoughts that what they are thinking isn't true is invalidating because it takes away the validity of that person's emotional experience.

In other words, it may be factually incorrect that that person isn't loved, and yet the emotion that they experience is real and is not readily dispelled simply by someone saying that they shouldn't feel it.

REMEMBER

Invalidation occurs when you tell another person that it doesn't make sense that they feel a certain way. Telling a person not to feel the way they feel rarely leads them to change their emotional experience, and it also tells them that the way they feel is out of proportion to whatever event elicited the emotion.

Reinforcement of strong emotions

Another feature of the invalidating environment is that it can *reinforce* displays of strong emotions. Reinforcement is any consequence that comes after a behavior that increases the likelihood that the behavior will either increase or be maintained at current levels.

TIP

Another way to think about a reinforcer is that it's like a reward. So, if a person is ignored when they are distressed at low levels of emotional expression but attended to when they have big emotions, and if what they want is other people's attention, then it makes sense that high emotions will show up more frequently.

Shame

Another feature of the invalidating environment is that when a person is told that their displays of emotional upset are unacceptable, unwarranted, or unjustified, they often begin to feel *shame* for having behaved in the way they did or even for having any emotions at all. The problem with this is that shaming someone doesn't teach them what to do when they are feeling strong emotions, and as such, they don't learn what to do the next time strong emotions show up. It also prevents a person from learning how to accurately name and label their emotions.

Imagine that a person could not name and label vegetables and that they were told to go buy vegetables but instead came back with bread and milk and were then ridiculed for not having bought vegetables. Shaming this person wouldn't teach them what they had to do, and long-term shame can cause significant psychological damage. In such situations, what the person actually learns is to oscillate between going to great lengths to prevent the display of big emotions for fear of being punished and then having big emotional eruptions without knowing how to manage them.

Dismissal of problems and reactions

Finally, the invalidating environment tells emotionally sensitive people that their problems are *easy to solve.* "Oh, just calm down. That's what I do," a parent might tell an emotionally sensitive adolescent. Whereas this may be easy for the parent, it might not be for the child. When people who are emotionally sensitive and, according to the biosocial theory, have a biologically hard-wired temperament or disposition toward being emotionally vulnerable, they have a relatively low threshold for responding to factors in the environment that are emotionally arousing.

It would be like a child having been born with a peanut allergy and being sensitive to peanuts in the environment. Telling the child not to have a reaction to peanuts would ignore what the child's biology is. Similarly, telling a person with emotional sensitivity not to have the reaction they are having ignores their neurobiology.

REMEMBER

When other people ignore, dismiss, or punish emotionally sensitive people's reaction or oversimplify the ease of coping or solving the problem they are experiencing, over time that person is left without adaptive coping mechanisms. Instead, they turn to quickly executable and often self-destructive ways of coping, including behaviors such as self-harm and drug use.

Focusing on the Functions and Goals of a Comprehensive Treatment

Based on the conceptualization of disorders characterized by difficulties in emotion (see the earlier section "Beginning with the Biosocial Theory"), DBT specifically focuses on helping people regulate their emotions in more adaptive ways. And so, DBT includes many behavioral skills that specifically aim to teach patients how to recognize, understand, label, and regulate their emotions.

A comprehensive treatment is needed to help people who are emotionally sensitive. For any treatment to be comprehensive, it must address five essential functions, and DBT is no different. A comprehensive treatment must accomplish the tasks in the following sections.

Motivating the patient and the therapist

A comprehensive treatment motivates a patient to participate in and complete the treatment, and various strategies are used to keep both the patient and the therapist in the therapy. Motivation comes from understanding the person's goals while at the same time identifying their relevant strengths and relative weaknesses. The therapist works to ensure that they themselves are clear as to what the patient's goals are, that they have explained how DBT can help the person attain their goals, and then that they and the patient can collaborate in the process. Motivation goes beyond just the patient. It also targets the therapist's motivation, particularly when then are finding the work to be frustrating. We review motivational strategies in greater depth in Chapter 19.

Teaching the patient new coping mechanisms

A comprehensive treatment teaches the patient new ways of coping with life's challenges or enhances a person's existing capabilities. In DBT, therapists hold the assumption that people who are struggling aren't doing so out of choice but rather that they lack, or need to improve, several important life skills, including the following:

>> The ability to regulate emotions

>> The ability to pay careful and accurate attention to the experience of the present moment

>> The ability to tolerate difficult moments

>> The ability to effectively negotiate relationships

REMEMBER

The idea is that maladaptive or ineffective behaviors are replaced by healthier, more effective, and longer-lasting ways of managing difficult moments. The teaching of these skills usually takes place in a weekly skills group session, which usually has up to ten patients and two co-leaders. The group generally lasts 90 minutes and has a didactic component where skills are taught, and homework is assigned and is reviewed in the next skills group. We cover skills therapy later in this chapter.

Incorporating new skills into the patient's daily life

Comprehensive treatment generalizes the new skills and new ways of coping to a patient's daily life. If the skills learned in therapy sessions don't apply or transfer to patients' daily lives, then it would be difficult to say that therapy was successful. This function is accomplished in two ways:

>> In the skills training group, the therapist provides and then reviews the weekly homework assignments given in the skills group.

>> The patient is allowed to contact the therapist between sessions so that they can get help directly from the therapist in situations where the patient doesn't know what to do or how to apply the skills. (Find out more about phone coaching later in this chapter.)

Supporting the therapist

To be effective in the work they do, therapists delivering DBT treatment must stay motivated to work with patients, particularly those patients whose behaviors they find challenging. Many therapists find the work with patients who have BPD and related conditions to be very rewarding, while at the same time, their patients' intense emotions and at times self-endangering behaviors can lead to therapist burnout and despair.

Therapists who provide DBT are required to sit on a *consultation team*, which is a group of other DBT therapists who meet on a weekly basis to help each other by using the same techniques that they use with their patients. Therapist burnout is essential to deal with and is applied by using consultation with the therapist, problem-solving, validation, and ongoing training and skill-building, as well as encouragement to persist in applying compassionate care. The typical consultation team meets once per week for one to two hours. We talk about consultation teams in more detail later in this chapter.

Structuring the patient's environment

Structuring the environment, when necessary, in a way that maximizes the chance of success includes the use of reinforcement of adaptive behavior and not reinforcing maladaptive behavior. Structuring also includes helping patients modify their environment. For example, patients who use drugs might modify their circle of friends. People who use dating apps that have led to abusive relationships may be coached to delete the apps. Patients who struggle by staying up late at night might need to modify their nighttime routine to promote better sleep hygiene.

Patients may need help in finding ways to modify their environments. Typically, the patient is coached as to how to make the modifications, but for younger or less skilled patients, the therapist may need to take a more active role in helping structure the environment. Get the scoop on structuring the environment in Chapter 16.

Checking Out Modes of Treatment

How can the five essential functions in the preceding section be attained? There are four modes of treatment in the standard model of DBT to ensure that the treatment can be comprehensively applied. Not included in these four modes are other modes of treatment, such as medications and services like case management. These other modes can be added to DBT, and often; however, they aren't core to the treatment.

Skills training

REMEMBER

The mode of treatment most frequently implemented in DBT is the skills group. There are various reasons for this. Pragmatically it's easily implemented and structured. It can meet the needs of many patients because it teaches more than one patient at a time. It has a set curriculum, handouts, and homework, so it appears very much like a typical classroom setting. Further, many mental health settings don't have enough DBT-trained staff to have every patient be assigned to an individual therapist, and in this context, a therapist working with a co-leader can, at a minimum, introduce a larger number of patients to the treatment. It's important to note that there is strong evidence that the use of skills training alone is effective in helping patients with many of their mental health symptoms.

In this mode, patients focus on learning new skills in a classroom-like atmosphere. The skills are then enhanced through practice exercises, as well as generalized to other aspects of the patients' personal lives by the assignment and review of homework. The specific skills that are taught are the four DBT skills modules: mindfulness, emotion regulation, distress tolerance, and interpersonal effectiveness. The modules are typically taught over six weeks, although this can vary, depending on the needs of the patients and how quickly they learn the material. The specific skills are reviewed in depth in Part 3.

In a group meeting, the typical structure is once per week, lasting somewhere between two and two and a half hours. The first hour is devoted to a review of the homework assigned in the previous session, and the second hour is dedicated to the teaching of new skills. Homework is then assigned as the last task of the group.

Note: There are certain circumstances when skills are taught in individual sessions. For instance, a person may have work limitations that don't allow them to participate at a particular time, or they may have language limitations or learning disorders that don't allow them to keep up with the pace of teaching in a large group.

Individual therapy

Individual treatment in standard DBT is conducted weekly or biweekly in 60-minute sessions, and it's focused on understanding, exploring, and targeting the behaviors that a patient wants to change. It does so by keeping the patient motivated to complete the treatment and encouraging them to apply the new skills they have learned in the group. A variety of techniques, which are covered in Part 4, are used by the DBT therapist to address motivation when it has started to wane.

Phone/skills coaching

The skills of DBT are of little value unless they are put to use in the moment that they are needed. When times are calm and emotions are better regulated, it's easy to see how the skills can be useful, and many patients can explain how the skills would work in their day-to-day life. However, in times of emotional turmoil, the more familiar, often maladaptive, behaviors are the ones that tend to show up first. When the urges to self-harm or use substances show up, the more intense the emotions, the more likely the unskilled person is to use these old forms of dealing with the urges.

Dr. Linehan recognized that life's most challenging problems tended not to happen when patients were in therapy. They could happen at any time, day or night.

She emphasized the importance of intersession coaching to help patients generalize the skills they had learned in the skills training group to their everyday life. The duration of a skills-coaching call is intended to be a brief call of typically no more than 15 minutes to offer patients support and ideas to deal with an in-the-moment situation.

WARNING

One of the major concerns that new therapists worry about is that spending time out of session on the phone with their patients might reinforce life-threatening behavior. In other words, they worry that if patients feels supported during a call when they are feeling suicidal, it's possible that they may then express more suicidal thoughts to be able to speak to their therapists more frequently. Therapists are taught how to deal with this eventuality (see Chapter 14).

A therapist consultation team

One of the more difficult aspects of working with suicidal patients is that it's common for therapists to become discouraged and burned out. Dealing with suicidal people every day can make therapists feel much of the despair that their patients feel. Behavioral change can take time, and many therapists worry about their patients' safety during episodes of emotional distress. The therapist consultation team is intended to be *therapy for the therapists,* supporting them in their work with patients who have severe, complex, and often difficult-to-treat disorders.

REMEMBER

In the same way that individual therapy helps the patient stay motivated for treatment, the consultation team works to ensure that the therapist remains motivated in order to provide the best treatment possible. Teams typically meet weekly for an hour to an hour and a half, and are composed of individual therapists, family therapists, group leaders, and anyone else providing DBT therapy. It's such an essential component that a therapist can't say that they are providing DBT therapy if they aren't on a consultation team. Chapter 17 covers therapist consultation teams in more detail.

Incorporating Dialectics

REMEMBER

The fundamental principle underlying the practice of DBT is the recognition of and emphasis on the *dialectical process.* The dialectical philosophy at the core of DBT is that seemingly opposing experiences such as thoughts, emotions, or behaviors can coexist, and both make sense. In other words, two ideas that are seemingly in complete opposition to each other can both be true at the same time. This requires that a therapist and a patient be able to look at a situation from multiple perspectives and find a way to synthesize the seemingly opposite ideas.

Within this framework, reality consists of opposing forces that are in tension, not dissimilar from a game of tug-of-war. As it pertains to therapy, in many cases the push to apply change-oriented treatment strategies often creates a resistance to the recommendations. The therapist pulls in one direction and the patient in another. This is because the prospect of facing the emotional turmoil and suffering that many people with conditions like BPD experience during therapy feels more painful than they are willing to bear. Dialectical philosophy also recognizes that opposing forces are incomplete on their own; you can't have a tug-of-war with only one team.

Practitioners noted that it was by moving into a collaborative and accepting stance, rather than one solely focused on trying to get their patients to change, that the possibility of change occurred. And so, when the therapist balances and synthesizes both acceptance and change-focused strategies in a compassionate therapy, the patient experiences the freedom they need to heal. In many cases, prior to DBT, patients experienced the opposite. They either noted locking horns with their therapists, who insisted that the patients had to change, or they experienced passive, though caring, therapists who simply listened and didn't offer ideas that could help. In some cases, individual therapists would swing between the two extremes, another style that was unhelpful to patients who themselves would tend to swing between extremes.

Another way that this manifested in traditional therapies is that frequently the therapist would feel that their formulation of the patient or their interpretations of the patient's behavior was "right." In DBT, the therapist lets go of the need to be right and is open to the idea that there are other possibilities in the moment. Finally, in DBT, there is an emphasis on moving away from a rigid style of therapy, and so there is often a lot of movement, speed, and flow within a therapy session. This is achieved by the therapist using various strategies to increase or decrease the intensity, seriousness, lightness, or energy of the therapeutic interaction, and then in so doing assessing what works best for any one particular patient, rather than assuming that a single style works equally well for all patients.

The following sections delve more deeply into the dialectical process. Flip to Chapter 15 for even more information.

Searching for multiple truths in any situation

The core dialectic in DBT is that *acceptance* and *change* coexist. This is best illustrated by an example. Imagine that you're stuck in very heavy traffic. You can't get out of the car, there are no nearby exits, and your mobile app tells you that you're at least an hour away from a meeting that you should have been at

30 minutes ago. What can you do? For some people, there could be rage, for others resignation, and for others an attempt to solve the problem a different way, like calling in to the meeting. The reality of that moment requires the *acceptance* that the moment is as it is.

So, if there is acceptance of the moment, where does change come into the picture? Because a traffic jam can be so aggravating, it can lead to persistent suffering. Another way to consider it is to say, "I cannot make the traffic be anything other than what it is, but I can change my reaction to the heavy traffic. I can learn to relax when I am in intolerable situations." Imagine that your identical twin was traveling in the car next to you and you were both in the same traffic. Imagine that you were not accepting reality and fighting it all the way, feeling that it was unfair that the traffic was so bad. What would your state of mind be? On the other hand, if your twin were practicing to see that change coexists in the moment and that the one thing that they can control is their state of mind and their reaction to the stressful situation, they would be in a far more relaxed state of mind. What research shows is that the more emotionally regulated a person is, the more capable they are of solving problems, and that the more dysregulated a person is, the fewer options come to mind.

From a philosophical perspective, we have the *thesis* on one side and an *antithesis* on the other side. Then comes what Dr. Linehan termed the *dialectical synthesis*, which is the integration of the two perspectives: "I can be in a situation that I don't like and yet accept it, and by doing so, I can make the changes necessary to be more effective. As a result, difficult moments are opportunities for me to learn to be more capable and skillful." For example, a thesis might be "I can't bear being stuck in traffic." The antithesis to this is "I can bear being stuck in traffic." The synthesis is finding a way to bear the unbearable by finding a different route, changing the reaction to the problem of being stuck in traffic, or learning to accept being stuck in traffic.

Moving from contradiction to synthesis

For people who enter DBT, life is much more complicated than being stuck in traffic jams. Often intense emotions lead people who are struggling to behave in self-destructive ways, and self-injury like cutting is a very common behavior in people who have intense emotions. Many people, when seeing self-injurious behavior, would say, "Cutting yourself is a serious problem!" However, people who cut don't always see this as a problem. Instead, they see self-injury as a solution to the problem of intense emotions. So, the behavior is both a problem and a solution? This appears to be a contradiction. From a dialectical perspective, however, both positions are true.

The synthesis is that people who have intense emotions that lead to significant psychological suffering want the suffering to end, and that self-injury is a quick way to solve the problem of emotional suffering. People who self-injure have been found to have higher activity in the amygdala, the part of the brain that experiences emotions, in response to emotional images. Higher activity in the amygdala is associated with a feeling of distress. Although for many people, self-injury would increase amygdalar activity, paradoxically, in people who for whom self-injury is regulating, there is a reduction in amygdalar activity, and this in turn leads to a reduction in negative mood and an increase in positive mood.

And yet self-injury is only a short-term solution that doesn't solve the problem of long-term emotional distress. When we move the focus from the self-injury to the problem being intense emotions, we develop a new perspective on the various points of view as having validity. The contradiction has become a new way of seeing things through the synthesis of seeing the perspective of each.

Another seeming contradiction is that DBT therapists hold the assumption that in the absence of other information, a person is doing the best they can. The contradictory position that the therapists also hold in mind is that a person in DBT can do better. So, how can a person be doing the best they can, and also be able to do better? Here the contradiction is explained by the consideration that if a person is incapable of managing intense emotions, either because they don't have the skills to do so or because they are flooded by the magnitude of the emotional storm under those circumstances, then it's the best that they can do. The synthesis between the two positions is that the person is doing the best they can in the moment and needs to try harder and be more motivated to change.

TIP

An analogy would be to consider that a person has just learned how to swim. They get into a shallow pool and paddle around just fine. If they are then taken to a stormy ocean with big waves and thrown in, they have great difficulty managing the situation. Given that they are a beginning swimmer, it's the best that they can do. However, our swimmer must learn how to manage more difficult swimming conditions if they ever want to leave the shallow pool, and the way to do this is by learning the skills necessary to become a better swimmer.

REMEMBER

For the emotionally flooded patient, their behavior at the moment of heightened emotion may be the best that they can do, and yet it's also the case that they must do better if they want to live a life with less suffering. The way to do "better" is by learning new ways of coping when strong emotions threaten to overwhelm the mind. And so, the seeming contradiction that a person is doing the best they can and that they can do better coexist, and the synthesis is that the learning of new skills makes the person more capable of managing more complicated situations, whether intense emotions or swimming conditions. This is the nature of dialectics.

Chapter **3**

Accepting Multiple Points of View

S eeing multiple points of view isn't always easy, and for some it can, at times, feel nearly impossible. At the foundation of DBT is the concept of *dialectics,* the idea that two opposing viewpoints can be true at the same time (see Chapter 2 for details) — that is, we can hold multiple points of view or truths. For example, in DBT we wouldn't necessarily say that the opposite of the truth is always a lie; we would say that the opposite of the truth can be another truth. When you think about it that way, you can begin to open your mind to other points of view, even when you feel very strongly about something.

While people's thinking can be more or less flexible, one of the things that most strongly gets in the way of seeing another point of view is our own emotions. We know that the more emotional we get, the narrower our thinking becomes. When your thinking narrows, seeing perspectives other than the one you feel most passionate or certain about becomes hard. It can be as if you have tunnel vision.

If you're someone who feels emotions strongly and intensely, this may be a familiar struggle. Sticking too strongly to your own perspective means you can miss important information, damage relationships, and be less effective at getting what you want or being heard.

In this chapter, you discover how to pay attention and evaluate your first reaction, broaden your awareness to other points of view, and find compassion for yourself as you begin this process.

Questioning Your First Reaction

REMEMBER

Our first reaction doesn't always come from a wise place; instead, it can be powerfully driven by emotions. In DBT, we say that these reactions come from your *emotion mind.* When you're in this state of mind, you see the world and react to it based solely on how you feel in the moment, with little consideration about the facts of the situation. When first reactions are problematic, they are driven too much by how we feel and lead to an equally problematic sense of certainty that we are right or that there is only one possible option or perspective. We can forget that there may be other possibilities, and our thinking can become rigid. Along with this chapter, the mindfulness skills discussed in Chapter 9 will help you become more aware of strong emotions, learn to step back, and more purposely (instead of reactively) move forward with broader awareness and curiosity.

Questioning your first reaction is a challenging and wonderful practice. When you do so, you're more able to act with an open mind and in a way that is consistent with your values. The following sections discuss some important aspects of questioning your first reaction to a situation: realizing that it may be exaggerated, matching it to what's in front of you, and stopping yourself from taking action.

REMEMBER

It's important to note that when you feel absolutely certain about something, you may be missing important information. That can be a helpful cue that you should consider other points of view.

Realizing your first reaction may be exaggerated

When you feel passionately about something, it's easy to react strongly when you feel misunderstood or when someone disagrees with you. If you're an emotionally sensitive person, you may have been told that you have big reactions to things. It's important to understand that sometimes reactions — the ones that happen quickly — are exaggerated or too big. This is simply something to know about yourself. That knowledge will help you assess when you feel like your reaction fits the situation, or when it may be driven too much by your emotions. Again, the more you practice mindfulness (see Chapter 9), the easier this practice will become.

People are often judged by others for having exaggerated or larger emotional reactions to things, and this can be very painful. That being said, it's important to realize that at times our reactions are too big and that this can be due to a range of things, including our own sensitivity to vulnerabilities such as being sick, feeling stressed at work or school, having financial stressors, dealing with relationship problems, being hungry, or simply not getting enough sleep.

The first step to opening your mind to multiple points of view is to accept, with compassion, that your initial reaction may in fact be exaggerated, too big, or too rigid and certain. This involves knowing that this reaction is a problem and wanting to change it. It can be helpful to remember that you are not letting go of your position or belief, but instead, holding onto it while also being open to other information or hearing other perspectives. That is dialectical thinking.

Matching your reaction to what is in front of you

When you're in the moment, before you can expand your awareness, you must regulate whatever strong emotion is coming up. Emotions like fear, anger, shame, jealousy, and envy can be particularly challenging to work with. Sometimes you'll need to use another approach, such as employing DBT distress tolerance skills (see Chapter 11), to decrease the intensity of how you feel, and then it will be much easier to open your mind to new or other information.

TIP

If you're an emotionally sensitive person, sometimes trying to match your level of emotion to the situation in front of you can be hard. This makes a lot of sense, because emotionally sensitive people tend to feel things longer and more deeply than the average person. Here are some skills you can work on:

>> **Think about someone who reacts to situations in a way that you would like to react.** Ask yourself how they would react in this situation, and compare your reaction to theirs.

>> **Use self-validation by recognizing how your emotions make sense, and stay away from judging yourself.** This will help you decrease the intensity of your emotions and access your inner wisdom to assess your reaction. It's often self-judgment, self-blaming, and self-invalidation that continue to drive up the intensity of your emotions and make it hard to think (see Chapter 5 for more on self-validation).

>> **Take five mindful breaths to help you decrease the intensity of your emotions.** Just taking a few breaths will help begin to calm both your body and your mind.

> **»** **Be aware of topics or situations that prompt your reactivity.** This awareness will help you know that certain situations leave you at a higher risk to be reactive so that you can plan ahead for them. Some people find it helpful to identify these topics or situations as "red flags" and then make a skills plan or cope ahead plan to use when they come up. If you can identify these red flags, you can catch yourself before you react and instead use your skills.

REMEMBER

Matching your reaction to what is in front of you is a skill, and skills improve with practice. As you master this skill, you'll find that what now feels reactive and almost automatic will become deliberate and filled with choices.

Holding off on taking action

One of the three functions of emotions is to motivate action. In some cases, that is exactly what needs to happen; however, in other cases moving into action too quickly can get you into trouble. When the goal is to open your mind and be able to see multiple perspectives, you'll often need to observe your urge to argue your point of view, ignore or dismiss another position, or get stuck in a state of certainty that there are no other options.

Simply observing, which is discussed more in Chapter 9, means having awareness that moving into action isn't necessarily going to be helpful or effective. Sometimes you may find that awareness after you have charged ahead; in those cases, your task is to observe with compassion and remember that in many cases, it isn't too late to slow down, breathe, and work to open your mind.

Expanding Your Perception

Once you have the willingness and skill to observe your first reaction (as we describe earlier in this chapter), you'll have the opportunity to expand your perception and consider alternative points of view. The wonderful thing about developing this type of awareness is that you can give yourself some choices about what to do next. You can decide to stay stuck in your perspective, but it's more likely that your mind will become more open and less certain, and that you'll find it easier to consider different possible perspectives. Expanding your perception and awareness can be very helpful when you are stuck feeling like you have only one option to solve a problem or are in a conflict where it feels like you can't understand the other person and they can't understand you. Often strong emotions blind us to alternatives that are really helpful.

Being able to expand your perception is critical to nurturing and maintaining important relationships. Many relationships end when one or both people can't slow down and see alternative perspectives. Simply seeing another perspective doesn't mean that you'll necessarily agree with it, and if you can see and understand where the other person is coming from, you can validate their emotions and become more curious and non-judgmental about how they got to their position. If the interaction is becoming escalated, this can decrease the emotional intensity for everyone involved. By approaching it in this way, you'll help the other person be curious about your perspective, allowing for a more effective conversation.

The following sections walk you through the main steps of expanding your perception and considering other points of view.

REMEMBER

Seeing multiple perspectives doesn't mean that you give yours up; it means that you can be more understanding and open. You may keep your perspective or position, you may adopt theirs, or you and the other person may come up with some unique synthesis of the information together.

Considering your therapist's point of view

As we discuss earlier in this chapter, sometimes the hardest thing to do is to *not* move into action to make a decision, to continue a conversation or debate, to get in the last word, to quit a job or school, or even to end a relationship. Due to the very direct nature of communication in DBT, clients sometimes have difficulty seeing their therapist's perspective. It may be that the therapist is holding a firm contingency that was part of a behavior plan or is giving you difficult feedback. When this happens, sometimes it can be hard to see your therapist's point of view.

REMEMBER

When you're struggling to see your therapist's point of view, it's helpful to ask yourself whether you're confused or you're noticing strong feelings about what they have said or done. Keep in mind that interpersonal challenges are best addressed when both people are regulated. The stronger your emotions are, the more difficult it is to see other points of view. Here are some ways to remain effective and see your therapist's points of view:

>> Take a few deep breaths, and make sure your breathing and heart rate are regulated.

>> Note that your therapist is trying to help you reach your goals; ask yourself how your therapist's perspective may be helping you achieve those goals.

>> Ask yourself: What is the wisdom in your therapist's position?

>> Ask yourself: Do you want to be right or effective in this interaction?

Coming to an agreement

In close relationships, feeling misunderstood or angry can be very painful. So, how do you move forward when this happens with your therapist or someone you care for? One of the biggest barriers to coming to an agreement is that you're unable to see another perspective, or you feel that if you change your position, you're giving up, giving in, or letting the other person win. Here are some useful questions to ask yourself in order to help you come to an agreement when you're stuck:

>> **Are you zooming out?** As you try to come to an agreement, it can be helpful to zoom out. Think about the other person's perspective. Does your therapist care for you? Is she trying to help you meet your goals? Could she have made a mistake? Is there wisdom in what she is saying? This technique can be very effective to use with other important people in your life when you feel misunderstood or are having difficulty seeing their point of view.

>> **Are you being effective?** It can be a helpful reminder to ask yourself whether you're being effective. Is the perspective or the point you're making helping you get what you need? Are you delivering it in a skillful way that your therapist or the other person can hear? Are you maintaining your integrity as you make your point?

>> **Are you acting from a wise mind?** As we discuss in the earlier section "Questioning Your First Reaction," sometimes when you struggle to hold multiple perspectives, it's because you're acting from an emotion mind. Can you take a few breaths and connect to your wise mind? Your wise mind is the state of mind in which you have access to both what you feel about something and what you know or understand about something (see Chapter 9).

>> **Are you thinking the best of the other person?** While you may be feeling strong emotions, this will help you refrain from forming negative judgments about the other person. Judgmental thinking tends to drive up already intense emotions.

REMEMBER

People disagree with one another. It's okay to skillfully disagree, and to see the wisdom in why the other person feels that way and then simply let it be. It is "agreeing to disagree," which isn't uncommon. You may also agree that one or the other person is correct. This can happen when you have both been able to be curious and open to the other person's perspective or information. A third option could be that you come up with a new perspective that somehow synthesizes each of your perspectives. What you'll notice is that throughout the process, you're continually looking to open your mind to see ideas or perspectives you may have missed.

Moving forward with a purpose

REMEMBER

Once you have come to an agreement, it's important to move on. For some, it can be challenging to let go of the experience and the emotions that came with it. We discuss this more in Chapter 10. Holding onto these challenging experiences can keep you in a past that has already occurred and can make it very difficult to stay in the present. Be mindful of judging the other person, and most importantly, be mindful of your own self-judgments or regrets.

Looking at Yourself with Friendly Eyes

Accepting multiple points of view isn't always easy, and when you get stuck, unable to expand your awareness, it can damage your relationships, interfere with work or school, and lead to you doing things that compromise your integrity or undermine your values.

While you learn to be more skillful and able to keep multiple perspectives in mind, it's critical to remember that we all make mistakes and get stuck thinking and acting from an emotion mind. To build this skill, you must find compassion for yourself and know that we all get caught in an emotion mind. For many people who are emotionally sensitive, these types of challenges can feed self-hatred and self-judgment, and when you practice that way of being, you feed the very feelings that make it hard to be skillful. If you're going to embark on this practice, it's inevitable that you'll get stuck and return to an old way of doing things. Being kind and forgiving to yourself will help you step back onto the skillful path.

TIP

For some, finding self-compassion is no easy task. We talk more about this in Chapter 10. A short practice that many people find useful is to think about a friend who you care for and ask yourself how you would treat them if they were in a similar situation. This can be a helpful exercise because most people are able to find compassion for friends and loved ones, but can't find that same compassion for themselves. Treating yourself as you would your close friend can help you be gentle with yourself and find you own inner friend.

» **Moving past your initial reaction**

» **Opening up to other possibilities**

» **Changing negatives into positives**

Chapter **4**

Moving from Impulsive to Spontaneous

mpulsivity is one of the main reasons why people come into DBT treatment. It's also one of the distinctive features of emotion dysregulation conditions such as borderline personality disorder (BPD). These impulsivity aspects of BPD encompass some of the most worrisome characteristics of the disorder, including suicidal behavior, self-injury, drug and alcohol misuse, dangerous sexual behavior, erratic driving, and difficulties in controlling anger. (See Chapter 2 for more information on emotion dysregulation.)

In DBT, we want you to move from impulsivity to spontaneity. In this chapter, you find out how to shift from impulsivity to spontaneity by moving past initial reactions, opening yourself up, and changing negative thoughts to positive ones. But first, we explain the differences between being impulsive and being spontaneous.

Distinguishing Impulsivity and Spontaneity

Impulsivity is a complicated behavior and considered to be both a personality trait and a component of chemicals and nerve cell connections in the brain:

>> From a personality trait point of view, impulsivity is a lack of restraint characterized by a disregard for social conventions and a lack of consideration as to the possible outcomes, particularly in potentially risky situations.

>> From a neurobiology point of view, impulsivity is seen as a lack of ability to inhibit certain actions.

Slightly different from impulsivity, which is the action of doing something without considering the impact of the behavior, is the related idea of spontaneity. Although in each case the outcome of behavior isn't known, spontaneity has a different quality. Spontaneity is behavior that tends to be joyful, expansive, and dynamic. Whereas impulsivity tends to have a narrow focus, spontaneity has a big-picture perspective. Even though the outcome might not be known, spontaneity is uplifting in its nature — for instance, calling a friend out of the blue and meeting them for lunch, taking a French language class after seeing it advertised in a magazine, and breaking out into dance while pushing your cart down the aisle of the grocery store when you hear your favorite music being played.

REMEMBER

In either case, the behaviors are impromptu. So, what makes one life-enhancing and another potentially destructive? One key element is the state of mind that you're in when you do the behavior:

>> Typically, if the behavior is coming from strong emotions like fear or anxiety and it's used to alleviate the discomfort of the emotion, it's impulsive. When there's fear of missing out on an activity, excessive boredom, or an insistence on needing something to happen right then and there, impulsivity tends to show up.

>> If, on the other hand, the decision comes from a sense of grounded stability, or when there is a recognition that there is an opportunity in the situation and we are in control of our behavior, that is the quality of spontaneity.

Moving Beyond Your First Reaction

REMEMBER

Impulsivity often leads to undesired consequences, and in retrospect it seems easy to consider that you could have done something other than what you did. At the time, you may have felt that there were no other options, and yet between an impulse and an action there is always a space, and it is when you linger in that space that other options unfold. Among the available psychotherapy options used to tackle impulsivity, mindfulness is especially helpful in changing impulsivity-driven actions, and so it is in the mindfulness module of DBT that impulsivity is most readily addressed (see Chapter 9).

The following sections provide pointers on how to effectively use the space between an impulse and an action in order to make different choices.

Taking a breath

Taking a breath to target impulsivity isn't some theoretical exercise; a research base shows that it helps. For instance, in one study, more than 500 teens aged 14 to 18 who went through a four-week program where they learned yoga-based breathing techniques had better impulse control than a comparison group of teens who didn't go through the program.

Taking a breath is an excellent way to deal with an urge to do something impulsive. A focus on the breath is a way to reach the gap between the urge and the action, and the more you practice this, the more you'll see that this gap exists. Also, the more you practice this, the bigger you will see that the gap is. Although you're breathing all the time, it's unlikely that you're paying attention to each of your breaths. This is particularly true when an impulsive action is about to happen in the context of high emotions.

TIP

Here is a way to focus on the breath:

1. Take a deep, slow breath in through your nose. This inward breath should last somewhere from four to six seconds.

2. Breathe out through pursed lips, as if you were blowing up a balloon. The outward breath should last longer than the inward breath — for instance, five to eight seconds.

3. Focus on breathing this way for about two minutes. After a few minutes, pay attention to the point when the inward breath stops and the outward breath begins.

In this book, you should practice all the recommended exercises when you don't need them, so that when you *do* need them, they are available. It's the same as taking practice tests before an exam, so that when the exam comes, you're ready, or practicing tennis before the match, so that when the match comes, you know what to do.

The next time you're likely to do something impulsive, practice this breath for five minutes. You might still decide that you're going to engage in the behavior based on your urges, but on the other hand, when you slow down, the pause might allow you to fully consider the consequence of your actions.

Finding your emotional balance

Experiencing stressful situations and having no time to unwind can lead to psychological distress. The thought of dealing with life's stress can feel impossible, and many people choose to ignore or avoid dealing with problems that come along. DBT teaches that avoidance of dealing with stress can lead to more stress, and so rather than avoiding the stress, finding emotional balance is a way to manage these situations.

But what is emotional balance and how do you achieve it? Typically, when in the heat of an unwanted situation, most of us react with strong emotions — typically anger, fear, anxiety, worry, or sadness. Having emotional balance is the practice of balancing these unwanted emotions using effective ways of dealing with them so that you don't end up stuck in them or spend your time ruminating about how terrible and unfair life is. Finding this balance is also a way to increase happiness, improve motivation to do things differently, and help you get a good night's rest.

Specific steps can help you practice, build, and maintain emotional balance. *SUN*, *WAVE*, and *NO NOT* are ways to do this, as you find out in the following sections. You can also practice gratitude and use behavioral activation.

In finding balance, you can use emotion regulation skills (see Chapter 10) along with distress tolerance skills (see Chapter 11). When you use emotion regulation skills, you focus on dealing with difficult emotions without acting on behaviors that might have adverse consequences. On the other hand, distress tolerance skills are used for the tolerance and momentary acceptance of difficult situations without making the situations worse. Using all of these ideas on a regular basis is the DBT way to find emotional balance.

Identifying the emotion: SUN

TIP

Many people who struggle with emotional intensity and reactivity recognize that they don't know precisely which emotion they are feeling, and so it makes sense that they might not know what to do when they are feeling unbalanced. One way to identify the emotion is to use the acronym SUN:

>> **Sensations:** Focus on what you feel and the physical sensations in your body. Notice whether there is tension in any part of your body.

>> **Urges:** Do you have any urges to do anything in particular? Most emotions come with an action urge. For instance, people who are angry have the urge to attack, while people who are sad have the urge to cry or isolate.

>> **Name (the emotion):** When you put together the body sensations and action urges, it's easier to name the emotion.

Riding out the emotion like a WAVE

Emotions are like waves: They will start to form, peak, and then come crashing down before petering out on the beach. The idea is to focus on the emotion, to notice it as it peaks, and then to ride it down until it is more manageable before acting on the urges.

NO NOT

Here, the task is to remind yourself that you are not your emotion. So, rather than saying "I *am* sad," say "I *feel* sad." By doing this, you aren't making yourself and sadness equivalent. Also, if sad is who you are, then you can't change that; however, if sadness is how you feel, then that is something that you can change. The task here is also not to enhance or suppress the emotion, because doing so makes a stressful situation even worse.

Practicing gratitude

REMEMBER

Another way to find balance, besides SUN-WAVE-NO NOT, is to practice finding gratitude for things in your life. There are always things in life that we can be thankful for. Many people think that this isn't true because they don't have "big" things. And yet there are often little things for which we can have gratitude: a kind smile from another person, a silent moment, the sound of birds in a garden, the end of a busy workday. By following this practice, you remind yourself that life isn't made up of a series of unfortunate or unwanted effects.

Behavioral activation, a.k.a "get moving!"

Physical movement is a way to tackle emotional lows. Behavioral activation is based on the observation that, as a person becomes depressed, they increasingly engage in isolating and avoidance behaviors. The goal of behavioral activation, therefore, is to work with people who have unwanted mood states like depression by engaging in activities that have been shown to improve mood. Often, these are activities that a person enjoyed before they became depressed. These activities don't need to be excessive. If a person enjoyed running before their depression, they don't have to run a half-marathon to get moving. They might jog around the block or go for a 30-minute walk. The task is to make movement a part of their daily routine.

Opening Up

Opening up — the topic of this section — means realizing that you're open to seeing other possibilities as a way of understanding situations and open to other ways of solving difficult problems. Rather than acting on impulse as a sole solution, when you open up, life becomes less one-dimensional and allows you to take greater control of your life.

Seeing different perspectives

The shift in perspective-taking is a powerful way that DBT uses to help people transform the way they see something. This can happen in various ways:

>> If a person feels that they have screwed up and are unlovable, the therapist might ask them what they imagine their best friend would say.

>> A person may reflect on whether the way they are treating themselves is consistent with their wise mind. *Wise mind* is the dialectical synthesis of rational mind and emotion mind — where these two states of mind integrate into a single state that leads to a more intuitive, values-based, and holistic course of action.

>> In some sessions, therapists might take a more concrete approach to perspective-taking by switching seats with their patient, so that the patient literally has a different point of view.

>> Other techniques go beyond simply imagining another person's perspective by imagining what a person's younger self would say about a certain situation, or what their future self would say about their current actions.

The following sections dig deeper into different methods of seeing different perspectives.

Projective and reflective perspectives

Perspective-taking is considered to be projective or reflective:

>> *Projective* perspective means projecting a point of view into the future; for instance, a therapist, or you yourself, might ask the question: "How do you imagine you will look next year after you have completed therapy?" Of course, you can't actually know what you'll look like, so the only way to think about this is to project your feelings and thoughts onto what you imagine your future self might look like.

>> When perspective-taking is *reflective,* it requires the observation of the current experience. So, the therapist might ask, "If you viewed yourself after you had completed a course of DBT a year from now, and could remember yourself as you are today, how would you describe yourself?"

REMEMBER

The goal of projective perspective-taking is to help people broaden their awareness by looking outside of themselves. On the other hand, reflective perspective-taking focuses on getting a person to access insights about a current situation. Both of these styles of perspective-taking can be achieved within the person themselves, or they can take the perspective of another person to reflect on new ways of thinking. For example, they might ask, "What would I do if I were my therapist/parent/best friend right now?" Alternatively, imagine what you would say if you were your best friend hearing your own self-criticism.

The THINK skill

TIP

Another aspect to perspective-taking is to consider another person's point of view when you feel that you've been wronged by them. The DBT skill that is taught to move a person from an emotion-minded response to a wise-minded response is the THINK skill. This is typically used in a situation where there is an active disagreement between two people. Here's how it works:

>> **Think:** Think about the situation from the other person's perspective. How might they be interpreting the situation, including your words and actions? If you put yourself in the other person's shoes and hear what you're saying, what would you imagine?

>> **Have empathy:** What might the other person be feeling or thinking? Are they afraid of your aggression? Are they sad, feeling that you're drifting apart? Are they feeling misunderstood?

>> **Interpretations:** Can you consider alternative interpretations or explanations for the person's behavior? Make a list of alternative explanations, including positive or good reasons as to why the person responded in the way they did.

>> **Notice:** Try to reflect on how the other person has been trying to improve the situation. Notice attempts by the other person to be helpful and notice how they may themselves be struggling in their life in the present moment.

>> **Kindness:** In considering the perspective of another person, remember to be kind toward them in the way that you would hope that someone would be kind to you.

Widening your range of emotions

It's in our nature as human beings to feel emotions. For people who are emotionally sensitive, emotions are the very experiences that make them suffer, and often all they want to do is to get rid of their emotions. Because they want to get rid of their emotions, the last thing they want to do is to examine them deeply, but that is the very thing that DBT requests of people.

If you're emotionally sensitive, it's possible that you feel a huge range of different feelings in response to situations. So, for instance, if you're depressed, you may feel sad, but this sadness will often come with feeling lonely, misunderstood, hopeless, and so on. The reason why it is hard to identify exactly how you're feeling is that the emotions seem to come on really quickly and they are then blended with other feelings as well as thoughts. As a result, the experience can be confusing.

To deal with what is actually going on and to address the main emotion being experienced, DBT gets patients to recognize the emotional experiences that occur most often and to separate out primary emotions and secondary emotions. In so doing, you're more likely to describe how you are truly feeling:

>> **Primary emotions:** A *primary emotion* is the first emotion experienced, which is connected directly to the event that generated the emotion. The emotion is typically short in duration; however, as time passes and we get away from the event that caused it, the primary emotion rapidly dissipates and starts to take on other elements, such as thoughts or other emotions. Primary emotions are like a snowball that begins to slide down a steep mountain. Without slowing down, the primary emotion can gather steam and become an avalanche of secondary emotions that can be more overwhelming and harder to stop. It rarely stops and just stays as the snowball, and it is in the gathering of more snow and other things like rocks that it can become an avalanche.

Primary emotions are less complicated and easier to understand. From a DBT perspective, there are ten primary emotions, and we review these further in Chapter 10.

>> **Secondary emotions:** *Secondary emotions* are essentially emotional reactions to primary emotions. These are learned emotional reactions that we typically develop as a result of the experiences of early childhood and observing our parents and their reactions. There is a wonderful explanation of secondary emotions from the movie *Star Wars: The Phantom Menace,* when Master Yoda says, "Fear leads to anger, anger leads to hate, hate leads to suffering."

A way to know whether an emotion is primary or secondary is that if the emotion lingers long after an event has happened, it's likely to be secondary. If the emotion is complex and hard to define or identify, it's almost always secondary.

And so the new perspective is this: By paying attention to emotions rather than avoiding them, you not only widen your range of experience, but you also recognize that although they may be painful, they won't destroy you. In recognizing this fact, you can develop the skills needed to manage intense emotions.

Breaking free of rigid choices

People who have conditions like BPD often have the experience of black-and-white thinking or make rigid all-or-nothing decisions. For some people, this way of living can lead to a pattern of recurring automatic negative thoughts that become increasingly destructive. So, a thought like "I can't do anything right" can become "I am worthless" and then "I shouldn't be alive." The following sections help you break free of rigid thinking.

Moving from either/or to both/and

In DBT the key is to move away from a polarized position to a synthesized position, meaning that the truth in each position is acknowledged. The synthesis comes from what Dr. Marsha Linehan, who developed DBT, described as the recognition of truth in seemingly opposing positions, which she termed *thesis* and *antithesis.* Take the earlier example:

Thesis: "Because I make a lot of mistakes, I can't do anything right, I am worthless, and so I shouldn't be alive."

Antithesis: "Making mistakes is not a big deal. Everyone makes mistakes. I shouldn't really care about making mistakes."

These are either/or types of statements. The first one is extreme and filled with all-or-nothing type thinking, and the second one invalidates the truth about what a person might actually be feeling.

Dialectical synthesis is the integration of a thesis and its antithesis in a way that acknowledges that change is the only constant in the universe and that it's an enduring process. It further recognizes that all things are made of opposing forces, and particular to the context of DBT, dialectical synthesis integrates the most essential and core parts of two polarities in order to form a new meaning, a new understanding, or a new solution in a given situation.

Dialectical synthesis isn't compromise. Whereas compromise is typically an agreement that is reached by each side making concessions, in dialectical synthesis, the agreement is reached by each side integrating the wisdom of the other side's perspective, an understanding derived from genuine curiosity. The following is the dialectical synthesis of the preceding thesis and antithesis:

> **Dialectical synthesis:** "It is true that I make mistakes, and also that others make mistakes. It is true that when I have such an experience, I think that I am worthless and that I should not be alive, and it is also true that everyone who is alive has made mistakes and they are not worthless. So, by acknowledging that I make mistakes and committing to learn and improve on the situations that lead me to make mistakes, I become a more skilled person, and the mistakes that I have made do not diminish my value and worth as a person."

Choosing instead of reacting

WARNING

Many of our responses to events are reactions rather than choices. The problem is that these reactions aren't always the best course of action. The consequences of these reactions may be that they keep people stuck in misery or even worsen the situation, including adversely impacting the quality of relationships.

We often react without thinking. This is most likely an evolutionary response. If a snake were to cross our path, we wouldn't want to stop and ponder the nature of the snake and wonder whether it was poisonous. In many situations it actually makes sense to just react. However, if our responses are based simply on our fears and insecurities, then those responses are often not in our long-term interests.

Choosing, on the other hand, is taking all the elements of a situation into consideration before then deciding on the best course of action. This includes integrating values, long-term goals, emotions, current circumstances, and so on.

A more concrete example is that your best friend goes to a party and doesn't mention to you that she is going. You immediately react by angrily calling her. Now both of you are upset. You have worsened the relationship, which is likely inconsistent with your values and relational goals.

If instead you choose your response, you'll notice your anger reaction. You can then use the STOP skill (see Chapter 11), which essentially asks you to pause, take a breath, and reflect on the situation. Do you know all that was going on with your friend? Do you know her intentions? Was it her goal to reject or disregard you? Does it help you to dwell on what happened? The choice might then be to call her and say that you were feeling hurt about not having been told about it, or to let her know that you were confused. Or you may even just let it go, knowing that your best friend may have had a good reason for not having invited you, and that she cares deeply about you.

REMEMBER

The DBT practice of mindfulness (see Chapter 9) is key to the practice of choosing. This is because it entails noticing our reactions to the things that happen in our lives. The task is then to pause without an immediate reaction. The fact that we have an internal reaction doesn't mean that we have to respond to it. We can notice the urge without acting on it. And then, on noticing it, we can decide that in fact it was the wise choice or that it was not, or that we can simply notice the urge. Choice is sometimes the choice to not do anything at all.

After the pause, pay attention to the reaction urge. You'll notice that it passes. Everything always passes. It is the nature of impermanence that it will pass. Eventually it will go away altogether. Think about all the urges that you have ever had in the past. Where are they now? They have all passed. Once the urge has passed, the task is to consider what the wise and — if dealing with another person — compassionate response would be. Ask yourself: "What response will help my relationship?" and "What response will help me stick to my values and reach my long-term goals?"

TIP

The practice of *choosing* rather than *reacting* takes time, because it requires the observation of the reaction urge without actually reacting. The best way to do this is to set an intention and then practice with little urges to get the feel of the practice before tackling bigger urges.

Transforming Negatives into Positives

DBT often uses metaphors to teach. One type of metaphor is known as a *short*, which is similar to a parable, a short story that illustrates a point. One that we use is the story of the farmer and his horses, which goes like this:

> An old farmer had worked his crops for many years. He was considered wealthy by his neighbors as he had ten horses. One day, during a terrible storm, his horses ran away. Upon hearing the news, his neighbors came by to commiserate: "What bad luck you've had," they said sympathetically. "Maybe," replied the farmer.

The next morning, the horses, hungry from being out in the wild, returned and brought with them ten wild horses. "How wonderful! You are a rich man!" the neighbors exclaimed. "Maybe," replied the farmer.

The following day, his son tried to tame one of the wild stallions. The horse bucked the boy off and he broke his leg. The neighbors again came to offer their sympathy. "Your son won't be able to help you in the fields. What bad luck!" they said. "Maybe," said the farmer.

The next day some military officials came to the village looking to draft young men into the army as they prepared for war. On seeing that the son's leg was broken, they passed him by. The neighbors again came out and congratulated the farmer on how well his circumstances had turned out. "Maybe," said the farmer.

REMEMBER

The point is that we never know exactly how things will turn out, and it's possible for positives to be seen as negatives and negatives as positives. For many people who struggle with conditions like BPD, positives are often seen as negatives, and turning negatives into positives seems like an impossible task. The following sections can help.

Setting new thinking patterns

Many people who come for DBT treatment struggle with negative thinking. Some have a judgmental inner critic or repeat loops of worry thoughts, low self-worth, or even self-hatred. Negative, or unhelpful, thinking patterns can have a strong and often adverse impact on work, family, and relational life.

There are ineffective ways to deal with negative thoughts. If you struggle with these thoughts, you might try distracting yourself from them or avoiding them altogether. Some people use drugs and alcohol or other short-term self-destructive behaviors to try to prevent the negative thinking from repeating over and over, and it makes sense that they would, given how painful the negative thoughts can be.

Negative thought patterns are repetitive, unhelpful, unwanted thoughts. These thought patterns typically leave a person feeling worse off about themselves and their situation. Through analyzing the pattern of thinking, DBT teaches people to recognize and then fully identify the pattern as it occurs. This process of stepping back from thoughts is called *cognitive defusion.* It's the act of noticing thoughts rather than being caught up in them as if they were something other than thoughts. When people get caught up in acting as if their thoughts were real, this is known as *cognitive fusion.*

Cognitive defusion includes the practice of letting thoughts come and go rather than holding onto them. In cognitive defusion, you learn to recognize that thoughts in your head are simply thoughts. If you instead fuse with your thoughts, your tendency will be to take them seriously as if they were true. You believe them, particularly when there is no, or little, factual basis to the substance of the thoughts.

REMEMBER

When you are *not* fused with your thoughts, you can step back into cognitive defusion. You then hold the thoughts lightly, and this makes it easier to let them go. This is the first step in letting go of negative thoughts. Simply turning them into positive thoughts is not the goal, if the positive thoughts also have no basis. The positive thought is recognizing that you don't have to live believing that your negative thoughts are real and that you can recognize them simply as thoughts that you don't like, and thus don't have to spend too much time dwelling upon them. We look further into how to deal with difficult thoughts in Chapter 7.

Switching self-destructive behaviors to healthy ones

Self-destructive behaviors are those that a person engages in that are likely to cause harm to the self, whether physical or emotional. The types of self-destructive behaviors that people bring to DBT when they are looking for therapy include suicide attempts, cutting, binge eating, dangerous driving, gambling, dangerous sexual behavior, substance abuse, and others.

WARNING

In the short term, people who use these behaviors say that the behaviors bring them some relief from the pain of emotional suffering. This likely happens because certain chemicals are released into the brain. For instance, when people cut themselves, research shows that the brain releases a chemical that is a type of opiate. Drinking alcohol can lead to sedation because of alcohol's effects on the brain. Driving dangerously is a risk-taking behavior that can cause the brain to release dopamine and cause the person to feel elated. All these dangerous behaviors can temporarily change how a person feels, but those who use them tend to discover that the effects are short-lasting and often leave them feeling worse in the long run, as many of these behaviors are ones that cross their values.

DBT focuses on the formation of healthier habits such as avoiding drugs and alcohol, getting to bed on time for a full night's sleep, exercising, and focusing on healthy eating habits. What people who practice these healthier behaviors discover over time is that although these behaviors don't have the immediate impact that the self-destructive behaviors have, they last longer and have an overall positive impact on general well-being, mental and physical health, and relationships. We dig deeper into addressing behaviors in Chapter 6.

Increasing your trust in your responses

Ultimately, if you rely on others to tell you whether you have made a good choice, you'll never learn to trust yourself. If you can't trust yourself, you won't learn to make effective choices, or if you do make a choice, you won't know whether it was the right choice. The only option you have then is to make choices based on the opinions of others, or what others pressure you to do. The problem with even a well-intentioned other giving you advice is that it doesn't teach you to make decisions based on who you are and what you need. Also, what will happen when they are no longer there? Because of the impact of repetition on the brain, if you spend years not trusting your ability to make a choice, you'll end up with a life made up of others' advice. Many people who don't trust themselves experience chronic unhappiness and depression.

How did you *not* learn to trust yourself? For many people who are emotionally sensitive, being punished for having had big displays of emotion meant that they learned that they were bad or wrong for having displayed these emotions, and so they look around to see what other people do. There is a huge problem with this approach. Here's a slightly different example: Imagine that a child was punished for being allergic to peanut butter, that their body had a huge allergic response when they were exposed to peanuts. And if in their situation no one else had such an allergy, and they were teased by others for having it, it makes sense that they might feel bad about themselves and try to make excuses for the reaction they have.

Similarly, if certain situations trigger a big emotional response in you, that is your nature. There is nothing wrong with being sensitive. It is only when you don't know how to deal with being sensitive that you get into trouble, and this is made worse by others having reacted negatively, judgmentally, or punitively to your response. Children who don't learn to trust their experience grow up to be adults who don't trust their experience.

The key to learning to trust yourself is built into your body and your brain. Your body gives you physical and emotional signals all the time; however, some of us haven't learned to pay attention to these signals. A slightly trivial example of this is that we are given the sense of temperature. When we touch something that is hot, a message is sent to our nervous system telling us to pull our hand away. We trust in our body's experience. We don't need to question this. Similarly, when you're about to do something that is inconsistent with your values and long-term goals, your body and brain will send you a signal warning you. Maybe that signal is a spike in anxiety, maybe it's a feeling in the pit of your stomach, maybe it's a headache. The first step to learning to trust yourself is to pay attention to these body sensations and emotions. When you don't pay attention and act reactively, you never give yourself the chance to truly know your experience, and without doing so, you'll never learn to trust yourself and your choices.

As you learn to branch out and pay attention to your mind and body, and you begin to make choices based on the signals your body is sending you, you'll almost certainly make mistakes. But here is the great news: They are *your* mistakes. The DBT therapist works with patients in a way that they are rewarded for trying and not punished for making mistakes. There can be no learning without making mistakes, and it is in making them and then realizing what went wrong that patterns can be corrected. Another vicious cycle happens when the fear of making any mistake prevents us from even trying, and that in turn can lead to more mistakes when a decision-making situation arises. The task is to begin to trust both your successes and errors along the way. Even trust your mistakes because you never know where a mistake might take you.

One of the risks that sensitive people face when learning to trust themselves is that they will be judged. How can you trust what you are thinking about yourself? Are you filtering your decisions through how you think others will respond? The truth is that most of the people in your life are probably so caught up in their own lives that they barely have time to go around judging you, even if it feels like that is what they are doing. As long as you care more about the opinions of the people in your life, you'll dismiss your own, just as valid, opinions.

Altering your behavior to please others is inconsistent with self-trust. Although it might temporarily feel good, if other people weren't true to themselves and altered their behavior to please you, how would you ever know if they were being honest?

REMEMBER

By being present in the moment through the practice of mindfulness, and being present to the emotions, thoughts, and sensations that your body is broadcasting, you tune into your inner wisdom, and there is no more powerful a tool to get to self-trust.

2

Gaining Understanding

IN THIS PART . . .

Recognize how strong emotions can lead to unhelpful behaviors.

Replace unhealthy behaviors with more helpful alternatives.

Notice how judgmental assumptions can lead to poor self-worth, and use thinking skills to address situations in healthier ways.

Improve your relationships with others by improving your relationship with yourself.

Chapter 5

Understanding Your Emotions

Being able to identify and label your emotions is the first step in understanding and making sense of your experience. This is really the first piece of the puzzle of integrating DBT into your life. It isn't uncommon for people to readily be able to identify the general state they are in, such as feeling overwhelmed, stressed, upset, good, or bad; however, for you to better understand your emotions, your description of how you feel must be much more precise. Furthermore, a precise description of your emotions will help you identify which DBT skills will be most effective in achieving your goal of increasing, decreasing, changing, or tolerating and accepting your emotions.

Many people come to DBT troubled by the intensity of their emotions. We have been asked by patients if we could simply make their emotions go away because the impact of their emotional sensitivity or reactivity has been so destructive to their lives that they believe living without emotions would solve the problem. If you've suffered this way, it's an obvious conclusion to draw; however, living without emotions would be hugely problematic. Emotions have functions, and when they are effectively regulated, they provide us with critical information. It's generally understood that emotions have three functions: to communicate to yourself, communicate to others, and motivate action. Think about how many interactions, decisions, and even thoughts are impacted by how you feel in a single moment.

In this chapter, you discover the value of increasing your emotional vocabulary. You find out how to identify and label your emotions, turn up and down the intensity of your emotions, and begin to pay specific attention to particular emotions that you may find challenging. Learning all of this will help you suffer less. Our hope is that in time and with practice, you can learn to love your emotions, even the ones that cause you pain.

Recognizing How You're Feeling

The first step to recognize how you're feeling is to pay attention. However, for people who struggle with intense emotions, the urge is to do just the opposite. Instead of paying attention, they tend to do things to avoid their emotions. Emotional avoidance can take many forms, from distracting yourself and never returning to the feeling, to telling yourself you should not or cannot feel that way, to using alcohol or drugs, sex, reckless behaviors, self-injury, or even suicide.

REMEMBER

If you can pay attention to what you're feeling and shine a light on the experience, as challenging as it may be, it will actually begin the process of decreasing the intensity of that feeling. It's a big ask, we know. Sometimes your emotions will be too intense to start observing; when that is the case, you'll start by using distress tolerance skills (discussed in Chapter 11) to decrease the intensity of the emotion before looking more closely at how you're feeling. It can be tempting to stop after using a distress tolerance skill, but when you do, you're providing a short-term solution to get you through, but not creating any enduring change in how you feel.

In the following sections, you begin to see how paying attention and using mindfulness will help you get to know your emotions and give you the power to control them. Recognizing your emotions takes practice, but once you're familiar with the process, you'll find that you can easily integrate it into your life in a way that will support your use of all of the other DBT skills in this book.

Distinguishing between primary and secondary emotions

One of the most frequent questions we get when we ask people to begin to pay attention to their emotions is how to do that. It does sounds daunting and abstract, especially if we are asking you to pay attention to something that you experience as aversive. Before you can pay attention to what you feel, you first need to know what you are looking for and how you would label it. The following sections discuss how to identify both primary and secondary emotions.

Primary emotions

REMEMBER

As you may have guessed from their name, primary emotions are the ones that you feel first. You can think of them as the first emotion that your brain produces after a specific prompt, an internal or external experience that creates the need for an emotion. Primary emotions are hard-wired and often have associated facial expressions that you can see across many cultures. (Note that one of the functions of emotions is to communicate to yourself and others.) In the field of study of emotion regulation, there is much debate about the number of primary emotions; some researchers believe there are four, five, eight, or ten. Dr. Marsha Linehan, the creator and founder of DBT, believes there are ten primary emotions; these are the ten that we will want you to keep an eye out for:

>> **Joy:** A feeling of pleasure, happiness, or contentment

>> **Love:** An intense feeling of deep affection

>> **Sadness:** A feeling of sorrow or unhappiness

>> **Anger:** A strong feeling of annoyance, displeasure, or hostility

>> **Fear:** A strong feeling that something or someone is dangerous or likely to cause harm or threat

>> **Guilt:** A feeling of having done wrong, failed an obligation, or crossed a personal value

>> **Shame:** A painful feeling of humiliation or distress caused by the awareness of foolish behavior or behavior that crosses societal norms and that leaves you feeling ostracized or different

>> **Envy:** A feeling of discontentment due to the desire to have a possession, attribute, or quality that someone else has

>> **Jealousy:** A feeling of uneasiness from suspicion or fear of rivalry, or fear of something deeply important to you being taken

>> **Disgust:** A feeling of revulsion or strong disapproval aroused by something unpleasant or offensive

TIP

Many of these emotions may be very familiar to you. We encourage you to look closely at two sets of emotions that are often less familiar and are frequently used incorrectly in common language. Look closely at the definitions of guilt and shame, and jealousy and envy. Better understanding the definition of these emotions will help you know how to label your experience.

Secondary emotions

Understanding your emotions would be a little easier if not for secondary emotions. Secondary emotions are where you may get tripped up. These emotions are most commonly the result of thinking about your primary emotion. Your beliefs, judgments, and attitudes about emotions move you into secondary emotions — for example, getting sad and then thinking that sadness is weakness and so getting angry. Sadness is the primary emotion, the one that makes sense in the context of what you just experienced, and anger is the secondary emotion resulting from your beliefs and judgments about sadness.

REMEMBER

A primary emotion lasts an average of 90 seconds if we don't apply a chain of thinking that turns it into a secondary emotion. The problem with secondary emotions is they can last a long time — hours, days, weeks, months. You can get stuck in secondary emotions, and those emotions tend to perpetuate themselves with ease. Feeling miserable is a great example of getting stuck in a mix of secondary emotions. One tricky thing about secondary emotions is that a primary emotion can, in fact, also be a secondary emotion. If your beliefs, judgments, and attitudes about sadness lead you to feel more sadness, then sadness is also secondary. Self-invalidation and invalidation from others is an easy way to land in a secondary emotional experience. So, if you experience an emotion lasting more than 90 seconds (before something else prompts it), then you're likely inadvertently making sadness stick around longer than it needs to. It's actually a great clue! This is why it's so critical to learn to pay attention and be able to identify, label, understand, and validate your emotions.

Paying attention to what you feel

Paying attention to what you're feeling requires an openness and willingness to shine a light on your emotional experience. We know that when you look directly at an emotion, the intensity of it begins to decrease. If you're doubtful, we encourage you to try this sooner rather than later. Identifying an emotion and validating it — recognizing how it makes sense and is valid — is a powerful and healing experience.

So, where do you start? In DBT we have a skill called mindfulness of current emotion, and we break it down into steps using the acronym SUN WAVE NO NOT. Using this skill will help you identify the primary emotion and label it. Follow the steps in this section to do so.

TIP

When you're just starting to use this skill, it can be helpful to write down your answers on a piece of paper. Take your time; it can be a slower process in the beginning, but once you practice, you'll be able to simply pause and identify your emotions much of the time without even using all of the following steps.

SUN

REMEMBER

The acronym SUN stands for *Sensations*, *Urges*, and *Name the emotion*:

>> **Sensations:** All emotions have associated sensations. Your body holds important clues about how and what you're feeling. Briefly scan your body, starting at your head and moving down to your toes. Do you feel a tightness or clenching of your jaw? Warmth in your cheeks? Throbbing in your head? Tears in your eyes? Tightness in your chest? Butterflies or a sinking feeling in your stomach? Tightness or clenching of your hands?

>> **Urges:** All emotions have associated action urges. This makes sense, as one of the functions of emotions is to motivate action. For example, when you feel fear, you may have the urge to run, fight, or freeze. When you're sad, you may feel the urge to curl up, cry, or isolate. When you feel shame, you may want to hide. When you're angry, you may have the urge to yell or hit or throw something; other people may cry when they are angry. We don't all have the same action urges, but they tend to be similar.

>> **Name the emotion:** Once you have identified your body sensation and your urges, you typically have enough information to name the emotion. We know that once you can name the emotion, it begins to decrease in intensity. That often occurs because it gives you some space between your own experience and what you're feeling. This also helps you find the primary emotions, which may have been hidden beneath a secondary emotion. (We discuss primary and secondary emotions earlier in this chapter.)

WAVE

Once you have named the emotion, your task is to ride it like a WAVE. When a primary emotion runs its course, you'll experience it like a wave, first lower in intensity, building up to the peak or the crest of the wave, and then slowing, decreasing in intensity until you return to baseline, or the waves settle on the shore. The way to ride the wave is to use your mindfulness "Observe and Describe Skills," which we cover in more depth in Chapter 9. What you'll do is notice and describe your sensations and your urges, which you've already identified in the SUN part of this practice (see the previous section). Notice and describe without judgment the facts of your experience. For example, you may notice your thoughts moving quickly, a sensation of butterflies in your stomach, your face feeling red, and tears running down your cheeks.

You'll notice that this is a somewhat boring process as there are no judgments or editorials about your experience that pull in the past or the future. This is what helps your emotions simply run their course. Repeat this process until the intensity of your emotions becomes more manageable.

NO NOT

The final phase consists of NO NOT:

>> **NO:** *No* suppressing your emotions. *No* enhancing your emotions. This means that you don't tell yourself that you can't feel something, and you don't do things that increase the intensity of an unwanted emotion such as judging and invalidating it. You can think about this phase as consisting of things to avoid when you are riding the WAVE from the previous section.

REMEMBER

>> **NOT:** As you ride the WAVE, remind yourself that you are *not* your emotions and that your emotions will *not* last forever. It may seem like a small semantic thing, but when you talk about your experience, it's important to avoid saying "I *am* depressed" and instead say "I *feel* depressed." When you indicate it as a feeling state, it signals to the brain that it's something that changes. By definition, emotions change and fluctuate. The first statement communicates, "I am a person who is depressed; it is inherent to me and therefore is less likely to change." It may seem small, but it makes a big difference when you're working on experiencing emotions and allowing them to move through you. Sometimes when emotions are very intense, you may feel like they will never end. It's important to note that primary emotions last an average of 90 seconds, which is far from forever, even if it feels like it.

Confronting Disproportionate Reactions

If you're an emotionally sensitive person, by definition you feel things longer and deeper than the average person and you have a much slower return to baseline. This is simply your biology. You can think of it like the engine of a car. The engine in a Porsche and the engine in a Prius are very different in their capability to rapidly accelerate. What this means is that it isn't uncommon for emotionally sensitive people to react more intensely and hold onto emotions longer. The problem with this is that it can increase your suffering and negatively impact your relationships.

People we work with have often said that they have been told that they are "too much" or that they always overreact. That kind of feedback can be very painful. If you struggle with this, the good news is that like a car with a fast engine, you can learn how to drive it; you can also learn to recognize when your reaction is too intense and regulate it. The following sections can help.

Realizing that your reaction may be overblown

If you're an emotionally sensitive person, you need to accept, without judgment, that you may often have overblown reactions. Accepting this about some of your reactions will help you recognize when it happens, and that is the first step. In DBT, while we don't love the term, we talk about two types of emotions, justified and unjustified. This may seem subjective, and in many ways it is. You'll be the one who determines whether your emotions are justified or unjustified using a few guidelines from DBT. Again, this is not about judging your emotions, but about helping you cope when your emotions are leading to misery and suffering, and to then figure out what skills you can use.

REMEMBER

To answer this question, you want to ask yourself three questions:

>> Does my emotion fit the situation, and does it make sense that this emotion is showing up right now?

>> Does the intensity to which I am feeling it make sense?

>> Does the duration that I am feeling it make sense?

TIP

Sometimes it's hard to answer these questions when you're filled with strong emotions. Here is a helpful trick: We often ask our patients to think about people they know who they feel experience and regulate their emotions well and would provide a reasonable metric for comparison. It could be your group of friends, people you work with, or even other close or extended family members. Try to compare your answers to the preceding three question to theirs. Pick people who you think experience and regulate their emotions in a way that you could use as a model. This is not meant as a comparison that leaves you feeling bad about your emotions, but instead as a means of comparison that will guide your choice of skills. In Chapter 10, we give you some specific emotion regulation skills that you can use once you have identified whether your emotions are justified or unjustified.

Getting from recognition to regulation

While some find that recognizing their emotions is the hardest part, others find figuring out what to do with them or finding the willingness to use a skill to be the most challenging part. We discuss more specific emotion regulation skills in Chapter 10. Once you recognize your emotions, you need to ask yourself what you want or need to do with them.

Validating your emotions

One of the most critical and sometimes hardest things to do is to validate your emotions. For many people who come to DBT, this is one of the hardest skills because for many years, they, and often their loved ones, have been invalidating their emotions. The key to validation is to remind yourself (and others if you're validating them) what makes sense about how you feel. The NO in your SUN WAVE NO NOT (covered earlier in this chapter) helps you avoid the self-invalidation that may have become automatic.

WARNING

Validation, by definition, helps decrease the intensity of your emotion by reminding you that your emotions make sense. Invalidation, or telling yourself you shouldn't feel a certain way, that you're stupid or weak for feeling something, or even that you should just get over it, are some of the most effective ways to enhance the very feelings that are already painful and leading to suffering. Invalidation is a main ingredient of generating a sticky secondary emotion. (We discuss primary and secondary emotions earlier in this chapter.)

Asking a few helpful questions

REMEMBER

Once you've recognized and labeled your emotions, you may want to ask yourself some questions to help you think through what skills will be the most effective. We recommend that you practice doing this so that it becomes a habit. Consider asking yourself these questions:

1. How can I validate my current emotion?

2. Do I want to tolerate and accept this emotion so I can ride it out like a wave?

3. Do I want to increase or decrease the intensity of this emotion?

4. Do I want to stay miserable?

5. Do I want to do something to make it worse?

We review many skills to help you tolerate, as well as increase and decrease, the intensity of your emotions in Part 3 of this book.

TIP

Often people get confused at question numbers four and five in the preceding list:

>> Sometimes, staying miserable for a period of time can be validating. It's okay to do that. That being said, we include it as number four because we want that to be a choice made with intention and not a state that you find yourself stuck in, not realizing how you got there. You can think about it like this: It's okay to throw yourself a pity party — sometimes we all just need that — but you need to know that you're going to the party, so that after a reasonable period of time, you know how to leave.

>> Number five is there for similar reasons; it will help you avoid falling into the trap of making things worse. Remember, you can almost always make your situation and emotions worse. Our hope is that you learn this as an option so that you can experience this emotion less. It isn't uncommon for this to happen in a split second and with little awareness. The idea is to slow yourself down. It may seem like an obvious example, but when you're angry and you punch a wall, it may feel good in the moment when you get a huge rush of adrenaline, but then you just have a hole in the wall that you need to explain and then fix. You have worsened your problem, and if you're like many people, you've piled on an intense feeling of shame.

If you can keep these questions in mind, you can build the awareness to decrease reactivity and increase your sense of choice of how to move on a skillful path toward regulation.

Identifying and Handling Problem Areas

We all have problem areas. In DBT we have a number of skills training assumptions, and two of the most important ones are that we are all doing the best we can, and we need to do better, try harder, and be more motivated to change. Problem areas, or areas of emotional vulnerability, are a reality. It can be helpful to not get lost in judgment about problem areas, but instead to embrace them as nuggets of wisdom that you know about yourself and that you can build awareness and skills to manage.

Looking at what causes you distress

Looking at what commonly causes you distress can help you anticipate challenging situations. When you can anticipate difficult situations or interactions, it gives you time to plan ahead so that you aren't continually experiencing distress in the same situations. Knowing your common areas of distress will also help you validate your experience, which, as we discuss earlier in this chapter, will help you keep painful emotions from building in intensity.

REMEMBER

A wide range of things cause people distress, and each of us has unique areas that we find harder to manage, based on our sensitivity and experiences. When you begin to think about this, some situations may be quite obvious and easy to identify, while others may take more time to figure out. Consider the following questions:

>> Is there something you do that repeatedly causes you distress (posting on social media, being with certain people, going to certain places)?

>> Are there certain relationships or interactions that repeatedly cause you distress?

>> Are there certain holidays or gatherings that repeatedly cause you distress?

>> Are there certain places you go (work, school, restaurants, people's houses) that repeatedly cause you distress?

>> Are there situations that repeatedly cause you distress (hearing the word *no*, receiving a compliment, receiving feedback at work or from a friend, saying no to someone)?

>> Are there certain emotions that are harder to manage and that frequently cause you distress?

Thinking about these experiences will help you narrow down specific areas that you can focus your skills on so that you don't keep finding yourself in similar painful situations over and over again.

Figuring out coping solutions

REMEMBER

In Part 3 of this book, we introduce the DBT skills that, with practice, you can use as coping solutions. Remember, sometimes the solutions are simply tolerating and accepting the reality in front of you, while other skills will help you solve problems, turn up or down the intensity of your emotions, or be more effective in your relationships or interactions with others. Being able to understand and identify your emotions is the first and very critical step in coping. Often, people skip over this step, and when that happens, they rarely choose the most effective skill to meet their goal.

Chapter **6**

Understanding Your Behaviors

Many of us in the mental health field find human behavior to be fascinating. Observing patterns of behavior and trying to predict what a person is going to do next can be useful in establishing what is helpful and what is not, and what interventions to use if behavior is to be changed. And yet in many instances, behavior is very predictable, because it's patterned through repetition. Take a behavior like walking. Because of repetition, it's predictable that a person will walk when getting from point A to point B. And yet walking is a relatively simple behavior. Behaviors that emanate from strong emotions can be very complex and much harder to predict.

People who are emotionally sensitive generally experience life with more intensity than those who are less sensitive. Typically, with more sensitivity comes a greater degree of behavioral variability.

There is nothing problematic with being more emotionally sensitive. Many artists, therapists, actors, musicians, and others recognize that being sensitive is helpful to their craft. However, people who have strong emotions can be at risk of behaving in ways that are dependent on their mood state. Mood-dependent behavior is often what causes people to request DBT therapy for two main reasons: The first is the person doesn't have the skills to effectively manage emotionally charged situations, and the second is the behavior that happens when a person acts on their feelings or urges without pausing to consider the consequences of the behavior can lead to suffering in the person's life. Often, mood-dependent behaviors seem automatic and seem to happen quickly, as if the person had no choice. They seem to come from nowhere and appear to be out of an individual's control, and because of this, they can seem hard to change given the powerful underlying emotions, urges, and often negative thoughts driving them.

In this chapter, we review the connections between feelings and actions, recognize the triggers that set off behaviors, and look at how we can link specific behaviors to specific reactions as a way to begin to change unhelpful behaviors.

Being Aware of How Your Emotions Manifest in Action

When you're engaging in mood-dependent behavior, you're acting on the urges caused by your underlying emotional state. An example of this is when, for instance, you have a low mood and have the urge not to get out of bed or see anyone. Staying in bed and not seeing your friends would be mood-dependent behavior. If you are feeling angry and lash out at your co-worker for a seemingly trivial transgression, that is mood-dependent behavior.

For people who are prone to such behavior, when the mood has passed, they can often feel guilty or shameful about their behavior. In the moment, however, the person acting on their emotions without thinking frequently feels justified and right for having done so. The alternative of stopping and reflecting on what to do, or even tolerating the discomfort of the emotion, can feel unbearable. Mood-dependent behavior can bring instant relief and feels great in the short run, only to cause greater harm in the long run.

REMEMBER

For any individual, every emotion has an action urge, and it's a core part of DBT for the person to know their typical behavior when they are feeling strong emotions. If you struggle in this way, being mindful is key to developing the awareness of how your emotional state in the present moment leads to these behaviors. Mindfulness is also key to then having a more deliberate response. This means that when a strong emotion arises, you should take the time to pause and ask yourself the following:

>> "Is what I am about to do consistent with my long-term goals and values?"

>> "Will this behavior actually get me what I want?"

>> "How likely is my behavior going to lead to regret, guilt, and shame?"

Identifying and Handling Emotional Triggers

Everyone's brain creates powerful associations between things that hurt them and the people associated with that hurt. For example, once you've been attacked in a dark alley, even walking by an alley can lead to a physical reaction. Interestingly, it's easier to recognize and forgive our own behavior and misbehavior because we understand the connection between our response and whatever is triggering that response. However, it's also true that other people have reasons for the reactions that they have. Just because we don't understand why they are doing what they are doing doesn't mean that they don't have their own triggers.

Particularly when someone has experienced trauma, abuse, and invalidation, this can lead to unexamined and unprocessed emotions that can be triggered by anything that leads to recollection of the events. The triggered person typically has a fair grasp on reality, but their emotional response fails to reflect the current situation; they may feel suspicious of the intentions of those around them or anxious around friends, or become very angry for a seemingly trivial slight.

REMEMBER

The point is that whereas you might understand your own reactions to triggers, it's important to realize that the reason a person is acting the way they are could be because they are triggered as well.

The most important reason to identify triggers is to either limit their disruption in your life or minimize the power they have in controlling your actions. The following sections provide more insight into identifying triggers.

Limiting their disruption

REMEMBER

To limit the disruption of emotional triggers, you have to know what they are. You can use the following process of examination to recognize them:

>> **What is the environmental trigger?** What was the thing that happened that led to the emotions now leading to your urges to respond in a particular way? For example, your partner told you that he was going to be home for dinner, and you become angry when your mother calls to tell you that she thinks she saw him having a drink with his friends at a bar.

>> **What is your internal mood state?** Label the emotion. In this example, you notice feeling jealous and then angry that your partner has been dismissive of you. You also notice feeling confused and then upset with your mother because she isn't actually certain that it was him.

>> **What is your short-term objective in the present moment?** In this example, you want to make sure that you're in a calmer state by the time your partner comes home so that you don't accuse him of doing something that he might not actually have done.

>> **What is your long-term goal?** You want to be able to trust your partner and have calm conversations with him — ones that are direct and full of curiosity.

>> **What actions will be consistent with your long-term goal?** Will your actions allow you to accomplish your goal? Will being upset help you attain this goal, or should you regulate to a state of being calmer and recognize that you have only a tiny snippet of information on which you and your mother may have come to unhelpful conclusions?

>> **If you act on your urge, will this help you attain your goal, or will it interfere with attaining your goal?** If you start yelling at your partner the second he walks through the door, accusing him of being uncaring and a liar, will this help you have a more trusting relationship with him? On the other hand, if he is being dismissive of you, will simply being angry without being curious as to what happened be consistent with how you value yourself?

>> **If you act on your urge, will you later regret having so acted?** What have past experiences taught you? Have you yelled at past partners, and if so, how did these relationships end up?

While these questions may seem obvious to a person who doesn't engage in mood-dependent behavior, they reflect the mindful path to limiting a trigger's disruption to one's quality of life and significant relationships.

Minimizing their power

There are several ways to reduce the impact of emotional triggers, as you find out in the following sections.

Reducing the size of the response

The first way to reduce the impact of an emotional trigger is to reduce the magnitude of the emotional response. There are various ways to do this:

>> **Having a *time delay*:** The simplest way to minimize the impact of strong emotions is to let time pass before making a decision. The reason this makes sense is because at a neurological level, unless the person keeps ruminating about the situation, emotions are short-lived. The physiological manifestations of any emotion are fleeting and fade quickly. However, because strong emotions compel people to action, letting time pass is easier said than done.

>> **Using *suppression*:** This would be the type of reaction where, for example, a person is asked to control their anger. Unfortunately, research shows that suppression is counterproductive. It often leads to the intensifying of the very emotional state that you're trying to suppress.

Reframing the trigger with reappraisal

A more helpful approach is the practice of *reappraisal.* Reappraisal means reframing the meaning of the triggering event that led to the emotional response. It's the strongest way to weaken the power of the emotional response. An example of reappraisal is, for instance, recognizing that failing a single test isn't the end of the world ("It's just one test. I can study more for the next one and get some help from my teacher.") or by noticing "the fact that I lost my job means that I can pursue some other long-term dreams."

This approach is consistent with the practice of *changing your relationship to the problem* in DBT problem-solving. In contrast to suppression, reappraisal not only reduces negative feelings as a response to triggering events but also reduces the body's and brain's biological responses. People who use reappraisal typically have more positive emotional experiences and show fewer episodes of unwanted emotions.

Using the concept of opposite action

Another useful approach is the practice of inducing a counteracting emotional state. The idea behind this is to counteract a maladaptive behavior caused by an intense emotion by inducing another emotion, one that triggers opposing or differing action urges or tendencies. For example, say that your best friend had promised to call you last night and she didn't. You're angry and all you want to do is rage at her and tell her what a terrible friend she is. If instead, you could conjure up the love you have for her and all the wonderful ways that she has been there for you in the past, you would be opposing hatred with love. This practice is consistent with the emotion regulation skill of *opposite action* in DBT.

Another way to think about this is that if an emotion has an action that follows, that means the emotion has caused the action. You can change the emotion by changing the action that follows. Here is the beauty of opposite action: Not only do emotions cause actions, but actions cause emotions, and so you can change your emotion by changing your action.

Opposite action works best when your emotions do *not* fit the facts of a current situation. If you're afraid of a rattlesnake in your living room in Arizona, then the fear fits the facts and it's justified if the snake is there. If the snake isn't there, then the fear doesn't fit the facts and is unjustified. If the emotion doesn't fit the facts, this means that its intensity and duration aren't effective in helping you achieve your long-term goals.

If you're going to use opposite action, it's important to throw yourself fully into the skill. Engage in behaviors that are opposite or different to the ones that you feel the urge to do, and then use opposite emotion words, thoughts, facial expressions, tone of voice, and body posture. For instance, consider these examples:

>> **Fear:** If you feel afraid, approach the situation or trigger that gives you anxiety. Try to face your fear. Engage in behaviors that increase your sense of control over your fear. You can repeatedly expose yourself to your unjustified fear in order to desensitize yourself. For instance, if you're afraid of speaking to your boss, then you can repeatedly practice approaching her with confidence.

>> **Anger:** If you are angry at someone and feel like lashing out, you can instead initially avoid them rather than attack them, and then practice empathy for them and the behavior that made them do what they did. You can try to find the *kernel of truth* in their actions. Something caused their actions. Be curious about what it was.

>> **Sadness:** If you're feeling low or depressed, rather than avoiding, isolating, or staying in bed, you can approach, engage, and get out of bed. You don't isolate, but instead engage in activities that connect and keep you active and busy.

>> **Shame:** If you feel shame over something you have done and the shame is justified, then apologize. If the shame doesn't fit the facts and is unjustified, then you need to engage fully in the situation that induced the shame by participating in social interactions, and even share your ideas and behaviors that led to the experience of shame.

>> **Guilt:** Similar to shame, if your guilt fits the facts, you need to apologize for the transgression. If your guilt is unjustified, then you must *not* apologize. Instead, change your body posture by walking tall with shoulders back and maintaining good eye contact while talking with a confident, steady, and clear voice.

Tying Specific Behaviors to Specific Reactions

Everyone has default and automatic behaviors. These behaviors can lead to specific and often automatic reactions, and how we handle these automatic responses can make the difference between effective and ineffective outcomes. DBT focuses on the careful paying of attention to these patterns of behavior with the goal of considering, if need be, alternative behaviors in order to create an alternative reaction.

Understanding physical responses and conscious feelings

Emotions are neurological phenomena that occur in response to a trigger event. The trigger could be an interaction with another person, a sight, a sound, a smell, a thought, or just about anything. Once the emotion has occurred, it causes us to take action. Every emotion is activating and hard-wired as a part of our evolutionary biology. This is so that when we experience an emotion or feeling, we act. Here are some examples:

>> **Thirst** tells us that we need to hydrate, and so it activates us to find water to drink.

>> **Hunger** tells us that our body is short on fuel and to find food to eat.

>> **Fear** tells us that there is a threat in the environment and to find safety.

>> **Extreme temperature** tells us that we are about to overheat or freeze and to find shade or warm clothes.

>> **Fatigue** tells us that our body needs rest and to slow down and get some sleep.

REMEMBER

Emotions are mediated by various brain circuits. Emotional states have two distinctive components:

>> **A pattern of characteristic physical responses:** Emotional physical states are the responses of our hormones, muscles, heart, bladder, stomach, and so on.

>> **A conscious feeling:** Conscious feelings are the thoughts we have that are associated with the situation.

When we're frightened, for instance, we not only feel afraid but also undergo unconscious body changes such as an increase in heart rate and respiration, dryness of the mouth, muscle tension, and sweaty palms. The conscious part of the experience consists of the thoughts we have about the situation.

In DBT, therapists work with the patient to connect the specific reactions and thoughts the patient has to the emotions they are experiencing. By mapping these out, they help the patient more easily recognize the emotions with a goal of realizing the automaticity of typical responses and the ideal of developing a greater repertoire of behavioral reactions. We review the impact of emotions and what to do with them in Chapter 10.

Establishing new pathways

There is an old saying that "you can't teach an old dog new tricks." If this were true, there would be no need for therapy and particular DBT treatment. DBT is all about teaching new skills (tricks) to replace old behaviors when the behaviors have been maladaptive.

So, what does behavior change look like in the brain? Neural pathways are the bundles of nerves that connect one part of the nervous system to another. They are like the cable that connects your phone to its charger, or the TV to the cable box. These bundles of nerves are connected to each other by dendrites. Think of a dendrite roughly as the plug that goes into the wall or your phone. A big difference between plugs and dendrites is that the number of dendrites increases each time a behavior is performed. Another way to think about repetition is to consider the grooves that a car makes on a dirt road. The more cars that travel on the road, the deeper the grooves become.

The bundles of nerves communicate with each other via a process known as *neuronal firing.* When brain cells communicate frequently, the connection between them strengthens. Another process that happens is *myelination.* Myelin is the covering of the neurons. Think of it as the plastic sheathing around a copper cable. Over time, the more a behavior is repeated, the more myelin wraps around the nerve cells.

Over thousands of instances of the repetition of behaviors, myelination and dendrite formation leads to communication between nerve cells becoming faster and more effortless. With enough repetition, these behaviors become automatic. The behavior of walking is one example of this. When a child learns how to walk, they often fall and are clumsy. After thousands of repetitions, walking becomes automatic.

REMEMBER

However, just because we have created the neural pathways that lead to certain behaviors, this doesn't mean that we're stuck with those behaviors forever. If we want to change our automatic behaviors, we must participate in new activities. By engaging in new behaviors, we're training our brains and our brain cells to create new neural pathways. Just like our old behaviors, the new pathways get stronger the more we repeat the new behaviors. Eventually, the new behaviors can become the new normal.

If we go back to the behavior of the child walking, initially the child moves around by crawling, and crawling is the automatic behavior caused by the repetition of crawling and leading to the strengthening of the brain cells. When the child starts to walk, eventually the new "walking" pathways become stronger than the "crawling" pathways, and walking becomes the new normal. This can be done with all behavior, even though it can be more difficult if the behavior has lasted for a long time.

REMEMBER

It can be easy to give up, because it can feel like nothing is changing. Research shows that it takes somewhere from three to six months for a new behavior to become more automatic, although this varies a lot by person. If you're in DBT, your therapist will want you to persist until your new behavior becomes more habitual. This will include your DBT therapist providing you with ideas for over-coming obstacles that might interfere with engaging in the new behaviors. We delve more fully into these ideas when we review the skills in Part 3 of this book.

Chapter **7**

Understanding How You Think

DBT is a synthesis of two other treatments: cognitive behavioral therapy (CBT) and mindfulness-based therapy. This chapter focuses more on the contributions that come from CBT. CBT works to change your behaviors and how you feel by changing your thoughts and beliefs. It's a treatment that focuses heavily on thinking or cognition. In this chapter, we help you look closely at your thoughts — not only at what you think, but specifically at how you talk to yourself and how that impacts your reactions and behaviors. A lot goes on in your head!

Tapping into Your Self-Talk

While it may sound strange, everyone talks to themselves. In the world of psychology, this is called *self-talk*. Self-talk is your internal dialogue; it's made up of thoughts, beliefs, assumptions, questions, and ideas. Self-talk helps your brain make sense of your day-to-day experiences. Your self-talk can be positive or negative, encouraging or punishing, helpful or harmful. Self-talk happens a lot of the time, and sometimes you may pay more attention to it than at other times.

The fascinating thing about self-talk is how much it influences your behavior. Most people believe there are two main types of self-talk: positive ("I can do it") and negative ("I can't do it"). Some believe in a third type of self-talk called possibility ("What if I can do this"). You can see how strongly the way you talk to yourself can impact your behavior. The challenging thing about self-talk is that you're constantly practicing it, so you may be very skilled at maladaptive or problematic self-talk. If this is the case, we can help you learn to practice a more effective way of talking to yourself. Don't be fooled; this isn't about living a life of rainbows and butterflies in your mind. This is about paying attention to how you talk to yourself and making sure that how you talk to yourself is helping you move toward your goals and what is important to you, and not getting in the way.

How do you want to use your self-talk? When used effectively, your self-talk can enhance motivation, calm your anxiety, provide reassurance, and even increase your confidence. For example, there has been a lot of research to help athletes use self-talk to enhance their performance. When you get caught in negative self-talk, you can become overwhelmed with negativity and believe that you are not good enough, are undeserving, can never be successful, or are a failure. If you're stuck deep enough, you can get caught in a loop of continually attacking yourself. Depression can lead to very negative and problematic self-talk, which can become a dark lens through which you see the world. Many people who come to DBT find themselves stuck in this painful cycle of negative self-talk.

WARNING

Negative self-talk can get complicated. You may believe that you're being honest, that you deserve it, that it will protect you from disappointment, or that it will motivate you to do better. These are all very interesting beliefs; however, none of them are true. For some, being hard on themselves or beating themselves up may motivate them in the moment, but it's a poor long-term strategy with negative consequences.

REMEMBER

Begin to pay attention to your self-talk and see whether it may be hampering you. Consider the following questions as red flags that your thinking is getting in your way:

>> Does your self-talk get in the way of setting or achieving your goals?

>> Do you tell yourself that you are stupid, a loser, a failure, or worthless, or do you use other judgments when you think about yourself?

>> Before trying something or while you are doing something, have you already decided that you won't be successful?

>> Do you draw absolute conclusions or do you have black-and-white thinking?

>> Do you become absolutely certain about what other people are thinking, particularly what they are thinking about you?

Answering "yes" to any of these questions means your self-talk may be getting in your way. The good news is that, despite how you feel, you don't have to believe everything you think. In essence, we all have a lot of "fake news" going on in our heads a lot of the time. Take a moment and think about this. The idea that you don't have to believe everything you think is very freeing. To do this, you have to learn the skills to pay attention to what you're thinking and then to work with your thoughts. Three cognitive skills in DBT will help you do this: practicing mindfulness of current thought, using cognitive reappraisal, and checking the facts.

REMEMBER

Thinking about and changing the way you think can profoundly impact how you feel. Emotions can really tangle up your thinking and make it hard to look at situations objectively or make accurate interpretations. Being aware of your emotion-minded thinking and using mindfulness to step back and work with your thoughts will truly help you decrease your suffering. When you're too deep in emotion mind — when very strong emotions are dictating not only how you feel but how you think and act in that moment — working with your thinking can feel impossible. In those instances, try to use mindfulness (see Chapter 9) or distress tolerance skills (see Chapter 11) to decrease the intensity of how you feel so you're more able to work with your thinking.

Practicing mindfulness of current thought

Paying attention to your thoughts is the first step. You use the observe-and-describe skill that we discuss in Chapter 9 to do this. The challenge of this skill is to remain mindful and not get caught up in the very thoughts that are getting in your way. You must practice being the observer, which is more challenging when the thoughts you're having are leading you to feel strong emotions. It is as if you're watching your thoughts with an open mind and curiosity, and reminding yourself that they are simply thoughts and not necessarily truths.

REMEMBER

Follow these four steps when you are practicing mindfulness of current thought:

1. **Observe your thoughts.**

   Observe your thoughts like a wave or like clouds moving across the sky. Simply observe without engaging or adding to them. You can label them as thoughts, saying to yourself, "I notice the thought. . ." Don't judge or analyze the thoughts. Acknowledge the thoughts that are there. Don't suppress them; just observe.

2. **Adopt a curious mind.**

   Be curious and open. Consider where the thoughts could come from without getting too caught up in them. Remind yourself that they are just thoughts.

3. Remember: You are not your thoughts.

Remind yourself that your thoughts don't define you and don't need to result in behavior. Note that black-and-white thinking and catastrophic thinking are the results of emotion mind and that when you are more regulated and not suffering or intensely angry, you will think differently.

4. Don't block or suppress thoughts.

You find out in Chapter 10 that suppressing your emotions is one of the best ways to enhance your painful feelings; the same is true of your thoughts. Telling yourself that you can't think something only makes the thoughts come stronger and faster. Engage with your thoughts in a mindful and deliberate way. When thoughts are intense, you can turn your attention to sensations or emotions and ask yourself what your thoughts may be helping you avoid. This can help you connect with the primary emotions, which are often driving these problematic thoughts. Try appreciating your thoughts or even saying, "Wow, isn't that interesting that I am thinking this."

You can play with your thoughts if they become very sticky and repetitive, sing your thoughts, say them over and over as fast or as slow as you can, say them in a funny voice, or imagine them being said by a celebrity.

REMEMBER

Mindfulness of current thought is a deliberate mindful practice. We say this because at first glance, it can feel invalidating. Being able to observe your thoughts and at times take them less seriously will help free you from being captive to the thoughts in your mind and help you more mindfully choose what to believe. When you can do this, you will feel more in control of how you act or behave.

Using cognitive reappraisal

Cognitive reappraisal is a skill from CBT that helps you regulate emotions by reappraising your emotionally driven thoughts. Reappraisal helps you look at emotionally laden situations and how you can think about them in a different way by reframing your thoughts. Reappraisal can improve emotion regulation and increase psychological well-being. The meaning you make of something makes a difference in both how you feel and how you behave. For example, you could say, "Fall is coming," and a person could respond, "I'm so looking forward to the leaves changing," while a second person could respond, "Oh, Halloween and Thanksgiving are such wonderful holidays," and a third person could respond, "Summer vacation is over." What do you notice? The first two appraisals lead to feelings of happiness and excitement, while the third creates a sense of dread and perhaps anxiety.

You can see how mindfulness of current thought (see the previous section) will help you with reappraisal. Think of it as opening your mind to possibilities that will cause you less suffering. Your cognitive reappraisal will lead to a change in your emotional response. For example, you made it to a final interview and then didn't get the job, and you notice the thought, "I am a failure." How could you reappraise that? Is that an accurate thought? Reappraisal helps you more accurately assess an emotional situation. Another way to look at that situation is that you made it to the final two people and excelled beyond many other people, which is quite an accomplishment.

REMEMBER

The one thing to keep in mind with cognitive reappraisal is that it can be a very difficult skill to apply when you are very dysregulated. Sometimes, the most effective way to use this skill is to first use a distress tolerance skill (see Chapter 11) to lower the intensity of your emotions and then move on to reappraising when you aren't as deep in emotion mind. The more you practice this skill, the more able you will be to reappraise when you are in emotion mind.

Checking the facts

Checking the facts takes your cognitive reappraisal skill a step further. As we explain throughout this book, how you think about yourself and the things that happen around you impacts how you feel. These are the interpretations that you make. Sometimes your interpretations more than the event itself create suffering. What makes it even more complicated is that how you feel impacts how you think. Both how you think and how you feel then go on to impact how you behave. Examining your thoughts, and looking carefully at what you are thinking and what interpretations you are making, will give you the opportunity to decide whether that is an effective way to think and whether it's leading you to feeling how you would like to feel. While this is a cognitive skill, you can see how your mindfulness skills of observing and describing (see Chapter 9) will be very useful.

REMEMBER

There are six questions to ask yourself when you are using the checking-the-facts skill:

1. **What emotion do I want to change?** Be sure to use your SUN WAVE NO NOT skill (see Chapter 5) to identify your primary emotion.

   For example: *I am feeling sad and ashamed that everyone hates me.*

2. **What is the event that is prompting this emotion?** Nonjudgmentally describe what is happening. Watch out for emotion-minded thinking such as judgments, black-and-white thinking, or absolute certainty. Stick to the facts.

   For example: *I was not invited to the party on Saturday night and found out only because I saw pictures posted on social media.*

3. **What are my thoughts, interpretations, and assumptions about the event?** Pay close attention to your interpretations and assumptions. Practice having an open mind and looking at the situation from at least two other perspectives. Ask yourself, "Do my interpretations and assumptions fit the facts of the situation?" Here are some examples:

I am always being left out. This is the first time this has happened with these friends. Only two of my friends were in the pictures at the party, and when I think about it, they are newer friends who are also friends with another group. Two friends do not equal everyone.

My friends don't really care about me. My closest friends were not in any of the pictures. They have given me no reason to think they excluded me. I did tell them that I couldn't go out this weekend.

4. **Am I assuming a threat?** Identify the threat that you're fearful of. Consider how likely it is that what you are afraid of will happen. Open your mind to other possibilities. Ask yourself, "Could there be other possible outcomes?"

For example: *I am afraid I will lose more friends. I am afraid of being alone again. I think my fear is because I have lost friends in the past and I really struggle with being alone. Because of my fear, I make these types of interpretations. I think it is possible that this is something I struggle with and that my friends did not leave me out and have not changed how they feel about me.*

5. **What is the catastrophe?** Is the outcome catastrophic? If so, use your skills and cope ahead. Think about what you would do if that worst-case scenario came true. Make a plan for effectively managing.

For example: *Being left out and losing friends feels catastrophic. I have dealt with it before, and while it was painful, I could handle it. I always have my childhood friends who have always stuck by me.*

6. **Is your emotion justified (does the intensity fit the facts of the situation)?** Ask your wise mind — that place of inner wisdom where you can both think about the facts of the situation and what you know while also paying attention to and taking into account how you feel — if the intensity and duration of your feelings match the facts of the situation. If they do not, consider using opposite action (see Chapter 10).

For example: *I think my emotion is unjustified. I know I am feeling this more intensely and jumping to the worst-case scenario. I am thinking and feeling this way because I have lost friends in the past and it started by being left out. When things happen that resemble painful events in my past, I quickly go into emotion mind.*

Looking at Your Reactions

It's an interesting skill and practice to be able to step back and look at not only your thinking but also at the reactions that are prompted by your thinking. If you can chuckle a bit at some of the reactions that your brain produces, then you'll create a pause in which you can sit and decide how to proceed.

Many of us have reactions in our heads that are extreme, but if you can pause, take a step back, and look at them as coming from your emotion mind, then you're less likely to react in a way that is ineffective or problematic. For example, many people who come to DBT struggle with suicidal thinking. We know that the more you repeat ways of thinking, the more prominent they become. It is all about repetition. We have worked with patients who learn these skills and who tell us that they have observed that whenever they are faced with a problem, big or small, they observe suicidal thinking. One patient told us that she was in a long line at a grocery store and was going to be late for her appointment, and she noticed the thought, "I want to kill myself." She was able to observe it and practice just saying, "Wow, that is fascinating that I am worried about being late and suicide came into my mind." Before learning these skills, she would either get pulled deep into her suicidal thoughts or judge and blame herself as being so stupid for thinking this way. Now she has a much more balanced reaction.

REMEMBER

The reactions in your head are just that: They don't make you a good or bad person, because they are just thoughts that you can learn to observe. Many of your problematic reactions may come from long-standing judgments or assumptions about yourself and others. In the following sections, you look more closely at your relationship with your feelings, assumptions, and self-judgments. Remember, how you think about these things impacts how you feel and then how you act.

Recognizing what you feel about your feelings

Many people who come to DBT are emotionally sensitive, feeling things longer and more deeply than the average person and taking much longer to return to their baseline. Because of this, they struggle to regulate emotions, which in turn is exhausting. It isn't uncommon for us to hear, "Emotions are ruining my life." As we have said, we are often asked whether we can get rid of people's emotions. We obviously say "no," but what we can do is help you regulate and think about them differently. In Chapter 10, we review the emotion regulation module, where you learn that judging and suppressing your emotions only enhances the very emotions that you are feeling. Unfortunately, you end up inadvertently enhancing your suffering.

If you're an emotionally sensitive person, you need to accept and embrace that about yourself. We say that because it's something that will not change. What can change is how you regulate those feelings, but before you can really do that, you need to change the way you think about your sensitivity. Note that how you think about this will impact how you feel about your feelings. It's much more common for the way you think about your emotions to cause your suffering, rather than the emotions themselves. Consider the benefits of being an emotionally sensitive person. How does it make you a better friend or partner, or even better at your job? Take some time to open your mind to all the benefits that being sensitive brings to your life.

So, what can you do about the judgments that show up from day to day? The first step is to become very familiar with how you feel about your emotional sensitivity and your emotions. This will most likely show up in the form of negative judgments. Here are some examples:

>> *I'm so stupid for being upset.*

>> *I'm attention seeking.*

>> *This is so ridiculous that I even care.*

>> *What is the big deal anyway?*

>> *I should be over this by now.*

>> *I'm such a baby.*

>> *I hate that I am like this.*

>> *I'm weak.*

>> *I'm so dramatic.*

REMEMBER

Don't judge your judgments; just take stock of them for what they are. They are just thoughts you have about your emotions and likely show up in your self-talk as you make sense of what and how deeply you are feeling about something. Now that you're aware of these thinking traps, the nice thing is that everyone seems to have a handful of these judgments that show up again and again. Now you need to keep a lookout for when these thoughts show up. When you notice these thoughts, go back to basics and connect with how you feel. Managing how you feel in the moment is easier when you aren't enhancing the intensity of your feelings with your thoughts. Now try to practice staying with the feelings and using your skills to turn the intensity up and down. Then turn your thoughts to gratitude, and open your mind to the idea that you can connect with your emotions, that they will inform you, and that you can watch them without moving immediately into cognitive or physical action.

Assessing your assumptions

Most everyone has heard the saying, "When you assume, you make an ASS out of U and ME." The dictionary definition of an *assumption* is something that is accepted as truth or certain to happen, without any proof. You can see the problem. Making assumptions usually happens when you have incomplete information and when you cannot or do not want to ask the questions needed to get the missing information. You fill in the blanks. The problem comes from what you fill in the blanks with, and this usually comes from your own interpretations of what you have seen or heard, or even experiences from your past. You do this to fill in gaps and make sense of something that has happened.

The danger is that you may be connecting dots that aren't there. Your emotions make you vulnerable to making assumptions. Unfortunately, it's often the painful events of your past that fuel the interpretations that lead you to assume other people's motives and intentions, or how they will respond or even how a situation will end. The stronger your emotions are, the more certain your assumptions become. It can be hard to step back and even identify them as assumptions. Your assumptions are most likely rooted in past hurt, and when you act in the present based on feelings of the past, you can create a lot more trouble for yourself.

The following sections go into more detail about the problems with assumptions and how to look for your assumptions.

Picking out the problems with assumptions

Consider these problems with assumptions:

>> They are the path of least resistance, but they do not reflect the truth or challenge you to seek out the reality that is in front of you.

>> They keep you stuck in your painful path, blocking opportunities to see that the past doesn't always repeat.

>> They damage current relationships. People don't like always having the worst assumed about them.

>> They keep you always assuming the worst, which leads to feelings of anxiety, sadness, anger, and shame.

>> They cause you more pain.

>> They are always wrong. While on occasion, a part of your assumption could be true, the totality of what you assume is wrong.

Finding your assumptions

So, what are your assumptions? Keep a lookout for these especially problematic ones:

>> *They are better off without me.*

>> *No one will ever love me.*

>> *All relationships end anyways.*

>> *Things are easier for you.*

>> *You did that because you don't care about me.*

>> *I always get the short end of the stick.*

>> *No one is trustworthy.*

>> *If you get it wrong, you are a failure.*

>> *They are always happy.*

Some of these assumptions may resonate with you, but there are many more that you can find. You can use your mindfulness-of-current-thought skill to identify these assumptions and your checking-the-facts skill to work with the assumptions that you find. (We cover both skills earlier in this chapter.)

REMEMBER

Don't judge these assumptions; just notice them and be open to asking questions. These assumptions come from your painful experiences, so it's important to validate that it makes sense that you may fill in the dots that way; however, it is neither useful nor effective to hold onto them as truth.

Accounting for your self-judgments

In Chapter 9, we explain that judgments are shorthand or oversimplifications for a more complicated concept. A judgment takes an experience and condenses it down to one word: *good, bad, pretty, ugly, stupid/dumb, weak, strong, cool, loser,* and so on. Similarly, self-judgments sum up your own experience or who you are into one word. Negative self-judgments can permeate your self-talk and create suffering. Interestingly, they also move you away from your primary emotion and send you down a painful spiral of self-talk, assumptions, and ultimately, misery.

Leaning in, paying attention, and accounting for your negative self-judgments is the first step. Paying attention to self-judgments is no different than paying attention to your assumptions (see the previous section). The interesting thing about self-judgments is that they frequently repeat, and that repetition can be helpful in your hunt to find them.

Watch out — negative judgments can be hard to escape, especially if you're well practiced in using them. You may believe your judgments and be attached to them, holding onto them because they feel like a part of you. It can feel like if you let them go, you will be lost. If you believe you are stupid or a loser, you may feel lost without this quick way to make sense of an experience when you make a mistake or disappoint someone. The good news is that if you're open to working with these judgments, you can decrease your suffering, learn more about your experience, and learn ways to not repeat the things that make you feel bad about yourself.

TIP

Again, negative self-judgments are shorthand, inherently leaving out information. So, as with your assumptions, you need to start looking for what your negative judgments are leaving out. Use your mindfulness-of-current-thought skill (covered earlier in this chapter) to notice these judgments. Sometimes at the hospital, we give patients little clickers that are used at concerts or events to count the number of people attending, and we ask them to click each time they notice a negative self-judgment throughout one day. This is a great, and sometimes surprising, way to bring awareness to your judgments.

Once you notice your judgments, you can start to use your checking-the-facts skill (described earlier in this chapter) to get more information. For example, is it that you are stupid or is it that you got really anxious and couldn't remember the answer because when you are anxious, it is hard to think? Notice how we expanded the judgment to reflect the facts of the situation. Another benefit of this approach is that when you expand this judgment, you can more effectively problem-solve the situation so that it may not happen again. For example, it's good to know that anxiety got in the way; maybe you can cope ahead and think about skills to use the next time so that when you feel pressured to answer a question, you can regulate your anxiety, answer the question, and feel much better about yourself.

REMEMBER

We know that untangling your negative judgments isn't easy; however, we believe it is well worth the challenge.

Chapter **8**

Understanding Your Relationships

President Theodore Roosevelt once said, "The most important single ingredient in the formula of success is knowing how to get along with people."
Often, people struggle in relationships not because they are in conflict with
others, but because they either don't understand the other person's point of view
or don't have the skills to manage differences and difficulties as they arise. In this
chapter, we review how to understand the dynamics in relationships as they arise,
how to improve communication, and how to strengthen relationships.

Recognizing Relationship Dynamics

The word *dynamics* in the context of relationships pertains to the predictable pattern of interaction or communication between any two people, or between a person and a group of people. In this context, a person's development, life experiences,
interpersonal interactions, culture, and many other factors influence how they
engage with other people. In Chapter 12 we review the specific DBT skills that are
used to make interpersonal functioning more effective, but in this section, we go
over the two sides of relationship dynamics: yours and the other person's.

Looking at what you bring

At its most basic level, a *relationship* is the interaction that one person has with another. There are all types of relationships, including romantic, family, work, school, friend, teammate, and others. Each person in any dyad brings their own qualities to the relationship, and then there is the way in which these qualities interact. Many people who come to DBT do so because of difficulties in relationships, and often it's because the dynamics are hurtful.

WARNING

A familiar pattern is one where a person who is emotionally sensitive wants an emotionally intense relationship with another person. This typically starts off well, with the glow of a new relationship, but after a while the level of intensity dies down. The emotionally intense person starts to feel as if the other person is withdrawing, and then there is a cycle of repeated negative interactions, one where incorrect assumptions are made and the worst is imagined in the other person. If you're stuck in a negative cycle or destructive interactions, your relationship will suffer, and this pattern can eventually lead to a physical and emotional disconnect.

People who request DBT treatment often recognize this particular dynamic, and the aspect that can be most toxic is when there is repeated idealization and devaluation of the other person:

>> **What is idealization?** *Idealization* is the psychological process of attributing overly positive qualities to another person. Some people recognize that they feel safer and less anxious when they view someone as perfect, someone who only has positive qualities. During states of idealization, the person who is idealizing feels intense closeness toward the person they are idealizing, and that person can seemingly do nothing wrong. It's important to note that this state of idealization can quickly and at times unpredictably turn, and suddenly there is intense anger toward the idealized person, often followed by devaluation.

>> **What is devaluation?** *Devaluation* is the opposite of idealization. It's the process of attributing to themselves or another person the perspective that they are completely flawed, worthless, useless, and having only negative qualities with little hope of redemption.

These qualities are the most extreme of dynamics that people recognize in treatment, and they are the most destructive to relationships; however, other qualities are problematic as well, including the following:

>> **Overly controlling:** This behavior involves insisting that you make all the decisions, including what another person can do, who they can see, what they can wear, and maybe even what they can eat.

>> **Hostile:** Hostility occurs when you fight with another person in such a way that they change their behavior because they want to avoid conflict. This is connected to being overly controlling.

>> **Lying:** Lying is an interaction between two parties: the deceiver and the one who is targeted for deception. The deceiver intentionally communicates false information, and the one targeted for deception either believes the lie or sees through it. There are various forms of lying:

- Pro-social lying occurs when the liar tries to protect someone else.

- Self-enhancing lying intends to avoid consequences such as disapproval.

- Selfish lying is used for self-protection, often at the expense of someone else, in order to hide misconduct.

>> **Excessively dependent:** This behavior occurs when the emotionally sensitive person feels that they can't live without the other person and might even threaten to die if the other person ends the relationship.

>> **Intimidating and threatening:** These behaviors are an attempt to control elements of the other person's life by using threats that make the other person afraid.

The following sections dig deeper into the dynamics you may bring into a relationship. Acknowledging your initial emotions and fully accepting the other person are key.

Acknowledging your initial emotions

The most powerful elements to initiating and sustaining relationships are emotions. Emotions make us want to spend time with the people we love. They spark passion and the secure feeling of belonging. They generate pride in the achievements of loved ones, and the security of feeling understood.

The other side of emotions is that the negative ones can make relationships difficult. They can make you lash out and say things that you wish you hadn't; they can shut you down and lead you to isolate; they can leave you feeling out of control.

Many people with an intense emotion are often unclear about what emotion they are feeling. One of the tasks of DBT is to know and acknowledge their emotions in order to be able to get a handle on their feelings as a way to preserve the relationship. Because of this, it's important to consider what role emotions play in relationships. (We discuss emotions more in Chapter 5.)

A *primary emotion* is the emotion you first feel in response to an event or situation. In many situations, however, your primary emotion gets covered over by your secondary reactions to the initial emotional response. These comprise your secondary emotion.

Here's an example: When Rebecca was looking forward to spending the night with her boyfriend, she felt hurt when he told her that he was going to visit his friends. Sadness was her primary emotion. Her secondary emotion might vary:

>> **If she then felt *guilty*** because she didn't think that she should need anyone and that she should have learned how to be alone rather than depending on someone else, guilt would be a secondary emotion.

>> **If she felt *shame*** for being pathetic because she didn't now know what to do, shame would be a secondary emotion.

>> **If she felt *angry*** that her boyfriend prioritized his relationships with his friends over her, anger would also be a secondary emotion.

In DBT, the task is to focus on your initial or primary emotion; this is critical for avoiding pitfalls in relationships.

Adapting to what is

To adapt to what is, you have to accept what is, and in relationships this means loving someone fully for who they are. This includes loving them for not only all their wonderful qualities but also their flaws, shortcomings, physical and emotional imperfections, and so on. It's a love without judgment and filled with compassion. By accepting someone in this way, you begin to feel better about yourself.

If it's hard to imagine loving someone this way, think about it from your point of view, and imagine that a person you cared about loved you in that way. How wonderful that would feel! This doesn't mean that by adapting to what is by accepting what is, you resign yourself to the difficult behavior of the other person. Instead, it means that you approach these behaviors with kindness and compassion rather than with intense emotions. In doing that, in the context of calm, any one of us is more likely to be able to hear about what aspects or qualities of our personality are making it difficult for the other person.

Accepting another person's perspective

In psychology, the practice of trying to understand the perspective or mental states of others is a concept known as the *theory of mind.*

How does this perspective-taking work in a relationship? The ability to take perspective depends on our ability to think and our use of executive functioning. *Executive functioning* is the use of mental abilities that include flexible thinking, self-control, and shifting between mental sets. When you look at things from another person's perspective, you're shifting from your own state of mind to understand the other person's state of mind. When you're considering another person's point of view, you're using the parts of the brain that hold other people in mind.

REMEMBER

One significant benefit to recognizing another person's perspective is that you start to see the reasons why they did what they did and that they make sense. When you start to see that their perspective makes sense from their point of view, this increases your bond and connectedness with them and reduces a judgmental and blaming position.

Enhancing Communication

Of all the qualities that couples rate as important, communication is considered the most important. People are often not very effective in being clear about what they need, or how to express the impact that the other person's behavior is having on them. The following sections walk you through the basic process of enhancing communication in a relationship.

Checking in with your own dialogue

In DBT, the mindfulness skill gets people to become more reflective. As they become increasingly so, they begin to realize just how much their initial perception can be colored by so many elements. They begin to see how their expectations of others are based on things like past experiences, societal and familial expectations, and their own desires. Our own dialogue often guides us to conclusions based on our own needs and expectations.

REMEMBER

The first step to really listening to others is to identify any distortions and biases that might be filtering our own thought process and perspective. We have to practice listening to ourselves before we can really listen to and understand the dialogue of others. Such internal listening is particularly difficult in the heat of intense emotion; however, by slowing down, we can recognize the times that this dialogue interferes with accurate listening. See Chapter 9 for more about mindfulness.

Opening up to honest listening

Once you realize that your perception of an interpersonal situation might not be accurate, you face a significant choice. Do you actively explore your perception by asking the other person what they meant? Do you try to explain yourself further? Or do you become curious and continue to listen to the other person, allowing them to share their perspective, without interruption?

By recognizing your own internal dialogue and suspending your feelings, you allow for a deeper and more complete communication between you and the other person. This means that when, for instance, you are upset by what someone else says, you have the choice between initially voicing your reaction to what they are saying, asking them more questions to understand them better, or deciding that the effective option is to let things go. In DBT, people find it difficult to suspend their assumptions, particularly when they feel misunderstood or misinterpreted, and yet individuals in couple and family therapy find that by suspending their assumptions, they ensure that emotions remain low and the furthering of the conversation allows each person to share and clarify their point of view in a way that can be validated.

Accepting a range of perspectives

There is an ancient fable that goes like this: A group of blind men who have never previously encountered an elephant come across one and decide to conceptualize the creature by touching it. Each blind man touches a different part of the elephant's body — the trunk, the skin, the tail, the tusk, the leg, and the ear — and then share the experience with the others. In one version of the fable, the blind men believe that the others are trying to be dishonest and come to blows. In another version of the fable, the men still don't have a complete view of the elephant. When we don't accept that there are other perspectives, two significant problems can arise. The first is that we might believe that others are lying, and the second is that without integrating all the points of view, we end up with an incomplete view of an event.

REMEMBER

In DBT, the task of dialectical exploration is one of looking at a situation from the various perspectives of everyone involved, with the goal of getting a more complete perspective on the situation. From a single perspective, we are like the blind men trying to describe the elephant. By putting it all together, we not only see the whole situation, but we also see how another person came to the understanding that they did. Thus, because it's true that other people involved in the situation had reasons and perspectives that explain their reactions and behaviors, even when we don't completely understand the reasons, it becomes clear that they had their own triggers. Chapter 13 looks further at the dialectical process of examining multiple perspectives.

Making Room for More Possibilities

The goal of dialectics in DBT is to broaden perspectives so that new ideas can flourish. It also involves the idea that out of seemingly troubling ways of interacting, something helpful can arise. Think about sodium and chlorine. Sodium is a very volatile metal that explodes under almost any condition. Chlorine, on the other hand, is a poisonous, lethal gas. And yet when they are combined, they make sodium chloride, more commonly known as table salt. Allowing for more perspectives is a key imperative in DBT. The following sections provide more information on how to build a new relationship dynamic.

Being willing and able to create a new dynamic

Just as sodium and chlorine atoms can combine to make a wonderful molecule, the willingness to share and accept different perspectives is the way to create a new dynamic in a relationship. Without the willingness to create a new dynamic of communication and listening, things may go back to the previous ineffective and emotionally painful way of interacting.

Consider this example: Henry, a 17-year-old teen, desperately wanted to regain his parents' trust. They had taken away his car privileges because of months of his having missed curfew. However, one Saturday night, he went to a party, knowing that a girl he liked would be there. He was upset to find his "best friend" Jack — he had said in air quotes — flirting with the girl. Henry was so close to getting the car back, but he had promised his parents that he would be home at 11 that night. On the other hand, he wanted to keep an eye on Jack to make sure that nothing happened between him and the girl.

He missed his curfew and when he got home, he got into a big fight with his parents. Rather than go back to their old style of interacting — where his parents would become punitive and immediately prolong his curfew, causing him to become bitter and to fight, self-isolate in his room, and sneak out at night — they decided to keep things on hold until their next DBT family session. In family therapy, both Henry and his parents gave an account of the evening. They recognized how much he had been on top of his curfew. He shared the struggle he had had with speaking to girls and his concerns about Jack. Both he and his parents had been working on developing mutual trust and communication, and it was in this context that they were able to hear each other out. He was willing to believe that his parents were honest about wanting him to become more independent and get the car back, and they recognized that he had shared a difficult interpersonal conflict and then understood his missing the curfew in that context. Together they came up with a reasonable plan that kept them on track.

Enhancing good practices and letting go of hurtful ones

When you're in conflict with another person or in a frequent state of disagreement, it can feel particularly upsetting to think that a loved one's values are in opposition to your own. Letting go of the old, destructive ways of interacting is the key to a more harmonious relationship. Developing and then enhancing better interpersonal communication practices takes time and repetition, and is possible when you're committed to working on it.

Often, the other person's values are not all that different from yours, but their response means that they didn't have the same information that you did or they themselves were experiencing intense emotions. Here's a practice that can help. Initially, the DBT therapist might do this in session by trying to elicit everyone's perspective:

1. The DBT therapist gets each person to clearly state their perspective or account of a situation. They should do this without being interrupted by the other person or people in the discussion. Each person should be given enough time to share their narrative.

2. Once this has happened, the therapist asks what the goals of each person in the room are.

3. With these goals in mind, the therapist and the other participants in the therapy can ask clarifying questions if they don't understand what another person meant or if there is any confusion. This shouldn't be an interrogation with rapid-fire questions.

4. Once the situation is clear and everyone's perspective has been shared, the therapist then asks the participants to brainstorm possible solutions.

5. The discussion should center around the viability of each solution and consider how these solutions might be implemented. A hierarchy of the viable solutions should then be established.

6. The first solution should then be implemented, with an agreement to review how this went in a future session.

7. If the practice is successful, this should be the model for future problem-solving. If the solution doesn't work, then all participants can either troubleshoot what went wrong or consider the next solution on the list.

REMEMBER

By committing to new ways of interacting and to letting go of old maladaptive, ineffective, and hurtful interpersonal ways of transacting, you help the meaningful relationships in your life improve.

3

Exploring DBT Skills

IN THIS PART . . .

Strengthen your ability to pay attention with mindfulness.

Regulate your emotions by accurately labeling and validating the emotions, while recognizing and reducing vulnerability factors that intensify the emotions.

Tolerate difficult situations while preserving self-dignity and not making the situations worse.

Improve, enhance, and strengthen your relationships with the significant people in your life.

Discover how to walk the middle path — a special skill for adolescents in DBT and their families.

Chapter **9**

Thinking about Mindfulness

DBT has, at its core, the practice of mindfulness. Many people are confused by mindfulness and rarely think about it in the context of therapy. Instead, they often consider mindfulness and meditation to be practiced by people who are religious, cloistered in a monastery, or sitting in a cave on a high mountain. From the DBT perspective, mindfulness is considered a skill, one that can be acquired and practiced. Dr. Marsha Linehan, the psychologist who developed DBT, incorporated mindfulness into behavior therapy because she recognized that it was the most effective and enduring way to alleviate the suffering that many emotionally sensitive people experience.

If you take on the practice of mindfulness, it will be unlike anything you've ever done in therapy, and as with anything that is new, the unfamiliarity can make it difficult to practice at first. It's important to keep an open mind. Many people who struggle with intense emotions have found mindfulness to be the way out of the suffering caused not only by their emotions but also by their thoughts, behaviors, and relationships. This chapter delves further into mindfulness, and we give you more ideas for practicing mindfulness in Chapter 24.

Exploring Your Own Mind

REMEMBER

Before we can talk about exploring the mind in the following sections, it's important to consider what we mean by the mind. From a psychological perspective, the mind is the way that the brain perceives and experiences events, and that includes emotions, thoughts, sensations, urges, motives, and memories. It includes everything in a person's immediate awareness and also the stuff that isn't in their awareness. The thing to remember is that different brains do different things with information.

For example, look at a table. What do you see? "I see a table," you say. However, the table you think is there is not exactly the same as the table that is actually there. It is only a perspective. Here's what happens:

1. Information about the table enters your brain via your visual system.

2. Your brain creates a model of the thing you call the table. All brains do this, by the way. If you were a fly with compound eyes, you would see many tables. Each visual system has its own way of encoding information.

3. Your pre-frontal cortex, the part of the brain that deals with thought and labeling information, receives the model of the table that your brain has created.

4. You talk about the table. This seems very straightforward. Imagine that you were an indigenous person from the depths of the Amazon jungle and had never seen a table before. Certainly, you would receive the information from your visual system, but the rest of your brain would not know what to make of it.

The truth is that the brain does this with everything, including its own experience. And in almost all cases, the brain's quick-and-dirty model of its own experience is a simplification rather than a perfect representation of the experience. For example, say you have the thought, without any facts, that someone doesn't like you. If you're like many people who come to DBT, you claim that the thought is true. You think the thought is true because it resonates with things that your brain has created. And what the brain has created made you come to the conclusion that the person doesn't like you. No one can convince you otherwise. You're certain that it's true. But unless the person said, "I do not like you," whatever your brain is picking up on is not perfectly accurate, even if it feels that way. That information is almost certainly not perfectly accurate. Whatever awareness you think you have is different from the awareness you actually have, and it's in the practice of mindfulness that you get to have a more accurate picture as to the functioning of your mind.

Discovering mindfulness at its core

At its most essential, developing the skill of mindfulness is the purposeful practice of seeing the reality of the present moment and everything in it without judging it. This is actually much more difficult than it seems, and if you get too caught up in the definition, you realize that the present moment contains a huge amount of stuff, including everything that is going on within you and everything that is happening around you, as well as everything going on in the country and the planet and the universe.

REMEMBER

The essential task of DBT mindfulness is to begin paying attention to all the ways in which you do things automatically, and in particular to the things that make life difficult. Just because you have a thought doesn't mean that the content of your thought is true. Just because you have an urge doesn't mean that you're compelled to act on it. Just because you have an emotion doesn't mean that it will last forever. When you realize all of this, you realize that you have the freedom to choose what you're going to do. By not acting on the thoughts, urges, and emotions that lead to painful outcomes, you suffer less.

This type of exploration of the mind isn't usually how we spend our time. For most of us, even if we try to see our mind at work, we get easily distracted by other thoughts or events in the environment, and our attention begins to wander. Mindfulness practice is the way to tame this interference.

Surveying the three states of mind

Dr. Linehan recognized that people who initially came seeking DBT therapy were often struggling because of the impact of highly emotional states that would often get them into trouble. On the other hand, there were people who didn't struggle with emotion regulation. They didn't seem to be impacted by strong emotions and often acted from a place of logic and reason.

REMEMBER

Dr. Linehan observed the natural human tendency to operate from a place of logic and reason on the one hand and strong emotions on the other. The problem is that when you're viewing any situation through either the lens of logic or the lens of strong emotions, you miss out on a lot of nuance and information. It can feel cold and robotic to view events and relationships through nothing but facts, logic, and rational thought. Conversely, life can feel chaotic and disorganized if seen only through the perspective of emotions. Wanting to help her patients, she simplified the concept of states of mind by saying that people were either acting from their *emotion mind* or their *rational mind.*

It was, however, the third state of mind that was key. She termed this *wise mind* and recognized that we all have wise mind whether we realize it or not. When you act from your wise mind, you're taking a more deliberate and contemplative approach to decision-making; that is, you're using all of the mind's experiences — be they emotions, rational thinking, intuition, or goals — to direct you to a course of action. You don't have to be aware of having wise mind to actually have it. However, once you're aware, you'll be capable of experiencing wise mind. Again, awareness isn't the initial key to wise mind. This is true of many things. For instance, just because you aren't aware that you have a stomach or a kidney right now does not mean that your stomach and kidney do not exist and are not functioning. And so wise mind is there, and by practicing mindfulness, you can recognize it and use its power to not only reduce suffering but also enhance so many aspects of your life.

Practicing mindfulness with the WHAT skills

For many people, the thought of practicing mindfulness can seem impractical, even if they want to do it. Imagine a monk or nun meditating in a church or temple. You might wonder, "What are they actually doing?" Dr. Linehan realized that for mindfulness to be useful to her patients, it had to be accessible in a way that didn't necessarily require the person to be religious. Or, if they were religious, the practice could not be incompatible with their faith. To do this, she simplified the practice by breaking it down into skills that focused on *WHAT* someone had to do and *HOW* they should practice it. She then called these the WHAT and HOW skills. In Chapter 24 we give you some concrete practices.

There are three WHAT skills: *Observe, Describe,* and *Participate.* (You discover the HOW skills later in this chapter.)

Observe

The practice of observing is one of noticing. It is noticing things in the environment, sensations in the body, and thoughts and emotions in the mind. Notice your environment and what is around you. What thoughts, feelings, and sensations are you experiencing? Simply observe without having any reaction. Do not attach a label or judgment to your observations. The goal is to observe without words. This can be very hard to do, but you're trying to simply experience without labeling. Notice your emotions and your thoughts. Do not push any of these away; instead, be open to these phenomena as they arise. Use your five senses to improve your observation skills.

TIP

To practice the observe skill, do the following: Find five minutes when you can be away from your day-to-day distractions. Sit cross-legged on the ground, on a cushion, or on a chair. Turn off your phone, or maybe place it in airplane mode, and set your timer to five minutes. Take a deep breath in and say, "My intention. . ." and then breathe out and say, ". . .is to practice Observe." Once you're in a settled, seated position, start your five-minute timer. Then do the following:

>> Notice your space environment, the temperature in the room, and any sounds. Notice body sensations. Notice thoughts and emotions. Stay seated without reacting to any of these.

>> Avoid reacting to emotions and thoughts. Should one arise, simply notice the experience without doing anything other than observing.

>> Notice the emotions and thoughts showing up and then notice them going. All thoughts arise and all thoughts leave. That is because they are phenomena of an active mind. No thought or emotion has ever lasted forever, and none will, no matter how much you believe it will.

>> Don't avoid noticing, no matter how uncomfortable or painful the sensations are, and don't cling to any thought or emotion, no matter how enjoyable or pleasant.

Describe

The practice of describing is the practice of putting word labels onto the thoughts, feelings, sensations, and phenomena that are observed. There is an upside to this: It allows for ease of communication. For instance, imagine having to say, "So that we can have dinner, I want you to put these plates on an item of furniture, made typically out of wood, that has a flat top and that sits on one or more legs." Of course, a better option would be to use the word *table*. However, imagine that there were five people of different nationalities looking at the table. When asked what they are looking at, the English speaker says "table," the Spanish speaker says "mesa," the Zulu speaker says "ithebula," the Nepalese person says "tālikā," and the Samoan person says "laulau."

The point is that although everyone might observe a very similar thing, the second each person starts to put words onto the thing they are observing, it can become confusing or even adversarial because others may not share the observed experience in terms of the words used to describe. The description is important in that words don't completely convey the exact thing that a person is experiencing, but they are the only tools we have.

When describing an experience, it can be useful to say it out loud. For instance, if you're feeling anxious, you can say, "I am noticing that I feel anxious. I am having the thought that no one is going to invite me to the party. I am noticing that my heart is speeding up." Once again, be careful not to attach any labels or judgments to what you're describing.

TIP

To practice the describe skill, do the following: Find five minutes when you can be away from your day-to-day distractions. Sit cross-legged on the ground, on a cushion, or on a chair. Turn off your phone or place it in airplane mode, and set your timer to five minutes. Take a deep breath in and say, "My intention. . ." and then breathe out and say, ". . .is to practice Describe." Once you're in a settled, seated position, start your five-minute timer. Then do the following:

>> Notice your space environment. Label the chair you're sitting on as a chair, and the sounds you're hearing as a radiator, bird, or outside car noise. Label your body sensations as an itch, pain, or pressure. If you have a thought, label it as a thought. If you have an urge, label it as an urge. If you notice an emotion, label the emotion.

>> Avoid reacting to emotions and thoughts. Rather, place words on your experience and say to yourself, "I notice that I feel the emotion of anxiety," or "I notice the thought that people don't want me around," or "I notice the urge to run away."

>> Notice whether you're using judgmental language. For instance, if you have the thought "I am stupid and everyone hates me," instead describe the experience in this way: "I am having the thought that I am stupid and that everyone hates me." By labeling thoughts as thoughts, you're removing yourself from the *being* of the thought.

Participate

This is the practice of throwing yourself fully into the action that you are doing, and doing so by letting go of judgments, expectations, or any negative or self-critical thoughts. In other words, when you're eating, you just eat. When you're reading, you just read. When you're gardening, you just do that. The point is that by fully throwing yourself into the activity that you're participating in, you are fully present. Another element to fully participating is to let go of self-consciousness. This is difficult, but with practice you'll become better at letting go. If you're distracted by other things, you can't fully participate in the activity you are in. Consider the effect of a friend talking to you while they are distracted by also being on their phone.

TIP

To practice the participate skill, do the following: Set an intention to fully participate in some activity — for instance, that you will wash the dishes. Turn off your phone and turn off the TV. Take a deep breath in and say, "My intention. . ." and then breathe out and say, ". . .is to practice Participate." Once you're settled in front of the sink, start your five-minute timer. Then do the following:

>> Stack the dishes that need to be washed, and wash each one with warm water and soap. Then rinse each plate with clean water.

>> Avoid reacting to urges to check your phone, particularly if you receive some notification. Notice whether boredom arises and there is a desire to turn on the TV.

>> Pay full attention to the water, the soap, and the dishes. Be meticulous in the washing, the rinsing, and the drying as if they are the only things that you have to do.

Using the HOW skills in mindfulness

The HOW skills describe the way in which the WHAT skills are used. There are three HOW skills: *non-judgmentally, one-mindfully,* and *effectively.*

Non-judgmentally

This is the practice of letting go of judgments, and then if you find yourself judging, you don't judge yourself for judging.

Why let go of judgments? Most of us judge automatically and habitually. Because of this, we rarely know that we are judging. When we judge, we don't notice that judging increases our emotional pain and damages our relationships. For example: Imagine your child is late coming home and hasn't called. You might judge them as being selfish: "Here I am awake and waiting for them to come home, and they don't have the decency to call me and let me know what's going on." You can see how this judgment that your child is being selfish can make you feel worse and could damage your relationship with your child.

Deciding to practice being non-judgmental doesn't mean you can't acknowledge your feelings, thoughts, and preferences about a situation. You can rephrase your reaction in the following way and do so by sticking to the facts: "I'm upset that my child has not come home and that they did not call. It makes me worried, and it feels to me as if they are being selfish. My preference is that they call if they are going to be late, and yet I realize that I don't actually know what the circumstances are."

Can you see how removing judgments allows you to mark your experience as your own and be more in charge of the situation? Also, that by being less judgmental, you suffer less? By removing the emotional charge, it makes it easier to think of a plan and to decide how you're going to address the situation. By focusing on what led to the situation, you can consider various solutions, which is much more effective than judging.

REMEMBER

Letting go of judgments means not considering situations and interactions in terms of good and bad, fair and unfair, or right and wrong. When you use these terms, noticing that you have done so is the first step.

Next, stick to the facts of the situation. (You can read more about how to check the facts in Chapter 7.) Sticking to the facts is sticking to the who, the what, the where, and the when. By adding judgments to these elements, such as "My selfish son was out with his bad friends at a ridiculous hour, getting up to no good," and then acting as if those judgments were facts, you miss the truth of the situation and to suffer.

REMEMBER

It's important to note that the goal is not to replace negative judgments with positive ones, even if positive judgments don't cause as much suffering as negative ones. It is to not use judgments at all, because positive judgments can rapidly become negative ones. For instance, say that you judge your best friend as the most wonderful person on the planet, and then they then do something that upsets you — something that happens in all relationships. The positive judgments can rapidly turn.

When it comes to judging yourself, let go of thinking that you should be different than you are. Self-judgment is often the most painful and the type that most people have the hardest time letting go of. Don't judge yourself as stupid or lazy or insignificant. By practicing non-judgmentally, you stop beating yourself up and instead start accepting yourself exactly as you are in this moment. This doesn't mean that you have to let go of wanting to change certain aspects of your behavior, but you can recognize these elements as unhelpful or ineffective or inconsistent with your long-term goals and make a decision to tackle these aspects.

REMEMBER

Reducing judgments takes practice, so it's important to be gentle with yourself as you work on noticing your judgments and replacing them with non-judgmental statements based on facts.

One-mindfully

Doing things one-mindfully has two elements:

>> The first is being fully present in the moment, without dwelling on the past or thinking about the future.

>> The second is doing one thing at a time rather than dividing your attention between things — like having a conversation on the phone while checking your email.

Many people believe that they can multitask, but research shows that very, very few of us actually can. Doing one thing at a time is the solution to the delusional belief that we can multitask. Imagine trying to do four things at the same time. When you try to juggle four things at once, you have to divide your attention in four, and the brain isn't built in a way to effectively do this. Or imagine that you have a lion coming at you from the left and another from the right. You can focus all your attention on one or the other. The second you start moving back and forth between the two, there will be gaps in your attention.

TIP

Take an everyday task and focus your full attention on it. For example: When you're washing your hands, notice the temperature of the water, the feel and the scent of the soap, and the sensation of your hands rubbing together. Notice as you rinse the water off your hands, and then notice the feel of the towel as you dry your hands. Then notice the feeling of having clean hands.

Effectively

REMEMBER

This is the skill of doing what the situation needs. It means doing what works versus wishing that reality was different from what it is. It's the act of asking yourself: "In this situation, would I rather be right in arguing my perspective, or would I rather be effective and do what the situation needs?" In DBT, being effective is about shifting the focus away from concepts such as what is fair and unfair, and who is right and who is wrong, and instead focusing on what works.

The first step in practicing the effectively skill is to figure out what you want. To act effectively, you have to know what you want out of a situation. Articulate your goal, and then once you know it, you can consider the most effective means to reach it.

For example: Imagine that you're in a parking lot with many spaces when you see that there is an opening right near the store where you plan to do shopping. You head to the space when someone speeds up and swings right into it. You notice judging them as selfish and how unfair it is that you were waiting your turn when someone took your space. You might be tempted to lean on your horn in response or to block their car so that they can't get out, and to then yell at them when they leave their car.

This example might seem extreme, but would getting into a fight be effective and save you time in pursuit of your goal? Would you rather be right that you deserved the parking space rather than be effective and take a slightly farther space and get your shopping done? Being effective in this example would be to not escalate the situation. Instead, take a mindful deep breath. You're taking care of yourself and accomplishing your tasks without punishing another person, and you don't actually know their circumstances.

Making space and setting a routine

You want to practice WHAT and HOW skills every day. Making time and setting a space and a routine are an ideal way to start.

Making space

There are two considerations in making space. It makes sense that you have to make physical space, but you also have to make mental space. When you're stressed, you can often feel as if pressure is coming from everywhere. Even your body can feel constricted, and you might feel as if you're unable to breathe. Having a space that brings you calm is an important first step.

For a physical location, an important aspect to creating your space is setting your intention for that area. Different practices require different attributes. For example, if you're doing a walking meditation, you want an outside space where you can walk. If you're doing a sitting meditation, you might find that a small, quiet room is best.

Once you have decided on your practice, decide on the space. For sitting mindfulness, you'll want a space that is quiet and where you won't be disturbed. If you're going to practice sitting meditation, make sure that you have a cushion or a reasonably comfortable chair to sit on. If you're doing a walking meditation, find a space where you can walk slowly for at least 30 seconds before having to turn around and walk back.

REMEMBER

The initial mental space is best achieved in relative silence. A silent space in meditation has the benefit of reducing the number of sensory inputs that bombard you. However, silence is not only about being in a silent space. It's also about not speaking. We spend a lot of our awake time talking to others, and so committing to even a few minutes of intentional silence can give us a break from having to fill silence with words.

Setting a routine

There are many benefits to setting and maintaining a mindfulness routine. For people with high-stress jobs, starting the morning with a routine can be a way to create a positive mindset for the rest of the day. For people who struggle with depression and anxiety, a morning mindfulness routine can be a way to establish a healthier habit.

Other people prefer a nighttime routine. A routine is *not* vegging out after a hard day's work and focusing only on your social media apps or relaxing while binge-watching some new TV show until you fall asleep. Mindfulness is about taking care of your mind and often following a routine that sets you up for a good night's sleep.

There is no universal way to set the routine; it's specific to the individual. The important thing is to set one. Also, the form of your routine doesn't need to be the same every day. Imagine that you committed to exercise each day. The form of exercise is less important than actually doing it. So, in the same way that you might run one day, walk the next, then swim or do push-ups, the goal is to exercise. Once you have your mindfulness routine, you can decide that you'll practice loving compassion one day, focused meditation the next, and open awareness the day after.

Understanding Types of Mindfulness

The practice of mindfulness has no aim other than non-judgmental awareness of the present moment, and from this come all the benefits of such a stance. Just like different types of exercise are good for the body, different types of mindfulness enhance the mind's capacity for awareness, and each type of mindfulness has its own form. Broadly speaking, there are four main types of mindfulness practice:

» Concentrative mindfulness

» Generative mindfulness

» Receptive mindfulness

» Reflective mindfulness

Concentrative mindfulness

The aim of this practice is to focus your attention, and a typical way of doing this is to consider some object and then to focus all your attention on that object. There can be external things to focus on, like a candle flame or a spot on a wall, or internal things like the breath. Many meditators choose to focus on the breath. Concentrating your attention in this way is like holding a magnifying glass and focusing it on one particular object in order to recognize all of its aspects.

Focusing on the breath is the concentrative practice that most meditators use and the one that most beginning mindfulness students can understand. This is because the breath is portable and always with you. It can be quite mesmerizing to look at a candle flame, but imagine trying to do this in a plane on a cross-country flight. The airline personnel wouldn't be all that happy! The breath is also a nice practice in that breathing is something that is shared with all living entities.

Now, although focusing on the breath is the most accessible of practices, one with a natural rhythm, any of the five senses can be used. In DBT we might ask our patients to listen to the sound of a singing bowl, to focus on the taste of a raisin or piece of chocolate, to feel a certain texture, and so on. The task in this practice is to slowly and gently bring the focus of your attention to the object you've decided on, and then when you get distracted, to gently bring your attention back to the object of focus while noting to yourself, in a non-judgmental way, that you have been distracted.

TIP

Here is a common version of concentrative breath practice:

>> Follow your breath as you inhale and exhale naturally. Once your attention is on your breath, start a count after each out-breath. After the first breath, silently count "one"; after the second, "two"; and so on until you have reached ten. Then note that you have reached ten and go back and start again from one.

>> Once you can focus your attention in such a way that you can get to ten and then repeat it without being pulled away by distractions — or if pulled away, then easily being able to return to your breath — a next variation might be to ladder down from ten. That is, start at ten and go to one.

>> Once you have mastered this, your next version of the practice could be to simply attend to the experience of the air entering and leaving your body.

>> Then, you might focus your attention on the tip of your nose and notice the air entering as you breathe in and then on your lips as you breathe out.

Generative mindfulness

The goal of generative mindfulness is to intentionally generate positive emotions and thoughts. This type of practice strengthens the quality of *intention*. The best-known practice in generative mindfulness is that of the generation of *loving-kindness*, also known as *metta*. It's a method of developing compassion for others and yourself. The way to practice this is through developing an attitude of loving-kindness using images of people in your life. What is tricky with this practice is that although you may feel that others deserve love and kindness, you may also feel that you yourself are undeserving of love and kindness. Two wonderful quotes embrace the spirit of this practice:

>> "Darkness cannot drive out darkness; only light can do that. Hate cannot drive out hate; only love can do that." — Dr. Martin Luther King, Jr.

>> "In this world, hate never dispelled hate. Only love dispels hate. This is the law, ancient and inexhaustible." — The Buddha

Here is a version of loving-kindness as a generative practice. Because you might find it difficult to do this for yourself, it may be more effective to focus this practice on someone else at first. Here's an important aspect to metta: It has no conditions, and it doesn't depend on whether you think that you or someone else "deserves" it or not. Ultimately, you should be able to extend it beyond yourself and those closest to you and include all beings, even those you struggle with and those you don't know. Loving-kindness is a practice in unconditional, inclusive love, a love with wisdom. You should expect nothing from others after you practice it. It's the practice of a pure love. Begin with yourself and then move onto others with the help of the following sections. (As mentioned, if this practice is difficult, you can start with someone else before moving onto yourself.)

REMEMBER

The practice is a way of softening your mind and heart toward yourself and others. It is without the desire to possess another, and it isn't some sort of sentimental feeling of goodwill. It doesn't depend on how another person feels about you.

For yourself

Here's a practice: When you know that you'll have, say, ten uninterrupted minutes, sit somewhere comfortable. Slow your breath. Anchor your attention on your breath. If it helps, place both your hands above your heart.

TIP

Continuing to breathe in and out, use some of these traditional phrases (you can also create your own). Think or say each of them slowly a few times before moving on:

>> "May I be free from danger."

>> "May I be safe."

>> "May I be free of mental suffering."

>> "May I be happy."

>> "May I feel ease."

>> "May I be healthy and strong."

>> "May I find peace."

For someone you're close to

Next, move on to a person who you feel closest to. This is typically someone you consider a mentor, and it could be a family member, a benefactor, or a close friend. It could be your grandparent, a teacher, or anyone toward whom it takes no effort for you to feel respect and kindness.

Say the same phrases as in the previous section, but instead of *I*, use that person's name.

For a neutral person

Next, move on to a more neutral person, someone who you neither strongly like nor dislike — perhaps a co-worker or neighbor, or a casual acquaintance. Hold them in mind as you practice, and replace the *I* with that person's name.

As you repeat the earlier phrases, notice genuine tenderness toward these people, truly wanting them to experience each of the feelings or conditions.

For someone you have difficulty with and for all beings

There is one final step in this practice, and here is where it can get difficult: Move on to someone with whom you are struggling or having difficulty with.

TIP

Repeat the earlier phrases, and replace the *I* with that person's name. If you're really struggling with this, then go back to the person who you care about so that you can feel the kindness you have for them and then return to your more difficult person.

When you have practiced this for some time — say a few weeks — extend the practice to all beings. Include your pets and other animals. Your ultimate goal is to replace anger and unkind feelings with loving ones.

You may have the following questions, particularly when you're practicing with a person that you don't feel good about:

>> "How can I be kind to someone who has hurt me?"

>> "If I let them off the hook, they get away with what they did to me."

>> "If I practice kindness toward them, they win, and I lose."

>> "I want to stay angry at the person as a reminder of what they did to me."

>> "They need to suffer as much as I have suffered."

REMEMBER

This is a mindfulness practice and the purpose is to produce ease of mind. If you think nice thoughts about a person 20 miles away, they have no clue. If you have judgmental thoughts about another person, they don't know either. You aren't doing the practice for them; you're doing it for yourself. Your mind's attitude is the key. It's the attitude that is present, and if it's an angry, hateful attitude, you'll feel angry and hateful, even if the other person is completely unaware.

Interestingly, in some circumstances, when you practice loving compassion, you might notice that you start to wonder why hurtful people have acted in the way they did. You might also notice that you're starting to consider that the hurtful person must have had a very difficult life for them to have behaved how they did toward you.

Receptive mindfulness

Receptive mindfulness fits in the space between concentrative and generative meditation. The idea is to attend to, and be receptive of, whatever experience is arising during the practice. There is an attitude of open, choiceless, non-judgmental awareness as the focus of the receptive type of mindfulness practice. In the Japanese Zen tradition, it is known as *zazen* or "just sitting."

The task here is to find the space to sit calmly. Next, you start to notice all the experiences in the moment, including the events outside the body, such as sounds and sights, and those inside the mind and body, such as thoughts, emotions, and sensations. All the senses are at play, and the noticing is done without judging, or if judging arises, then noticing that judgments have arisen. Be kind to yourself during this practice by not judging yourself and instead simply noticing phenomena as they arise and without trying to change them.

TIP

This type of practice should be done with your eyes open. This is important because we spend most of our lives with our eyes open, and from a DBT perspective, one of the functions of treatment is to practice doing the skills the way you live your life, and hopefully, that is mostly with your eyes open.

Reflective mindfulness

Reflective mindfulness is the practice of repeatedly turning your attention to some theme or topic. The task is to have that topic in mind, perhaps some subject that is worrying you, and then to be open to the thoughts, emotions, and sensations that arise from reflecting on the topic. This practice can be tricky to introduce too early in mindfulness training because you might spend too much time reflecting on how your life has been too hard. More experienced practitioners of this type of mindfulness recognize that all reflections and events are impermanent, and so even difficult moments will come to an end. This practice is a double-edged sword. On the one hand, impermanence is desirable because whatever is hurting you won't last forever, and yet on the other hand, you might conclude that if life is impermanent, then "Why do I need to struggle?"

REMEMBER

This practice should be reserved for more experienced practitioners in the context of DBT.

Realizing the Benefits of Mindfulness

Improving your ability to practice mindfulness increases many life qualities that contribute to a life of satisfaction and contentment. A more mindful way of living allows for the ability to fully savor life's pleasures as they occur. It helps you become fully engaged in activities and relationships, and it improves your capacity to deal with adversity as it arises.

Enjoying greater focus

One benefit of mindfulness practice is the ability to focus the mind. This ability to stabilize and direct the focus of the mind is particularly important in moments when you feel distracted or overwhelmed.

TIP

One specific mindfulness practice that can help you is focused attention training. Here's how to do this practice:

1. Sit on a chair in a comfortable posture. For this practice you can close your eyes. Notice your body on the chair seat, your feet on the floor, and your arms at rest on your lap. Just keep your focus on your seated position. Note that the more you practice focusing, the better your mind will become at focusing.

2. Switch your focus of attention. With your eyes still closed, after a few minutes switch your focus of attention to sounds in the environment. Some may persist, like an air conditioner, and some may be brief like a passing car. Keep your focus on the sounds.

3. If you're like most people, your mind will wander. The brain has evolved to pay attention to more than just one thing, so it isn't surprising if the mind wanders. However, because you're practicing increasing your ability to focus, you should notice that your mind has wandered to something else and bring it back to focus on your seated posture, to sounds, or to your breath.

Easing into relaxation

Mindfulness can help you relax in various ways; however, it's important to note that mindfulness and relaxation are two different things. There are instances when mindfulness isn't relaxing, such as if you're reflecting on a hurtful moment. Nevertheless, many people do experience relaxation with regular practice.

One practice in mindfulness meditation is a *body scan*. This is a practice in mindfulness where you focus your attention on various parts of your body. One way to do this is to start with your feet and then work your way up. As you focus on each body part, observe how each part feels without labeling the sensations as either "good" or "bad." Here is a step-by-step approach:

1. Lie on your back, legs uncrossed, with your arms relaxed by your sides. Start by slowing your breathing, and then focus on your breath for a few minutes until you start to feel relaxed.

2. Turn your focus to the toes of one of your feet. Notice any sensations you feel in your foot. Keep your attention on your foot while breathing slowly.

3. Move your focus to the sole of your foot, and again notice any sensations while breathing slowly. Move slowly up your body and repeat focusing on the sensations in that part of the body while maintaining a slow breath.

4. After you've scanned your entire body, bring your sole attention to your breath and continue to lie on the floor and relax for a while in silence.

If for some reason, such as body pain, this practice doesn't bring relaxation, don't force it. This might not be the practice for you.

Creating healthy space in your psyche

We like to divide our body into many different parts, and in some ways, this makes a lot of sense. If you have a heart problem, you don't want to go to a skin doctor. On the other hand, the body is completely interconnected. We can't live without a heart or without our skin, and taking care of one component means taking care of all of your body. A healthy mind and a healthy body are interconnected.

The other issue is this: Although technology has done wonders, it has also caused us to use less of our mind and body. Having a car means that you don't have to ride a horse or walk to work. Having an app means that you don't have to get out a physical map to figure out where you're going.

Mindfully and intentionally participating in the following are key to a healthy mind and body:

>> **Exercise daily.** Set the mindful intention to exercise for at least 30 minutes, five days a week.

>> **Do something different.** Set the intention to do something different every day. Brush your teeth with your non-dominant hand, wear something unusual, take a different route home.

>> **Do something creative.** Set the intention to be creative. Get out your camera and go take some photos. Buy some drawing materials and challenge yourself to draw. Make a meal you've never tried making before, with unusual spices.

>> **Stay connected.** Set the mindful intention to stay connected to the important people in your life, particularly the ones that you might not have been in touch with recently. Give someone you care about a call.

>> **Connect to your faith.** If you have a faith practice but are just going through the motions of attending services, make the intention of connecting to your faith's core truths.

Calming your emotions

Everyone has emotions. Some people have stronger emotions than others, and that is just a part of diversity, in the same way that some people are taller than others, more athletic than others, or more creative than others. Strong emotions aren't a problem unless you're unable to manage them very well, and many people who come to DBT do so because they have a hard time managing their emotions. When a person can't control their emotional reactivity, things can spin out of control and lead to potentially destructive behavior.

TIP

Here is a practice in calming your emotions:

1. Sit comfortably on a cushion or a chair. As you can see, many mindfulness practices include sitting! Now bring your mind to focus on something that you're struggling with. Try not to start with the most difficult situation you're facing. Once you have mastered calming your emotions with less agitating things, you'll move to the more difficult ones. Focus on your urge to push away difficult thoughts or any urge to make the situation easier (drugs, your phone, a piece of chocolate). Don't access any of these.

2. Turn toward the difficult situation and face it. Breathe in deeply through your nose to the count of five seconds (just like sitting, breathing features frequently in mindfulness), and breathe out even more slowly through pursed lips. Do this a few times.

3. Focus on compassion to yourself, and create in your mind a blanket of compassion and strength that surrounds you. Imagine a person who cares deeply about you, standing or sitting by your side.

4. Face the difficult situation full on. In this moment you don't need to be scared. If you feel fear, let the emotion of fear arise and fall. Observe and label the situation that is bringing up the strong emotion. For instance, "I am noticing

fear that someone does not like me." This may take a while, but the emotion will fall. Be kind to yourself and validate that this is difficult for you. Focus on facing the emotion while you breathe slowly, and have an attitude of compassion toward yourself.

5. If you notice yourself reaching for avoidance or some external object that makes you feel safe, turn away from avoidance or the object and turn back toward the thought that causes strong emotions. The more you train the mind to observe and name whatever the difficult emotional situation is, the more you'll be training the emotional centers in the brain to handle these situations. As an added benefit, you'll be sending a message to the rest of your body that it can start to relax.

Chapter **10**

Regulating Your Emotions

n Chapter 5, you get the nuts and bolts of emotions: how to name your emotions, which emotions are primary and which are secondary, whether emotions are justified or unjustified, and the overall function of emotions. Understanding all of this creates the building blocks for what we teach you in this chapter. Read on to discover more skills to regulate your emotions.

REMEMBER

In DBT, emotion regulation is about learning the skills you need to intentionally turn the intensity of your emotions up and down.

Turning the Keys of Emotion Regulation

In Chapter 5, you find out that emotions have three functions: to communicate information to yourself, to communicate and influence others, and to motivate action. Your emotions are obviously very powerful!

There are a few ways in which we tackle emotion regulation skills in DBT, as you find out in the following sections. There are skills that you will learn how to use in the moment, and then there is the very important skill of learning to reduce your emotional vulnerabilities so that as emotionally difficult things come your way, you have as steady an emotional foundation as possible.

Decreasing emotional vulnerability with ABC PLEASE

There are many things in your life that you can't control. One of the wonderful things about the ABC PLEASE skills is that while you can't control all these things, you do have some control over your ability to find some balance despite that. Think of this skill as creating the building blocks for your emotional base, the sturdy foundation that keeps you steady when the emotional hurricanes and tornados rage outside. To be effective, this skill must be a steady practice in your life. We know this isn't easy, and the impact on your ability to regulate your emotions is great.

This skill has two parts: The first part, ABC, includes more psychological behaviors that you can perform over time to reduce your emotional vulnerabilities, while PLEASE is focused on skills that are more physiologically based, ways in which you can take care of your body. We look closely at the second skill in the following sections.

TIP

The ABC skills consist of *Accumulating* positives, *Building* mastery, and *Coping* ahead of time with difficult situations. The PLEASE skills have to do with *Physical* illness (the *PL* in PLEASE comes from the first and last letters of *physical*), balanced *Eating*, avoiding mood-*Altering* substances, balanced *Sleep,* and *Exercise.*

REMEMBER

Applying ABC PLEASE skills is no easy feat, and yet they give you the opportunity to build a strong emotional foundation to help you support yourself so that you're as steady as you can be when life gives you challenges. As you read through the following sections, you may notice one of the challenges of ABC PLEASE skills, which is that when one or two of your PLEASE skills fall off, the others quickly come tumbling down after. For example, when you don't sleep, you don't have energy to work out or cook a healthy meal, so you order a pizza and drink a glass of wine because you're tired and stressed out. The good news about PLEASE skills is that as quickly as they fall off and you feel the negative impact, you can just as quickly begin to find balance and feel the positive impact. One or two nights of good sleep can get you back to the gym and accumulating positives. So while it's easy for these skills to get out of balance and leave you vulnerable, you can also quickly find balance and steadiness again as long as you're aware and paying attention.

Accumulate positives

Dr. Marsha Linehan, who created DBT, has always said that you need to live an antidepressant life. You need to actively look for what brings you joy and incorporate it into your life. Don't wait for good things to happen to you, but seek out these things and the experiences that bring joy into your life. When you're suffering, paying attention or doing things that bring you joy can be very challenging. These can be small things, but having positive experiences each day will build emotional resiliency. Think about values, experiences, or things that are important to you. Set a goal and work on achieving it step by step.

Build mastery

Having a sense of accomplishment makes a big difference in how you feel. Try to do something each day that is challenging so that it gives you a sense of accomplishment. You want to make sure that the task you're choosing not only provides a challenge but is also something that you can achieve. This could be related to work or school, a new skill to learn, a project around the house, or even something that is posing a challenge that you've been avoiding. Don't worry if it's a small task; if it's a challenge you can tackle, then you've been skillful.

Cope ahead of time with difficult situations

When you can anticipate and prepare for difficult situations, you'll be less vulnerable to strong emotional reactions that are problematic. For this skill, follow these steps:

1. Describe the facts of the situation. You must do this mindfully and non-judgmentally, and stick to the facts of the situation you're worried about. When you're clear on the nature of the problem, you can go to the next step.

2. Decide what skills you will use to tackle this problem. You probably need to use a chain of skills, as it's unlikely that a single skill will suffice. It's important to think about making a plan that involves at least three different skills. You may want to start with a distress tolerance skill to decrease the intensity of your emotions (see Chapter 11), and then depending on your goal, try a skill that is more focused on acceptance (if it is something you cannot change) or a change skill to move you closer to your goal of changing a situation or problem. Write your skills plan down if that is helpful.

3. Imagine the situation with as much detail as possible. Then imagine executing your skills plan and your effective skills use over and over. While you're imagining this, consider situations that may arise that are challenging, or new problems that may arise as you practice your skills.

4. Think of the worst-case scenario; this is usually something that you've been worrying about, and it may look like a lot of "what-ifs" circling around in your head. Now, rehearse your plan to address this scenario. Be open, as this can be very challenging. If you need to modify your plan for the worst-case scenario, then do so.

REMEMBER

The cope-ahead skill is very useful if you find yourself stuck ruminating about a problem and not moving into action. That behavior is emotionally depleting. When you notice it, begin a cope-ahead plan, moving deeply into the very anxiety you have been avoiding (most commonly by getting stuck in the what-ifs) and the details of the worst-case scenario; now make a plan. More often than not, the worst case doesn't happen, so having a plan allows you to stop generating multiple terrible outcomes without having a solution. It's also true that once you have a plan for the worst-case scenario, parts of that plan often help with the less catastrophic outcomes of the situation, and if the worst case does occur, then you have a plan to begin to deal with it.

Physical illness

When you don't feel well physically, it impacts your mood. You may notice more sadness or irritability and increased urges for target behaviors, or you may just find that you feel more sensitive or reactive. When possible, treat your physical illness. When you have a headache, take something; when you don't feel well, stay home, rest, or go to bed early. Go to the doctor if you need to. Be proactive and think about it as a way of also taking care of your mood. Be aware that physical illness leads to emotional vulnerability. It's important to keep that in mind, to self-validate, and to do what you can to get some extra support.

TIP

A number of patients at 3East (where we work) decided to enhance this part of the acronym by identifying some additional parts for the "L" that we think are very useful. They liked the idea of adding "*Lather* rinse repeat." They pointed out that when your mood is low, it can be difficult to do what are commonly called activities of daily living (ADLs), and that when you shower, it can be helpful in changing the way you feel and decrease additional vulnerability to an already low mood. They also, albeit begrudgingly, added "*Limit* screen time."

Balanced eating

The link between eating and mood starts almost immediately. When babies are hungry, they get upset, and that continues to adulthood. For many, the word *hangry* captures this experience. When we're hungry, we become more irritable and reactive. Parents manage this in young children all the time by pulling snacks out of every bag. It isn't just about eating or not eating, though; for many, it's important to be mindful of the frequency of meals, the kinds of foods they eat, and the quantity. Pay attention to the impact that your eating has on your mood.

Avoid mood-altering substances

REMEMBER

As their name states, mood-altering substances impact your mood. We are talking about drugs, alcohol, nicotine, caffeine, and even sugar. Whether you use them in a legal and responsible way or not, the end result is that they leave you more emotionally vulnerable. If these substances impact your mood in a negative way, think about how you can reduce their presence in your life.

Balanced sleep

Sleep has one of the most powerful impacts on mood. Healthy adults need between seven and nine hours of sleep per night, and adolescents need eight to ten hours of sleep per night. It's amazing how differently you experience the world on a day when you have slept compared to a day when you have not. When you don't sleep, it's hard to function, and yet many people who come to DBT struggle profoundly with the ability to sleep. Do your best to balance your sleep, consider sleep hygiene plans, work with your doctors to see whether medication or protocols for nightmares could help, and most of all, know that when you don't sleep, you're more vulnerable. Be kind to yourself; problems with sleep can take time to solve.

Exercise

There is a large body of research on exercise and mood. Study after study finds the benefits of exercise on mood, but when your mood is low, exercise can feel impossible. Get into a routine and work to make your exercise independent of your mood, meaning that you follow your exercise routine regardless of how you feel on any given day. Find a type (or types) of exercise that you like; for example, you may like walking, running, team sports, dancing, or going to the gym. There are many types of exercise. See whether you can start with 20 minutes a day, and pay attention to how that makes you feel. Think about what gets in the way of exercising and see whether you can resolve those barriers.

Practicing opposite action

While ABC PLEASE is a skill that we would like you to be aware of and practicing all the time to support long-term decreased emotional vulnerability, opposite action is a powerful emotion regulation skill to use in the moment when you need to change how you feel. You can use opposite action when acting on the emotion you're feeling isn't effective.

Sometimes your emotions don't fit the facts of the situation (unjustified), and when that is the case, acting on their urges is ineffective. All emotions have action urges — that is, they make you want to do something or, in some cases, to avoid doing something. As we discuss in Chapter 5, emotions are either justified or unjustified:

» **Justified emotions** fit the facts of the situation, as does the duration and intensity of your response to that situation.

» **Unjustified emotions** do not fit the facts of the situation — or more commonly in DBT, it is the intensity and duration of the emotional response that does not fit the facts and renders the emotion unjustified.

For example, you may feel very anxious about going to work because you worry that you'll get some difficult feedback from your boss. You are so afraid that you feel like you can't get out of bed, and so you decide not to go to work. It certainly makes sense that you're afraid or anxious about going to work; however, the level of fear is unjustified, as staying in bed and not showing up for work will only make your situation worse, especially if you're getting feedback about your work performance. Moreover, you aren't even certain of when you may be receiving the feedback or what kind of feedback it will be. As you can see, being anxious and following the urge to avoid work will be very ineffective. This skill asks you to act 110 percent opposite to that urge to stay in bed. When this happens, we're coaching you toward the opposite action skill.

REMEMBER

The following steps will guide you through the practice of opposite action:

1. **Identify and name your emotion.**

   You can do this by using your SUN WAVE NO NOT skill in Chapter 5. To follow up on the earlier example:

   Fear that my boss will fire me. Shame because I can't tolerate anything and am weak.

2. **Check the facts and determine whether your emotion is justified or unjustified.**

   My emotions make sense as it is hard for me to get feedback and I have been fired twice before. However, the intensity of my emotions is too high and I have been in bed since my alarm went off four hours ago.

3. **Ask yourself: What is my action urge? What do I want to do as a result of how I feel right now?**

   I want to stay in bed and never talk to my manager again.

4. **Connect with your wise mind — both how you feel about this situation as well as the facts of the situation — and ask yourself whether acting on these urges is effective. Does it move you toward or away from your goal?**

Acting on these urges is not effective. I like my job, and my manager has been supportive in the past. Also, in the future, he could be a good reference for another job or school.

5. **If your emotion is unjustified and it is ineffective to act on your current urges, identify some ways that you could act opposite to your current urges.**

   I can get up, shower, get dressed, and go to work; I can text my manager that I would like to check in with him; or I could go to work and speak to my manager directly.

6. **Act opposite 110 percent.**

   Throw yourself into this new action. The more your throw yourself in and act opposite, the more powerful the impact will be on how you feel.

   I will get up, shower, dress up a little for work, practice being assertive and confident when I see my manager at work, and I will ask if we can find some time to talk over the next day or two.

7. **Continue the process of acting opposite until your urges and emotions decrease.**

   I will continue to act confident and assertive at work until I am able to talk with him.

REMEMBER

Opposite action is a skill that takes a lot of willingness, often at a time when you may be very stuck. This is a challenging skill with powerful results. One of the helpful things about opposite action is that it can lead to longer-term changes in how you feel, compared to the shorter-term distress tolerance skills that we cover in Chapter 11. Effective use of opposite action can lead to a powerful sense of mastery that helps make the skill very self-reinforcing, meaning it helps you the next time you are stuck to be motivated into doing the hard task of acting opposite.

Being kind to yourself

For many people who come to DBT, it takes little effort to be unkind to themselves. Critical and self-hating thoughts have been practiced without awareness for years as a result of many painful things that have happened to them along the way. However, those thoughts feed into already-existing challenges with emotion regulation. Learning to be kind to yourself will support more effective emotion regulation.

TIP

Here are three ways that you can begin to practice increased kindness to yourself in a way that will support your ability to regulate emotions:

>> **Taking "me time":** If you're an emotionally sensitive person, you may find that you're easily overstimulated by the world around you. It may be the pain and suffering, the stress, the demands from others, or even joy and

excitement. Sometimes, you need a break. This isn't isolation or withdrawal, but time that you can set aside for yourself. Maybe it's doing something you love with the goal of accumulating positives, or maybe it's just giving yourself time to decompress.

» **Cheerleading statements:** We often don't get a lot of enthusiasm when we initially suggest practicing cheerleading statements. However, this is often because people mistake this for some sort of "way to go, you are great" self-talk. Cheerleading statements are unique to each one of us. You need to find what works for you. Think about what you would say to yourself if you were eight miles into a ten-mile race and needed to effectively urge yourself on. This type of encouraging self-talk helps you regulate and stay on course. The more commonly practiced negative self-judgment and criticism does the opposite. Help yourself stay regulated. Think about three things you could say to yourself to help you persist when things get difficult.

» **Making self-care an everyday practice:** Making something a practice means making it a routine. Try to do at least one thing that is focused on self-care each day. Think about ways to take care of yourself. For example, find a time to take a break; if you're feeling overwhelmed, make a checklist to help organize yourself; go for a brief walk to break up a day of sitting at a computer; buy yourself a nice cup of coffee; or make yourself your favorite meal. Take some time in your day to prioritize your well-being while still doing what needs to be done.

Being Your Own Emotional Support

Finding balance between being your own emotional support and relying on others is often difficult. It requires you to find a dialectical balance and move away from the all-or-nothing thinking of only being able to completely rely on yourself or on others. Healthy emotion regulation requires both. Some people are easily able to find balance, while others may either land solidly on the extremes or bounce back and forth. The more you practice your DBT skills, the more confident you'll feel in your ability to find balance and consistency in your life. In the following sections, we look at a few ways that you can practice being your own emotional support.

Reappraising your feelings

REMEMBER

Throughout this book, we discuss ways in which your thoughts and emotions can lead you off track. Use your mindfulness skills (see Chapter 9) to step back and look at your thinking and feelings. Get familiar with the errors that you make or the problematic reactions that you have, notice them, find compassion, and take control of your reactions. Have a gentle touch with yourself so that you become less reactive and thrown around by your emotions. Keep in mind that you don't have to believe everything you think, and you don't have to act on every urge. Build the skills you need to be at the helm, and make the choices that move you effectively toward goals and relationships that are important to you; have compassion when you veer off course, and don't lose time and emotional energy beating yourself up.

Adopting healthy self-soothing practices

Self-soothing is a way to treat yourself when you're trying to tolerate or regulate your emotions. Self-soothing is something you do on your own and for yourself. As babies, we use repetitive self-soothing behaviors such as thumb sucking, stroking or holding blankets, or attaching to stuffed animals that help us calm down or feel better when we're upset.

WARNING

Self-soothing may not have come easy to you as a young child, or it may be a skill that you haven't practiced in many years. You may have also replaced healthy ways of self-soothing with unhealthy ways such as drinking alcohol, excessive TV watching or video gaming, shopping, nail biting, leg shaking, over- or under-eating, or overworking, to name a few.

While most teens and adults no longer suck their thumbs or use blankets, they have come up with other ways to self-soothe. Being able to self-soothe is an important part of emotion regulation. Think about how you self-soothe. What do you do to soothe yourself when you're upset? Is it effective in the short and long-term?

TIP

It's easy to remember ways to self-soothe if you think about using your five senses. Here are some ideas:

>> **Touch:** Take a warm bubble bath; get into soft, comfortable clothing; get a massage.

>> **Taste:** Drink some relaxing tea; have hot chocolate; eat a warm bowl of soup.

>> **Smell:** Use aromatherapy, essential oils, or a scented candle.

>> **Sight:** Look at pictures of your favorite places; watch an episode (just one!) of your favorite show; go outside and look at the clouds or the stars.

>> **Sound:** Listen to your favorite music; listen to a sound machine with white noise or nature sounds; go outside and listen to the sounds of nature.

REMEMBER

This is just a short list to give you a few ideas. Take stock of what you already do that is effective and skillful self-soothing. If you're working to develop a self-soothing practice or want some more ideas, pick a few from this list or come up with some that you want to try. Make sure you're practicing at least one self-soothing skill each day. Self-soothing helps calm you down, and we know that when you are calmer, you can think more clearly and will more skillfully be able to regulate your emotions.

Chapter **11**

Building Your Distress Tolerance

The ability to manage stress effectively is a hallmark of mental health. There are times when a person is in a situation that they can do nothing about in that moment. In DBT, distress tolerance skills are taught for these moments. *Distress tolerance* is a person's ability to manage distress. For emotionally sensitive people, emotional distress is often the most difficult to manage. The focus of the distress tolerance skill set is on getting through stressful moments without getting stuck in misery or making the situation worse. If your ability to tolerate difficult moments or intense emotions is poor, you'll notice that you have a tendency to become overwhelmed and then at times to turn to unhealthy, maladaptive, or even destructive ways of coping.

Everyone's ability to deal with stress, of course, depends on what the stressful situation is. We all experience stress. Some situations cause minor aggravation. Others are major life stressors. Whether the stressful situations are minor or major, being able to go through these moments is key to maintaining stability in your life. Distress tolerance skills can make a positive difference in your ability to handle difficult emotions and are often the ones that people find most useful at the start of DBT therapy.

In this chapter, you find ways to survive and deal with difficult moments without getting stuck in a cycle of suffering. You also see how by understanding that all things are caused by the events that preceded them, that instead of getting stuck in feeling that things are unfair or shouldn't have happened, you can instead work on reducing the impact of such events should they arise in the future.

Managing Difficult Moments with Crisis Survival Skills

We all experience difficult situations. Some might be more aggravating than anything else: You might be sitting in a traffic jam, already 20 minutes late for an important meeting, or you might have missed a flight home for a much-needed break, or you may realize that you're out of coffee on a morning that you desperately need a cup. There are times, however, when the distress is much more than that: the loss of a job, of a relationship, or of a loved one. For people with conditions like borderline personality disorder (BPD), some distress can feel more unbearable than others could imagine. Waiting for a call from a romantic partner, especially in the context of feeling abandoned, can lead some people to feel as if they might die. That is the nature of intense emotions. They distort time, and it can feel as if a moment of suffering has lasted forever.

Interestingly, DBT therapists and patients with BPD weren't the only ones to recognize this. Albert Einstein once famously said, "Put your hand on a hot stove for a minute, and it seems like an hour. Sit with a pretty girl for an hour, and it seems like a minute. That's relativity." The point is that strong emotions influence the perception of time, and difficult moments can seem to take forever. This is often confusing to others who feel as if the person with BPD is making a big deal of nothing.

Another curious aspect of the experience of suffering is that it seems to emanate from the body's core, even though there isn't one specific body part to point to. Under such stress, if people with BPD haven't learned healthier and more adaptive coping skills to tolerate the distress they feel, they often resort to less adaptive, though immediately effective, behaviors like self-harm, substance use, dangerous sexual behaviors, eating behaviors, or other impulsive behaviors that seem to offer an immediate solution. In the long term, these solutions make problems and psychological pain even worse.

REMEMBER

DBT founder Dr. Marsha Linehan and her team developed various ways to deal with such moments. The first set of skills in the distress tolerance module are *crisis survival skills.* The time for crisis survival skills occurs when

>> You're experiencing intense emotional pain that doesn't seem to end.

>> You really want these emotions to end, and you consider using a behavior that will make things more difficult in the long run.

>> Your situation feels overwhelming, and yet there are demands and obligations to meet.

>> You're motivated to address a situation immediately, but you have to wait, perhaps until the next day.

REMEMBER

Crisis survival skills can be very helpful, but it's important to not use these skills for everyday problems or to solve all of the issues that may occur throughout one's life. These skills are not problem-solving skills; instead, they are ways to get through challenging times. A little bit of stress can be very useful, as long as it is manageable. Thus, crisis survival skills should be reserved for managing a crisis situation only. If you want to change an emotion, you should turn to the emotion regulation skills that are reviewed in Chapter 10.

REMEMBER

For many people who live in emotional turmoil, it can feel as if their entire life is in a crisis. So, what actually constitutes a crisis?

>> A crisis is typically a defined event, one that has stress or perhaps even trauma, and it contains a lot of strong and usually unwanted and painful emotions. Even though it can feel as if it will never end, a crisis has a beginning and an end. Dr. Linehan once quipped, "If it's something that lasts forever and you think it's a crisis, it's your life, not a crisis."

>> A crisis has the quality of needing to be resolved immediately, or that you have to escape it right now.

>> A crisis typically doesn't appear to have a ready solution. Of course, if you were in a difficult situation and could solve it in that moment, you would.

By definition, crisis survival skills are the skills necessary to get through a crisis. But how do you get through situations so stressful that the only solution seems to be to run and hide, or even consider something more destructive? Dr. Linehan described two sets of skills, the first where you try to distract yourself and the second where you soothe yourself.

Distracting yourself

Again, if you're in a difficult situation but one that you can solve, then you should solve it. Distracting isn't the skill for this moment. However, the solution should also not be one that makes the situation worse. Distracting is the act of taking your mind off the problem you're facing. It means putting your attention on something else.

As you see throughout this book, DBT uses a lot of acronyms, and for this skill set, Dr. Linehan came up with the skill called ACCEPTS:

>> **Activities:** The idea here is to throw yourself into activities. Don't do something that you can do mindlessly. If you do, then your mind will go to the problem. That defeats the purpose. Do an activity that will take your mind off the problem and onto the activity. For instance, it's hard to read and keep your mind on a problem. If that doesn't work, then maybe exercise or play a musical instrument.

>> **Contributing:** Contributing is the act of distracting yourself by focusing your mind on someone else or a cause that you help or contribute to. There are two benefits to this: The first is that you're distracting from the problem, and the second is that you're doing something good for someone else, and you'll notice that you feel better about yourself. Maybe you could volunteer for a non-profit, or you could make something for someone when they themselves are struggling. The thing that you need to do doesn't have to be big. The point here is that you aren't switching jobs; you're using this technique as a way to distract.

>> **Comparison:** The skill here can be applied in one of two ways:

  • **To compare yourself to someone who is in a worse situation than you are in:** Some people don't like doing this practice because they then feel as if they don't deserve a better life when people with less than what they have aren't complaining. Remember, they may not have had the situation that you have, and they may not be suffering.

  • **To compare yourself to a time when you were less skilled than you are now:** It's a practice in distracting by saying, "This could be worse," which puts your problem in relative perspective.

>> **Emotions:** Here, the skill is to distract yourself from one emotion by doing something that creates a different emotion. For instance, if you're feeling sad, you can decide to play happy music. Certainly, when you're sad, you don't want to put on sad music, unless you want to stay sad. You have to figure out what works for you, because the kind of music that makes you happy isn't necessarily the music that makes another person happy. Other ideas are skipping, dancing, or watching an emotional movie or video clip.

>> **Pushing away:** Pushing away is a skill you apply to distract yourself when you just can't cope with what's going on. You first make a list of the main problems in your life. Then you ask yourself of each one, "Can I do anything about this problem right now?" or "Is this the time to work on the problem?" If the

answer is yes, then work on the problem. If the answer is no, then skip it and go to the next problem.

One thing that happens to people in DBT is that after a day spent struggling, they stay up late ruminating about the day's problems. Well, now it's the middle of the night and there often isn't anything they can do at that point in time. The best thing is to push it away, get a good night's sleep, and then let a more rested mind deal with the situation at a time when it can more likely be addressed. By going through each item on your list, you decide whether you can deal with it now or you can push it away until later. It's about recognizing that this isn't the time to do so, and that trying to deal with the problem right now would be ineffective.

» **Thoughts:** This is the practice of distracting yourself from a crisis by focusing your mind on some thought, like the thought of counting to ten, naming countries from A to Z, or naming the things in your room that are blue in color. Just keep your mind busy. One thought that works very well for some people is to think "wise" as you breathe in and "mind" as you breathe out.

» **Sensations:** This is the practice of using sensations to distract yourself. It's one of the better skills to use when you're in extreme emotional pain or when you're overwhelmed by an urge to do something that is not in your best long-term interest. For example, take a hot bath or a cold shower. Hold a piece of ice until it melts. Suck on an intense mint. Smell a strong scent. It should be intense. Whatever you do, don't do something that will harm you. If you're holding ice, for instance, it shouldn't be to the point that it freezes your skin.

Soothing yourself

This crisis survival skill is about soothing yourself by focusing on your five senses. In doing this, you're shifting the focus of your mind from the stressful situation to something entirely different. It gives you a short break and allows you to reconnect with the world outside of your *self*. Use your sense of

» **Sight:** Stimulate your sense of vision by looking at something — for example, people-watching at a mall, focusing on the flames in your fireplace, or going to a park and observing nature.

» **Hearing:** Sit in a room and just listen to the sounds of your house. Or, go outside and listen to the wind blowing through the trees, the sounds of traffic, or the sound of people murmuring in the background.

» **Smell:** Light a scented candle and smell it. Peel an orange and smell the citrus scent. Take your favorite soap or lotion and enjoy the scent as you wash your hands and apply the lotion.

>> **Taste:** Slowly allow your favorite chocolate to melt in your mouth, or enjoy your favorite cup of tea. Focus only on the taste.

>> **Touch:** Rub your hand over your favorite material, or pet your dog or your cat. Wrap yourself in your favorite scarf, or wear your most comfortable pajamas.

Recognizing That Everything Has a Cause

Many people who suffer feel as if something bad is being done to them, and they often feel that it's being done with malicious intent. Another way they think about difficult situations is that things *just happen*, and they happen because perhaps they deserve these things that happen or that these situations *just happen* to them. "Bad things just happen." But things don't "just happen." Everything is caused.

Many times, we are asked, "What is the root cause of my (or my loved one's) problems?" DBT is very different from many other therapies in that we don't spend too much time looking into root causes. An important part of learning to accept reality, as you find out in the following sections, is to recognize that every event and every circumstance has a cause. When you see that everything has a cause, you'll stop saying, "Why did it happen to me?" Instead, because you'll recognize that events have causes, it will make perfect sense, whether you like it or not, that things happen in the way they do.

REMEMBER

When you say that things aren't fair and that they shouldn't be the way they are, you are in non-acceptance. Of course things are the way they should be. How could they not be? Because everything is caused, the reason why things are the way they are is because they were caused. Whether you like how things turn out is irrelevant. If you don't like the outcome, you don't like it. If you like it, you like it. The outcome won't change.

Checking out a real-life example

Imagine that your employer requires that each person on your team works on one of the federal holidays. The week before each holiday, if people can't decide among themselves, then they draw lots, with the person who has to work on that holiday then being excluded from the pool in the future. Thanksgiving, Christmas, and New Year's are left, and there are three of you. You've let people know that you don't mind which one you take, and the other two want Thanksgiving off. You then hear that your best friend from high school is coming home for Thanksgiving, a friend you haven't seen in years. You go to your boss and let her know, but she says that it has already been decided. You ask the other two employees, and they say that their plans are set.

You then ask that the decision be done by drawing lots, saying that was the protocol in case of a disagreement. The other two reluctantly agree, and your boss writes down the three holidays onto pieces of paper, folds them, and puts them into a box. Your chance is now two in three that you won't have to work Thanksgiving. You're excited because you were 100 percent going to have to work. Each employee takes out a piece of paper from the box and opens it. You open yours. "Thanksgiving!" You had been content prior to the draw, perhaps somewhat anxious. Your colleagues had been upset prior to the draw, feeling that they had been cheated. Now you're so upset: "It's not fair! My friend is coming after many years!"

You have forgotten that everything is caused. Had your company not had rules that someone needs to work each holiday, had you been assigned to another holiday earlier in the year, had your two remaining colleagues been happy to work on Thanksgiving, had you not suddenly heard that your friend was coming, had you drawn a different piece of paper from the box, then things would have been different. But that's not what happened. Your situation was caused by the events that preceded it. Your colleagues are happy, and you are upset. It makes sense that you are upset, but whether you like it or not, that was the outcome, and it was caused by everything that happened.

Changing your perspective

If you don't like saying that everything is as it should be, just say, "Everything is caused. Even the things that I don't like." Imagine that you're at the beach and the water is choppy. You're sitting with your child and you see a father with two young children, and he seems to be having a difficult time preventing them from running into the water. He is packing up and getting ready to leave, and in a moment of distraction, one of his children runs off toward the sea, jumps into the waves, gets pulled away, and nearly drowns.

You say, "That should never have happened." In DBT we say that it should have happened. The weather had churned up the waves, the father was having a difficult time controlling his children, he was trying to pack up and was distracted, the child didn't know how to swim and was intrigued by the water, and you had your own child and could not leave her to help them. It makes sense that things happened as they did. All the previous events led to that event happening. If the conditions had been different — if you hadn't been with your kid, if the father had just brought one child, if the water hadn't been choppy, if he hadn't been distracted — then things wouldn't have happened as they did, but we can't wish the conditions away. They were as they were.

We often only consider this when things don't go our way. Say that the water had been calm and the children had been compliant with the father and that nothing happened. We're willing to accept that nothing bad happened. The conditions for the child not nearly drowning were present and led to the child not nearly drowning. It makes as much sense that the child did not nearly drown when things were calmer, as it does that the child nearly drowned when the conditions were rougher. For things not to have happened as they did, you would somehow have had to go back in time and change the causes. And here's the thing: All those causes had causes of their own.

Accepting reality as it is also means accepting that everything is caused. This doesn't mean that you approve of the child nearly drowning, or that you think that it was good. If you were the child's father, you would do something different the next time you went to the beach in bad weather. Perhaps you would take another person, perhaps you would not go at all, perhaps you would take only one child at a time. However, whatever you choose to do next time, you can't change what did actually happen.

REMEMBER

Think about a situation in your life. Rather than saying, "It shouldn't have happened," can you think about the causes for the situation? What caused the event to happen? Once you realize that the event was caused, you realize that saying "it shouldn't have happened" makes no sense. You can definitely say, "I didn't like that the event happened," but not that it shouldn't have happened. Imagine that someone drops an egg and it smashes all over a hard floor, causing a mess. If you say that it shouldn't have happened, it would mean that you were on a planet where gravity doesn't pull things down, where the eggs have far thicker shells, or where floors aren't hard at all. You not liking something that happened doesn't change the laws of science. Certainly, changing your thinking from "that shouldn't have happened" to "I wonder what caused that to happen" will give you the opportunity to start tackling the causes if a similar situation should arise again.

Curbing Impulsive Behavior

When you're under intense distress, you're prone to head back to old behaviors, and the impulse to do something destructive can be strong. Without curbing the impulsive behavior, you slip back into repetitive patterns that keep you stuck. The following sections describe methods you can use to curb impulsive behavior.

Foregoing short-term gratification

Behaviors like self-injury, drugs and alcohol, dangerous and intense sexual encounters, and driving fast can provide instant gratification. All too often, however, that is all they do. They don't solve the problem you're dealing with, and often they are behaviors that leave you feeling worse for having engaged in them in the first place.

Say you feel that you'll never be loved. You meet some person on a dating app. They say that you look attractive and that they would like to date you. You say that you aren't going to have sex on the first date, and you go out with the person. You like them. They tell you that they want to have sex, and you're thrilled that they want to be with you. They promise you that they are interested in more dates, but that they want sex that night. You have made a commitment to yourself that you won't have sex on any first date, but you're desperate. You break your commitment and sleep with the person. Perhaps they aren't very considerate during sex, but you enjoy the feeling of attention. However, once the sex is over, they then ask you to leave. You feel terrible about yourself and notice a lot of shame for having violated your values and your commitments. Ideally, you should have stopped the moment they said they wanted sex that night.

REMEMBER

A situation like this is where you can use the STOP skill. As with many DBT skills, STOP is an acronym:

>> **Stop.** Don't go with whatever urge you're responding to. Stay in control of your body. Don't hit Send if you were intending to send a negative text or email or if you were going to self-injure. Remain perfectly still.

>> **Take a step back.** Remove yourself from the situation. Walk away from your device. Walk away from the person you want to yell at. Take a slow and deep breath. Don't act impulsively or based on strong emotions.

>> **Observe.** Take a moment to notice your thoughts, intentions, urges, emotions, sensations, surroundings, and environment. What is your current experience? Articulate this slowly to yourself.

>> **Proceed mindfully.** Once you have taken the first three steps, think about your goals in the current situation. Whatever you do, act with awareness. That doesn't mean that you aren't going to do what your urges told you to do; it just means that whatever you're going to do, you have examined your response and ideally used your wise mind to proceed. Ask yourself whether the action will make your situation better or worse, and then act in the interest of your long-term goals. Sometimes the best way to proceed is to do nothing at all.

Improving your situation

If you can't solve your situation in the moment and remember that the ideal thing to do is to solve your situation if you can, and if you're in a crisis, you can consider the situation that you're in and try to improve it. By improving the moment, you're attempting to make the situation better, at least in your mind. Dr. Linehan often uses acronyms to teach, and here again, the IMPROVE skill is one:

>> **Imagery:** This is the practice of changing a situation in your mind. Imagine a situation different than the one you are in. Perhaps if you're stuck on an airplane that has been stranded by bad weather, you can imagine the nice beach that you'll be on once the plane eventually takes off and you get to your destination. Another way to use this skill is to imagine being experienced in your current situation.

Ideally, and this is true of all the DBT skills, you practice these skills when you don't need them so that when you do need them, they are there. This is true of most life skills. The time to practice swimming is when the water is calm and you have a teacher. Jumping into a raging ocean is not the best first time to practice swimming.

>> **Meaning:** This is the practice of making meaning of the situation you are in. It can be particularly difficult to have to face a multitude of problems and then want to give up, feeling that life isn't worth living. By making meaning of what you're going through, you find a purpose in your suffering. If you're a person of faith, you can ask your spiritual leader to help you with this. Perhaps you meet a person in a group that you end up caring about and then your suffering was useful because without it, you wouldn't have met that person. The idea here is to think of some positive reason for things being as they are.

>> **Prayer:** Not everyone is religious or a person of faith, but if you are, prayer can be really helpful in a crisis. There is a famous wartime aphorism that goes, "There are no atheists in foxholes." The idea is that in times of crisis, people often have an increase in faith. But if you do have faith, prayer can be a wonderful way to see you through the crisis.

>> **Relaxation:** Often, when we are in a crisis, we tense up and our muscles tighten. You can't relax under these circumstances. It would be nice if you could "just relax" when someone tells you to do so, and as it happens, you can. The first step is to tense your muscles. This may sound counterintuitive, but by over-tensing, your relaxation of the muscles will be more obvious. Tense and let go, tense and let go. This even works in public. If you tense your leg muscles, for instance, and then let them relax, who's to see?

>> **One thing in the moment:** One thing in the moment is very similar to the mindfulness practice of one-mindfully (see Chapter 9). It's the practice of tolerating distress by focusing on one thing that you're doing right now, in this present moment. Doing one thing in the moment can be helpful in that by focusing on that thing, it can give you time to settle down in a distressing situation. It is not, however, avoidance in that eventually you need to get back to face the thing that you're distressed about. Another way to practice this is

to consider that often our suffering intensifies when we spend too much time dwelling on memories of past events. By staying in the present moment, we recognize that those past events aren't happening now — they are simply memories that are being remembered now. If we can stay focused on the present, it takes our mind out of the past, and our suffering reduces.

>> **Vacation:** If you could take a vacation whenever you needed one, that would be ideal, but that is rarely the case. The practice here is to take a mini-vacation from your worries. Perhaps you can take a 30-minute walk in a park, or shut your office door, lie on the floor, and close your eyes. Or, you can treat yourself to some popcorn and watch a movie on TV. Sometimes all it takes is stopping whatever you're doing and taking five minutes to relax.

WARNING

If you're going to take a mini-vacation, don't do anything that will harm you. For example, if you need to finish something at work by a certain time, make sure you do that; you can take the vacation afterward. Taking the vacation before and not getting your job done, and then getting fired, wouldn't be in the interest of your long-term goals.

>> **Encouragement:** The practice of encouragement involves encouraging yourself by saying things like "I can do it. I'll get through this. I am more skillful now. I am not a failure." It can be very difficult to do this in the middle of a crisis, and so the practice requires that when you do this, you say it with all the belief in the world. In other words, don't make it wishy-washy. Saying something like "Maybe I can get through this moment" is not the practice. When you're doing something hard, just continue to encourage yourself. When you're climbing to the top of a mountain, don't complain about how hard it is; encourage yourself. "You can do this! You can get to the top!" Of course, you have to be realistic. If you see an elite marathoner running by you, it would be foolish and discouraging to say, "Come on, you can do it, you can run as fast as she can."

REMEMBER

Using this practice can be really helpful, and research shows that people who encourage themselves can actually increase their ability to perform the action they are focusing on.

Using pros and cons

The skill of using pros and cons is the practice of evaluating the advantages and disadvantages of a particular course of action or doing certain things in a situation. The specifics to this approach are that you consider the *advantage* of engaging in some behavior and then the *disadvantage* of that behavior. Then you consider the *advantage* of *not* engaging in the behavior, and then the *disadvantage* of not engaging in the behavior.

There are three steps in doing this practice:

1. **Articulate the behavior or course of action that you are considering.**

   You can simply write it down.

2. **List the pros and cons.**

   There are four parts to this: the pros of doing the behavior; the pros of *not* doing the behavior; the cons of doing the behavior; and finally, the cons of *not* doing the behavior.

3. **Decide what is important to you.**

   Circle the items on your list that are consistent with your long-term goals. That will tell you what the best course of action is.

Doing Your Own Crisis Management

Some people seem to be destroyed by very difficult situations, while others are not only not destroyed by these moments, but instead seem to tolerate them and even get stronger. In DBT, people often call their therapists and ask for help. The therapists suggest various crisis survival skills (covered earlier in this chapter). Even still, how is it that some suffer so, while others don't? It can be easy to feel defeated by life's challenges, and yet once you have mastered the skills taught by your skills teachers and coached by your therapist, you can do your own crisis management.

Say that you're applying for a job and your application gets rejected. One option is to not apply for another job. Another is to keep on trying. For people who give up, the reason they do so is less about what happened and more about what they say about themselves. So, rather than say, "I didn't get a job and that is disappointing," they might say something like, "I am a useless person that no one wants to hire. It's pointless applying for another job. Everyone can see I'm a loser."

To deal with a difficult situation, you have to first accept it as it is. The following sections walk you through the process of acceptance and provide some helpful tips.

Acceptance of your situation

One approach is to say that you didn't get the job you were applying for, which is factually correct. A very different approach is to conclude that you are a loser who no one will ever want to hire. Those are simply destructive thoughts, conclusions, and assumptions. But how do you accept reality, especially if that reality is hard? Dr. Linehan said that reality acceptance has three components: radical acceptance, turning your mind, and willingness.

Radical acceptance

REMEMBER

Here is the single most important thing to know about radical acceptance: Radical acceptance is the acceptance of *this* moment. You aren't radically accepting yesterday or tomorrow. All you have to do is accept this moment. This is easy to say, but you'll see that it is difficult to do.

So, what is acceptance of this moment? Think about something that you can't imagine accepting, something really serious: a significant medical condition, a terrible trauma, the loss of a beloved person. How are you going to deal with any of these? One way to address this is to think about your options: Certainly, one choice is to stay miserable and spend endless hours thinking about your painful situation. Another option is to accept that it is your reality. The issue is that not accepting your reality will never change your reality.

Say that you were badly hurt as a child. Refusing to accept that the hurt happened won't make it not have happened. The situation happened, sure. It was painful, that is certain, but you have to ask yourself how continuing to think about it helps you. This doesn't mean that you have to be happy about what happened or deny that it happened, nor does it mean that you have to be miserable about something that isn't of this present moment. Radical acceptance is the complete and total acceptance of a situation; it means throwing your body, mind, and soul into accepting the situation. It means not denying or rejecting or fighting the reality of the situation.

It's easy to *say* that you have to radically accept something. It's much, much harder to do. Take a relatively trivial problem. You're stuck in traffic and you're angry that you're going to be late for a meeting. You start yelling at the traffic, and you notice that your blood pressure is going up. (By the way, it's interesting that we say things like "I am stuck in traffic," but we rarely say, "I am traffic." The truth is that you are just as much traffic as any other car in the jam!) Then you remember that getting angry isn't going to change the traffic, so you decide to practice radical acceptance. You take a few breaths and you just accept. What tends to happen after a few moments is that you start to get angry again and the cycle begins again. Radical acceptance is acceptance of this particular moment. It's the only moment you can accept! You can't accept tomorrow. It hasn't arrived.

People who practice radical acceptance find a sense of calm. It's not that they like what happened to them. It's just that they know that what happened has happened, and that rather than spending this moment ruminating about what happened, they can focus on anything else. If you're suffering because of some past situation — say that you didn't get a job that you had worked hard to get — try this exercise:

>> While sitting, close your eyes and in your memory go back to the moment just before you heard that you hadn't gotten the job. Hold that moment in your mind.

>> Imagine that you heard about the job, and that you accepted that you didn't get it. Have you ever had a moment like that? Probably not!

>> Imagine that you heard that you did get the job; you would feel happy and at peace.

Here's the thing: You can experience that kind of centeredness and peace whether you accept that you got the job or not. It's not about the job. It's about the acceptance. If you make it about the job, then you give up all the other things that might have happened. We imagine that we will be happy if we get what we want, but we don't actually know because we don't experience what didn't happen. (See the nearby sidebar "Getting back up after failure" for an example of someone who accepted failures and found success.)

One of the emotions that you might experience when you accept is sadness. However, many people who notice sadness, because they have accepted, have a sense that a heavy burden has been lifted and put aside. That's the freedom that comes with radical acceptance.

What about physical pain? How can you accept that? Pain is like any other experience, although most of us understandably don't like it. Imagine two people sitting next to each other, where one has a headache and refuses to accept it, while the other one also has a headache and accepts that in this moment, he has a headache. Who do you imagine feels more settled? Who would you prefer to be? Feeling that it's unfair that you have a headache, that you shouldn't have it, that you're the one who always gets headaches, simply amplifies your suffering. Now imagine that the headache ends for both of them. Each had pain, but one added so many other elements that led to suffering. Dr. Linehan wrote that suffering and agony are the result of pain plus non-acceptance. Radical acceptance removes the non-acceptance, and then all you're left with is ordinary pain.

GETTING BACK UP AFTER FAILURE

There is a narrative about President Abraham Lincoln's life that highlights many of his failures. It goes something like this:

- 1831: He lost his job: a failure.

- 1832: He was defeated in his run for the Illinois State Legislature: a failure.

- 1833: He failed in business: a failure.

- 1834: He was elected to the Illinois State Legislature: a success.

- 1835: His beloved Ann Rutledge died.

- 1838: He was defeated in his run for Illinois House Speaker: a failure.

- 1843: He was defeated in his run for nomination to the U.S. Congress: a failure.

- 1846: He was elected to the U.S. Congress: a success.

- 1848: He lost re-nomination: a failure.

- 1849: He was rejected for a land officer position: a failure.

- 1854: He was defeated in his run for the U.S. Senate: a failure.

- 1856: He was defeated in his run for the nomination for vice president: a failure.

- 1858: He was again defeated in his run for the U.S. Senate: a failure.

- 1860: He was elected president: a success.

Now, of course, this list mainly focuses on his failures, and certainly he had many successes, but the point of this narrative is that he got up each time he failed. What if he had succeeded in some of his failures? Perhaps he would have been happy with whatever situation he was in and his presidency would never have happened.

The setbacks in your life don't define you. They are moments in a journey.

Turning your mind

It would be wonderful if you could use radical acceptance all the time, but it's a hard skill to practice because it often feels as if you're being required to do something forever. Radical acceptance isn't something you do just once. It's something you have to do over and over and over. If you're sitting in traffic, it's not as if saying "I accept that I am sitting in traffic" once will make everything okay. Even if you notice the peace that comes with acceptance, you'll also soon notice the aggravation of being in traffic that comes once you stop accepting.

So how do you get back to accepting? This is where the skill of turning the mind comes in. It's the practice of turning the mind back toward acceptance. It's like wanting to hike up to the top of a mountain and getting to a junction on the trail, with one way continuing to the top and the other going back down the mountain. It's choosing to turn to the path up the mountain each time the option is there.

Heading up the mountain can be exhausting, while heading down can feel so easy. But if you don't turn your mind back to acceptance, you don't get to your goal, and often, along with refusing to accept the reality of the situation, comes old behavior and, with that, suffering. But accepting removes the suffering, and then you're down to ordinary pain. Ordinary pain is easier to bear than the same pain with non-acceptance. So, you start accepting, and then you're back at non-acceptance. What do you do? Turn the mind again, and again and again, back to acceptance.

But how do you turn the mind?

1. **Notice that you're not accepting the situation.**

   The clue that you aren't in acceptance is that you're angry, judgmental, saying that things shouldn't be the way they are, or engaging in a lot of repetitive and ineffective self-pity.

2. **Commit to yourself that you are going to accept.**

   This commitment isn't the same as radical acceptance; it's just making a commitment that you're going to turn the mind back to commitment. Notice that you aren't committing, and say, "I am committing to turning my mind back to committing." Now, do it again. Do it as many times as it takes, each time you're in non-acceptance.

Let's get back to the situation where you're stuck in traffic. You're going to be late for an important meeting, but the traffic is barely moving. You start noticing that you're having a lot of non-acceptance thoughts: "This is terrible," "What is wrong with these people?" "This is going to last forever," "I am going to be fired from work."

You notice all these thoughts, and you remember to practice turning the mind. Can you replace some of the thoughts you're having? For instance, you might say to yourself, "This is a difficult situation, but in the big scheme of everything, it is not a catastrophe." You could also say, "I don't like the situation I am in. This is a frustrating situation." You might also say, "I realize that everything has a cause. There's a reason that the traffic is moving slowly. The other drivers are not doing this intentionally to frustrate me." You notice that you're feeling calmer, but soon you notice that you're feeling aggravated again. You just repeat the practice over and over.

The key idea is that if you're trying to move from non-acceptance to radical acceptance, the first step is to turn the mind. But what if you don't want to turn the mind? This is where the third component of accepting reality comes in, and that is the practice of willingness. Keep reading.

Willingness

REMEMBER

So, what is willingness? *Willingness* is the practice of intentionally not fighting, allowing things to be as they are, and agreeing to participate in the world and all that is happening. Willingness, at its core, is an attitude.

Imagine heading up a mountain with two other people in your party. Both are relatively unfit. The first is complaining all the way. The second is willing to accept that it is hard. The first is really upset, saying that he wishes it were less steep, that he's going to quit, and that he doesn't like it. Does this person's attitude change the fact of the steepness of the mountain? No. The mountain, like life, will have its easier parts and tougher sections. You can get upset as much as you like, but each step will keep on coming.

So, what are your options if you have to keep climbing? You could go back down the mountain on your own. Or, you could just stand there and do nothing other than complain. Or, you could take a step up the mountain. Willingness is taking a step up the mountain.

Now imagine that if instead of you having a hard time climbing the mountain, it was a hiking companion. Imagine that hiking was actually something that you were fairly good at, and that instead of you, it was your companion who was saying, "I don't like this mountain. It's too steep. I am not going to do it." What would you think? Would you want to go hiking with that person again? Probably not. The person who is going to get to the top is the person who takes the steps that are necessary, no matter the conditions. That's willingness. Doing the opposite — that is, refusing to do what is needed — is willfulness. Fully participating in what is necessary with the conditions at hand is willingness.

REMEMBER

One thing that some people worry about is that if they are willing to accept, they are then in agreement, or they are giving in, or another person wins. It is none of those. Acceptance is a skill that says, "I am willing to accept that things are as they are and will participate in life anyway."

Willfulness is the opposite of willingness. It is forgetting that you're a part of the everything of life. It's a refusal to participate in life. Willfulness is a toddler's terrible twos, throwing a tantrum and saying "no" to everything offered, no matter what the situation is. Willfulness is not just something that emotionally sensitive people do. Each one of us has had the experience of, and participated in, willfulness. Any time we have refused to accept the reality of a situation, that is willfulness. The way to target willfulness when it shows up is to notice that it is there, then label it as willfulness. Accept that it has shown up, and then turn your mind to willingness.

TIP

Many people find that even though they want to turn their mind, they have a hard time doing so. One trick is to use a willing body posture. For example, rather than clenching your fists, you could sit and open your hands and then place them palm-up on your lap. You are telling your mind that you're willing, even when your mind isn't.

If that doesn't work, the next idea is to ask yourself, "What's the threat? What am I fearing? Why am I unwilling to do what I have to do?" Usually willfulness that won't budge is related to a threat and a perception that being willing is dangerous, and that perhaps we will lose something. If there is, in fact, a dangerous threat, then it's understandable that you might be willful, and in that situation, addressing the threat may be the task. Willingness is opposite-action to willfulness, in that being willing, you're acting opposite to the fear of the threat.

A quick TIPP

One of the complaints that some people have when trying to deal with distress is that many of the DBT skills don't work as quickly as some of the more self-destructive behaviors — and they are absolutely correct. Sadly, the reason some of the more self-destructive behaviors persist is that they work so quickly.

TIP

The TIPP skill is DBT's way of using the body's physiological response and, by rapidly changing its chemistry, of changing thoughts by changing the focus of attention. When a new patient, who might be in frequent crisis, enters DBT treatment and they are in extreme emotional pain, the TIPP skill is one of the best for reducing the intensity very quickly. Here is how it works:

>> **Temperature:** Fill a large cooking bowl with cold water. Add ice cubes to the water to make it even colder. Take a deep breath and put your face in the bowl of water, and hold it there for 30 seconds. If you need to, repeat two or three more times. This will almost always rapidly lower the intensity of your emotions.

>> **Intense exercise:** Do some exercise that will get you gasping for air. Sprint around a track until you can no longer sprint; do a plank until you can no longer hold it; lift weights until you can no longer lift them. Do this as fast as you can.

>> **Paced breathing:** Slow your breathing down. Take a slow breath in through your nose to the count of four or five seconds, and then breathe out even more slowly, through pursed lips, to the count of seven or eight. If you want, as you breathe in, say, "I breathe in to be calm," and then as you breathe out, say, "I breathe out to stay calm." Do this type of breathing for about two minutes.

>> **Paired muscle relaxation:** The most effective way to do this is with paced breathing, and then while breathing in, tensing all the muscles in your body. Notice how that feels. Then hold your breath for a few seconds, and as you breathe out, release all the tension in your muscles; notice how that feels. If you want, you can make this a progressive muscle relaxation by choosing different muscle sets — for instance, pairing the breathing with tensing the arms, the legs, or the abdomen.

Alternative rebellion

The skill of alternative rebellion was developed when Dr. Linehan recognized that one of the big draws of certain behaviors is that doing risky things generates excitement. Engaging in drug use, engaging in potentially dangerous sexual encounters, and driving way too fast often lead people to feel a thrill, which, though temporary, can be enough to make them feel alive. Although for many people, the reason or function for such behavior is not to get a rush, it is for some, and being a rebel who defies rules and stereotypes can be addictive.

For these people, the skill of alternate rebellion is the intentional focus on finding an alternative way to rebel, yet one that involves less risk than the original behavior. For instance, you might decide to get a tattoo, to color your hair differently, to wear casual clothes to an important interview, to get a piercing, to illustrate graffiti love-messages in impermanent paint. The exact form that alternate rebellion takes depends on the behavior that the person is trying to replace. The basic idea is that if some behavior is the manifestation of the need to be a rebel and stick it to society, then there are less self-harmful ways to be the rebel. For instance, say that you have to wear a tie to work. You hate wearing ties, and your boss is threatening to fire you because you refuse to wear a tie. You could decide to wear an outrageous tie to work, or one with a political message. In this way, you're keeping to the intent of the policy and yet rebelling within your nature.

Chapter **12**

Increasing Your Interpersonal Effectiveness

The last of the four modules of standard DBT is the interpersonal effectiveness module. It isn't uncommon for people who struggle to regulate their emotions to also have some difficulties with relationships. For some, it may be hard to develop relationships, and for others, it may be challenging to keep important relationships. In the interpersonal effectiveness module, you learn three DBT skills that will help you in your relationships: the DEAR MAN skill to help you ask for what you want, the GIVE skill to help you take care of your relationships, and the FAST skill to help you say no in a way that maintains your self-respect and respects the other person. (Check out Chapters 9, 10, and 11 for more information on the first three modules of standard DBT.)

Before You Begin: Being Aware of Obstacles

REMEMBER

Even if you don't struggle with emotions, relationships are hard. Many things can get in the way of you being effective at any given time. Because relationships are complicated and you bring your own vulnerabilities to each interaction, as does the other person, it's helpful to keep in mind what kinds of obstacles can show up. Dr. Marsha Linehan, the creator of DBT, came up with a list of the things that get in the way of being interpersonally effective. Note that these factors get in the way for everyone. Keeping them in mind can help you when you look back and wonder what went wrong or, on the flip side, what went right!

» **You don't have the skills you need.** Keep in mind that DBT is a skills deficit model. Many people who come to DBT are missing skills in very specific areas. Often, difficulty with regulating emotions can lead to difficulties in relationships for which you need specific types of skills to practice. DBT teaches these skills.

» **You don't know what you want.** It's hard to be effective when you don't know what you want. This can make it look like you're saying no to everything that is suggested — not because the solutions aren't reasonable, but because you aren't clear about your goal or the desired outcome. This situation is common when you're in emotion mind, when problem-solving is hard due to being driven so strongly by how you feel in the moment (see Chapter 3 for details). These types of interactions leave the other person feeling ineffective and frustrated, and you feeling invalidated and not helped.

» **Your emotions are getting in the way.** Emotions are one of the biggest, most common culprits for interpersonal ineffectiveness. We have all had those moments when we think, "I can't believe I said or did that." You did it because you were driven by how you felt and didn't stop to think. These are times when you damage your relationships and afterwards need to pick up the pieces, take responsibility for your emotions getting in the way, and apologize. In addition, we often hear that people we work with have been told by friends and loved ones that they are "too much." This is the toll that intense, unregulated emotions can take on relationships.

» **You forget or sacrifice your long-term goals for your short-term goals.** When you're overcome by strong emotion, it's easy to lose sight of your long-term goals and instead prioritize what you want to do in the moment. For example, when you're having a difficult time, you may cancel plans with your friends or simply not show up because you feel better staying at home, or going out feels overwhelming. However, in time, you may feel left out and your friends may feel you're unreliable and stop inviting you. You prioritized your short-term goal of avoiding an anxiety-provoking situation that may be difficult to manage due to how you're feeling right now over your long-term goal of maintaining important relationships.

>> **Other people are getting in your way.** There are times when you may start out being effective and then come across people who are more powerful than you are. This may be a boss, a teacher, a coach, a supervisor, a police officer, or someone else. There are times when you may start out being effective, but when you realize their power is getting in the way of what you had hoped for, you become ineffective.

>> **Your thoughts and beliefs are getting in the way.** Your thoughts have a significant impact on your behavior, and some thoughts get in the way of your relationships. For example, thoughts about deserving or not deserving things, believing you know how people feel and insisting you are right, or self-loathing thoughts — in which you are convinced and maybe even convince others that you are a terrible person — can really get in the way of your relationships. Over time, the behaviors that stem from these types of thoughts can make it hard to keep relationships.

REMEMBER

Think about this list and how it applies to you. Being aware of these barriers is the first step in doing things differently. Doing them differently will help you create and maintain the meaningful relationships that you want. Be sure to use this list as a tool and something to be mindful of, not something to beat yourself up about!

Mastering the DEAR MAN Skill

The DEAR MAN skill is used for effectively asking for what you want, or what we call *objective effectiveness.* It stands for Describe, Express, Assert, Reinforce, Mindful, Appear confident, and Negotiate.

Think about how many things you ask for, both large and small, in your relationships. If you notice that you're avoiding asking, this skill is also for you. You need to know how to feel confident asking for what you need. Now, you'll find some things easy to ask for, while other things may be much harder. This may have to do with not just what you're asking for but who you're asking. We frequently hear from loved ones that *what* the person is asking for is generally reasonable; however, *how* they ask for it is problematic and gets in the way of their request being granted. Emotion mind can turn your request from effective into demanding or threatening or, on the flip side, indirect with the expectation that the other people can read your mind. If you think about the barriers we just reviewed in the preceding section, almost all of them can get in the way of effectively asking for what you want. The following sections help you see the DEAR MAN skill in action.

You may notice that this acronym is rather long. There is a reason for this. When you're first learning and practicing this skill, you use this acronym as a script or guide. We ask that you write down the DEAR MAN acronym before you use this skill to ask for something. The act of writing it down first will help you not only organize your request but also slow you down. Slowing down will help you clarify exactly what you're asking for as well as how you want to ask. The length of the DEAR MAN is a wonderful barrier to emotion-minded asking as well as a way to keep you focused on what you want. As you practice DEAR MAN and become more skillful, you won't need to use the script. Ideally, like most things, with practice this too will become muscle memory as a way to ask for something.

At first glance, the DEAR MAN may seem a bit overwhelming. Take it one step at a time. Note that sometimes even the most effective DEAR MAN will result in a no. Just because you take a DEAR MAN approach doesn't mean that you're guaranteed to get what you ask for; however, if you hear no to your request, you can know that you asked in an effective way, stayed regulated, didn't damage your relationship with the other person, and walked away with your self-respect intact.

Describe

You begin applying the DEAR MAN skill by describing the facts of the situation. This may be a different way to start, as many people lead with how they feel. The DEAR MAN begins with the shared facts of the situation. You want to think about a few facts that you and the other person agree with. This has proven to be an effective way to bring the other person to the proverbial table and decrease the chance of initial defensiveness or arguing about the situation. You don't need too many facts, just a few of the most relevant ones.

For example, you can describe your situation like this:

Describe: It will be Andy's birthday in four weeks, and he has invited me and four of his friends to go skiing for a long weekend to celebrate. I have not seen Andy in six months. As you know, we have known each other since we were five.

Express

After you describe the facts of the situation, you express how you feel. Remember to stick with how you feel and be mindful not to tell others how they may feel. Again, don't get too lost in your feelings about the situation. Be clear and concise, as in the following example:

Express: I am really looking forward to seeing Andy and being with my guy friends. I will be really sad to miss out on celebrating with him as he has been so supportive this past year and always makes a big deal of my birthday.

Assert

TIP

The assert section of the DEAR MAN is where you ask your question. To have an effective DEAR MAN, you need to be very clear on what you're asking for. The most effective assert is a yes or no question. This way, the other person knows what you're asking for and in some ways is forced to answer you. Less direct or wishy-washy requests can lead to wishy-washy or unclear answers. Remember, your goal is to get a clear answer, and the best way to do that is with a clear and direct question, like the following:

> **A**ssert: Can I have your support to go away for the long weekend?

Reinforce

The reinforce is one of the most important parts of the DEAR MAN and definitely something that slows down the process and increases the effectiveness of your request. In simple terms, the reinforce focuses on what is in it for the other person to say yes to your request. This means you need to think about your goal but also to think about the other person and what is important to them. Why should they say yes to you?

You may know that a reinforce is something that makes a behavior continue (see Chapter 13 for details). A reinforce can be something that you gain or that removes something that is aversive to provide relief. For younger kids, reinforces are often tangible items; however, as we get older, the reinforces get more complicated and abstract, and include things like trust, freedom, friendship, and independence.

WARNING

A common and easy mistake is to say something like "If you say yes, it will make me happy." While that may be important to the other person, it's a weak reinforce because it really is more about you than the other person.

Consider the following example of reinforcing:

> **R**einforce: I know that me going away is hard for you and that this would be a wonderful opportunity to continue to build trust in our relationship, which is so important to both of us.

Mindful

The step of being mindful begins what we fondly call the style points of the DEAR MAN. When you're asking someone for something, it's easy to get off track. You may get distracted, or the other person may intentionally or unintentionally lead you off course, avoiding your question. While doing your DEAR MAN, it's important to stay one-mindful (see Chapter 9 for more details) and focused. When you're starting, your script will help you do this.

TIP

Don't get distracted by another topic or by talking about the past or the future. If you find yourself heading off course and straying from the question, gently return to your request. In DBT we call this *using broken record*. It isn't nagging, just repeating your request. It's okay if you get distracted, but use your mindfulness skills to catch that you are off course and get back to your question.

Here's an example of being mindful during your request in response to your partner:

> **M**indful: I hear that in the past and in other relationships, this has been very hard for you, and at the same time, I am asking about this birthday weekend and focused on our relationship and our relationship goals.

Appear confident

TIP

How you deliver your DEAR MAN makes a big difference. If directly asking for something is a new skill for you or you are anxious, you need to focus on appearing confident. Appearing confident when you don't feel confident can actually make you feel more confident. When you're working on asking in a confident way, you want to think about things like your posture, sitting up straight with your shoulders back, making eye contact, speaking up and not whispering, and using a confident tone of voice. All of these things will help strengthen your DEAR MAN.

Negotiate

The final part of your DEAR MAN is to negotiate. We often hear that a loved one can't tolerate hearing no, and when they do, they get very dysregulated and often leave the conversation in a problematic way. Negotiating allows you to cope ahead of hearing no before you enter the conversation. You can imagine what it would feel like to hear no to your request, and then think about what skills you'll use to stay regulated as well as a way to negotiate by coming up with a second request. Many times, we may initially hear no, but there are other options if we can stay in the conversation and think them through.

TIP

For every DEAR MAN, you should have at least one negotiate. The best case is that you won't need to use it, and in other cases you will need to, and it will help you stay in the conversation and not leave in a way that harms your self-respect or the relationship.

Here's an example of the negotiate step:

Negotiate: I hear that you don't support the trip yet, as three nights feels like too much. Since we have a month until the trip, can we try me going away with one friend for one night as a way to practice and get more comfortable?

Practicing the Art of Validation

On the surface, validation doesn't seem too hard, and it seems like a good practice to do with people you care about. Finding the wisdom or what makes sense in how another person feels, and letting them know, feels good. For some, the art of validation is easier to practice; for others, it's much harder to do. This often has to do with your own level of sensitivity and how much validation you received as a child. This also has to do with your state of mind: When your emotions are strong, or you are in emotion mind, it can be very hard to validate another person. One reason is that when you feel strongly about something, you tend to be more focused on your thoughts and feelings than those of another. While validation is important for us all, it's critical for people who are emotionally sensitive.

WARNING

As you find out in Chapter 2, most people who come to DBT have experienced many invalidating environments. In short, they have experienced parents, siblings, teachers, coaches, bosses, and peers who haven't recognized their emotional sensitivity, but instead did the exact opposite. It's important to remember that most invalidation is well-meaning, and we all get invalidated. For example, in an effort to help someone feel better, you might tell them to "let it go," or remind them "it wasn't that bad" or to "not make such a big deal of it." These short phrases, while often intended to help, are very invalidating. If you're an emotionally sensitive person, you often don't have the skills to "let it go" and instead hear a message that something is wrong with how you feel or that no one understands your pain or upset. Chronic invalidation is one of the experiences that lead to the symptoms that bring people to DBT and the deficits-regulating emotions.

Validation from others helps heal the wounds of past invalidation, and it can also help teach what makes sense about how you feel when understanding your emotions is challenging. Validation is critical for maintaining relationships, and you may have come to DBT because relationships are challenging for you. We also stress the skill of validation to loved ones of people with borderline personality disorder (BPD) because being validated by people you love helps teach self-validation, which in many ways is our ultimate goal. Being able to validate yourself helps you more skillfully navigate the invalidation of the world around you.

In the following sections, you get the scoop on different validation methods, validating when you disagree with someone, and the effect of problem-solving on validation.

REMEMBER

If validation is new to you and you aren't used to doing it, this will be a practice. Like all of our skills, the only way to get better at validation is to practice, and to be aware that you'll get it wrong. Sometimes it can feel rote or "canned"; you may even find that you get accused of trying to be a therapist or that you're speaking weirdly. Stay with it; in time you'll find your voice as you practice this concept with people in your life. You may also find that you're skilled at validation when you're regulated, but that when you are more emotional or with certain people in your life, it's harder for you to use this skill. If that is the case, practice with those people!

Discovering different validation methods

One of the most common questions we get is "So, what do I say?" Because we want you to find your own language, we can't provide a script. Instead, we want to share some different ways you can validate, and then you can apply these concepts when you use your GIVE skill, which we break down later in this chapter.

REMEMBER

Validation is not telling someone how they feel, but is tentatively seeing whether you understand their experience. We are all our own experts in how we feel. If we validate someone and that person says we are wrong or don't understand, even if we think we do, then we acknowledge that we must have missed something and try again. Some useful clues will help you know whether your validation has landed or whether you've missed the mark:

>> When people feel validated, one indicator is that the emotional intensity and speed of the interaction slows down. A second indicator is that they begin to share more about how they are feeling or what is going on that is making them feel a certain way.

>> When your validation misses the mark, the person will typically let you know in one of two ways: They will tell you, sometimes loudly, that you don't understand, or they will shut down, withdraw, and disengage. Paying attention to how the other person responds will be very helpful.

REMEMBER

Dr. Linehan offers six levels or ways to validate. These are not hierarchical, just different things you can do to practice validation:

>> **Pay attention.** Giving someone your full attention (putting your phone down, turning off the TV, and so on), making eye contact, nodding as they speak, and

asking clarifying (not interrogating) questions is one way to validate. By doing this, you're letting the other person know that you're interested in their experience.

>> **Reflect back.** When you're reflecting back, you're letting the other person know that you're following what they are saying, and you want to make sure that you understand or have it right in your mind. For some, this takes a little practice because you want to stay away from just saying "you are angry" if they are yelling, and it's very obvious. Instead of validating, that can feel patronizing. That being said, to say "you seem really sad" may work just fine. You want to let the other person know that you're listening, and then reflect the emotion that you think they are feeling back to them.

>> **Read minds.** This type of validation is what we call "high risk, high reward." When this lands, it feels great, and when it misses, you need to have a gentle apology in your back pocket. Reading minds is letting the other person know that you see how they feel without them telling you. You do this by paying attention to non-verbal clues. For example, when your roommate walks in looking down, drops her bag on the floor, and doesn't say anything, you could respond by saying something like "Tough day?" It can be wonderful to know that someone can sense how you feel without having to tell them. Now, if you get it wrong, you can acknowledge that and then ask a few questions to get a better understanding of what is going on.

>> **Understand.** Understanding is seeing how the other person's feelings or position make sense, given their own history or who they are. This can be a very useful type of validation to help make sense of an experience for yourself or someone else. For example: "It makes sense that you are anxious about dating, because you have had some really bad experiences in the past."

WARNING

One important note about this type of validation and the word *understanding* is that, in general, we suggest using the phrase "I understand" sparingly. Unless you're an emotionally sensitive person and have had the exact same experience, you really can't truly understand someone else's experience. Pay attention when you use that phrase; it works fine for some but is very problematic for others. When it's problematic, your well-meaning validation gets completely lost.

>> **Acknowledge the valid.** This is also a very helpful type of validation when the other person is having a hard time understanding their emotions. By acknowledging the valid, you're letting the person know that their experience is typical and shared by other people, and that you might feel the same way if it happened to you. For example: "It makes sense that you are anxious before your first job interview, because job interviews are stressful, especially your first one." While it isn't saying that everyone feels that way, it is letting the person know that their emotions and the situation are common and shared with other people.

>> **Show equality/radical genuineness.** This final example of validation relies much less on using words. Be yourself and very authentically recognize another's experience. This could look like recognizing someone's sadness and handing them a box of tissues, tearing up with them when they are sad, or joining them in their excitement. Be mindful that you aren't in any way hijacking their experience, but using your own to recognize what makes sense about how they are feeling.

Validating when you disagree

One of the hardest practices of validation is when you disagree with what is being said. The key to staying skillful in times like this is to remember that validation is about feelings and not about facts. Your task is to notice and regulate your own emotions and then think more about the other person's feelings and less about what you disagree with. When you think about it that way, it may be easier. That is, you can strongly disagree with their position and you can also recognize how they as an individual could feel so strongly about this.

For example, you could say, "I can see that if you felt like I excluded you, that you would feel hurt and angry." If you look closely there, you see dialectical thinking at work. You must hold your position of feeling like you didn't exclude them and their perspective that they felt excluded. Being able to validate someone when you disagree with them is a powerful relationship tool! It's easy to get polarized in disagreements, and validation is one of the tools that will help you tolerate disagreement without damaging a relationship.

Problem-solving and validation

Problem-solving and validation are an interesting combination when it comes to emotional sensitivity. For many people, problem-solving is validating: You recognize my problem and you solve it. However, for emotionally sensitive people, it doesn't work that way. Problem-solving before validation is one of the biggest traps for loved ones of people who come to DBT. For them, validation often needs to come before problem-solving. We've been told many times that when people immediately offer problem-solving, it feels as if they are telling them how easy their problem is to fix, leaving their pain completely misunderstood. Obviously, this isn't the intention, but it is the effect.

TIP

If you're a skilled problem solver, you'll find this a challenge as you rewire your brain to offer validation first. In fact, we often ask people to take it a step further and ask loved ones to validate and then ask whether the person would like some of their ideas, thoughts, opinions, or solutions. Many times, the sensitive person can solve the problem on their own once they get reregulated, and receiving validation can help that process.

Communicating with GIVE Skills

REMEMBER

Another interpersonal effectiveness tool is the GIVE skill, which is your relationship effectiveness skill. The main skill in this acronym is validation, which we cover in the previous section. Using your GIVE skill — Gentle, Interested, Validate, and Easy manner — lets the other person know that their feelings matter and that given who they are, they make sense. You can think of the GIVE skill as the skill that helps you take care of your relationships:

>> **Gentle:** This skill requires gentleness, which may sound easier than it often is. You want to do your best to refrain from attacks or threats. Be kind, caring, and curious about how the other person may be feeling. Stay away from being judgmental or black and white. Make good eye contact and have a relaxed body posture.

>> **Interested:** Show interest in the other person and what is going on for them. Ask open-ended questions. Open your mind to learning about them or what is important to them. Listen to their point of view and be prepared to see the value in what they are saying, even if you disagree. Don't interrupt; play the part of the listener.

>> **Validate:** Keep in mind that you can validate with words or by actions. Recognize how they are feeling and check in to see whether you're correct. Look at the situation from their perspective. We cover validation in more detail earlier in this chapter.

>> **Easy manner:** Smile, be a bit lighthearted, and avoid bringing intensity to the exchange. If humor makes sense and isn't invalidating, use some light humor. Be dialectical; see multiple sides or perspectives to the interaction.

TIP

You can think of the GIVE skill as adding some style or delivery pointers to your practice of validation. You'll find that sometimes you'll stick to validation while other times you'll combine your GIVE skill with one of the other interpersonal effectiveness skills. You can see how much more effective your DEAR MAN can be if you add a little GIVE, especially if you have to negotiate or ask someone for something that you know is going to be very difficult for them to do.

Staying True to Yourself with the FAST Skill

The final interpersonal effectiveness skill is the FAST skill: Fair, (no) Apologies, Stick to your values, and Truthful. This is recognized as the skill that helps you maintain your self-respect. We like to think of this skill as helping you walk away from any interaction feeling a sense of pride and integrity in the way you behaved, and feeling that you've upheld your values about how to treat another and how to make your opinion or position effectively known. This is the skill for effectively saying no or setting a personal limit.

WARNING

Some people struggle with self-respect more than others. Some struggle to assert themselves and their needs, while others may rely on threats or being overly aggressive when they assert themselves. You may find that your effectiveness with FAST skills is mood dependent or relationship dependent. In some relationships and when you're regulated, you're effective; however, when you are dysregulated or in specific relationships, you have a much harder time effectively setting a limit, saying no, or standing up for yourself. The FAST skill will help you master the skill of self-respect effectiveness.

REMEMBER

Here are the components of the FAST skill:

>> **Fair:** You must start out being fair. Step back and look at the situation, your position, and that of the other person. Move into a wise mind — the balanced place where you can keep in mind how you feel and what you know about the situation (see Chapter 3) — so that you can be fair to yourself as well as the other person. See the entire situation and multiple perspectives.

>> **(No) Apologies:** Keep in mind that apologies are called for when you've done something that crosses your values and that has been harmful to someone else. When you've done that, you apologize one time and make a commitment to do something different next time. Over-apologizing degrades your self-respect. Don't apologize for asking for something, for saying no to someone, or for being alive. Don't look ashamed or like you've done something wrong; instead, assert yourself. Apologize only when an apology is called for!

>> **Stick to your values:** Don't sell short what is important to you. Pay attention to your values and morals and stand by them. Sometimes this means you need to slow down before the interaction and identify what is important to you.

>> **Truthful:** Don't hide behind generalities or other people. Stay away from phrases like "everyone is doing this" and "it is what is appropriate." Your limit is your own, so make sure you take full credit for it. Don't make up excuses, exaggerate, or undersell your point.

Combining GIVE and FAST

We've found that the most effective way to use the FAST skill is to combine it with the GIVE skill. Most people would agree that you hear limits or no to something best when it feels like the other person has taken the time to think about how you'll feel. The GIVE skill (Gentle, Interested, Validate, Easy manner) is the perfect place to start.

Here are some examples of what we like to call the GIVE FAST combo. You use your GIVE skill, then the word "and" or "at the same time," and then your FAST skill — Fair, (no) Apologies, Stick to your values, Truthful:

> *I see that you are really worried about missing the party this weekend with your friends and that you came home two hours past curfew, so our agreement is that you stay in next weekend.*

> *I hear that you are very angry, and at the same time I am going to end the phone call if you continue yelling at me and calling me names.*

> *I know you really want to go out with your friends tonight and you made plans to spend the evening with me.*

REMEMBER

You'll notice in the examples that you begin with your GIVE skill and validation followed by the FAST skill. You place "and" or "at the same time" between them to create a dialectical balance. While they may seem to be opposing positions, they are given equal value. This is an example of dialectical thinking (which we introduce in Chapter 2).

Putting It All Together

Interpersonal effectiveness skills are some of the hardest DBT skills to put into practice. There are many variables in every interpersonal interaction: your emotions, the other person's emotions, your goals and their goals, and both of your skill levels.

Each of the skills addresses a different priority in a given interaction. The three priorities map to the three skills: objective (DEAR MAN), relationship (GIVE), and self-respect (FAST). In any given interaction, you're prioritizing one of these three skills. Many times, this prioritizing happens without your awareness. For example, sometimes the most important thing is to get what you want, while at other times, you may negotiate because it's more important that you support the relationship and come to a mutual agreement; at other times, the highest priority is asserting yourself and making yourself effectively heard, even if you don't get what you want. Thinking about your goal in the interaction will help you decide what skill you need to use.

REMEMBER

The best way to get more interpersonally effective is to practice. Initially you may require scripts for your DEAR MAN and practice sessions in front of a mirror; sometimes you'll have great success, while other attempts will be less successful. Keep practicing, as these skills will help you have better relationships and feel better about how you interact with people. You'll also feel more effective at getting your needs met and sharing how you feel.

Chapter **13**

Walking the Middle Path

When DBT was developed, Dr. Marsha Linehan originally had the treatment of adults in mind. As the versatility of the therapy became evident, it started to be applied to adolescents and their families. From this, adolescent specialists Drs. Alec Miller and Jill Rathus developed the Walking the Middle Path skill. This DBT skill was developed with teens and their parents in mind and helps bridge communication between them.

Walking the Middle Path means replacing an "either-or" stance with a more engaged and collaborative "both-and" stance. This comes from the observation that many people often make decisions using a black-and-white, all-or-nothing formula. Core to the practice of this skill is the family and their child understanding the concepts of validation, behaviorism, and dialectics. This chapter gives you an overview of Middle Path skills.

Finding the Balance

To maintain psychological balance, you need to consider various aspects of your nature and your goals. For instance, you need to balance what your emotions tell you with what your reason and logic tell you, what you want with what you need, and what another person is asking for with what you're asking for. In DBT three elements, or components, encompass and define how balance is considered and found: validation, behaviorism, and dialectics.

Validation

Validation is the practice of communicating to another person that their feelings, thoughts, and actions make sense and are understandable given the person's experiences and biological and genetic makeup. Validation is an essential part of communicating acceptance in your important relationships. It recognizes that another person's behaviors are caused, and that their emotional challenges and emotion regulation deficits make it difficult or even impossible to behave more effectively in certain circumstances.

REMEMBER

There are some essential features to validation:

>> It communicates to another person that their responses, which include feelings, thoughts, and actions, make sense and are understandable to you in a particular situation.

>> There is an acknowledgment, through non-judgmental observation, of a person's reality — for instance, a statement as seemingly obvious as "I can see how sad you are from what just happened."

>> There is an acceptance: "I know you are upset." (That's it — you don't need to say anything else.)

A close concept is that of *self-validation.* For many people who have had early experiences being told that they are weak for having certain emotions or that they shouldn't be feeling the way that they are feeling, this leads to the person believing that they shouldn't be feeling the way they actually are. However, because they do feel that way, they can end up experiencing enduring shame and self-hatred.

REMEMBER

Using the Middle Path skills teaches parents to validate their children, children to validate their parents, and then parents and children to validate themselves.

Behaviorism

DBT Middle Path skills teach effective ways to change behaviors, whether you're trying to increase positive/wanted behaviors or decrease negative/unwanted behaviors.

REMEMBER

The first task is for a person or loved one to ask what specifically is a behavior that they want to see changed. The more specific this is, the better. For instance, saying, "I want my child to be successful in life" is a valid desire; however, it doesn't say much about what that means exactly or what steps are necessary for that to happen. On the other hand, saying, "I want my child to do their homework every night" is a more clearly defined request.

DBT uses the following principles from behavioral science to focus on change. The most important concepts are those of reinforcement (primarily) and punishment (as a last resort) to target behavior change.

Reinforcement

Reinforcers are consequences (which are experiences including actions, feelings, and thoughts) that result in an *increase* in a behavior in a particular situation. There are two types of reinforcers:

>> **Positive reinforcers** are the *addition* of consequences that a person wants that lead to an increase in behavior. If praising someone for doing their homework increases homework activity, then praise is a positive reinforcer. However, if a person doesn't care about praise, then it's unlikely that praising the person will increase their homework-doing behavior. It's important to know that what is reinforcing is in the experience of the recipient and not the deliverer. One child or person may find praise to be reinforcing, and another may not. In some cases, the child may find the praise to be punishing (see the next section).

>> **Negative reinforcers** are the *subtraction* or *removal* of a consequence that is aversive to a person in order to get the increase in desired behavior. So, for instance, when you get in your car and hear the annoying seat belt noise and you put on your seat belt, you have been negatively reinforced because the annoying noise has been removed. Negative reinforcement provides relief. Another example is that when you take an aspirin to make your headache go away, if the headache goes away, then you're more likely to take aspirin in the future, and so taking aspirin has been negatively reinforced because the headache was removed.

Another behavior principle is that of *extinction*, which is defined in behaviorism as the reduction in the likelihood of a behavior because reinforcement is no longer given. So, if a child gets candy every time he goes to the store and cries, he has learned to cry because crying has been reinforced. If the parent then puts the behavior on extinction by not rewarding the behavior of crying, then the crying behavior will eventually be extinguished. However, because the child has historically been rewarded for crying, in the first stages of extinction there is likely to be an increase in the crying behavior before it's extinguished. This is classic in behaviorism and is known as a *behavioral burst*.

WARNING

If the parent gives in after having decided to extinguish the behavior and gives the child a candy, they will have a much harder task on their hands to extinguish the behavior in the future, because the child has now learned that all they need to do is to cry harder and that eventually the parent will give in. Most behavior is habitual, so even though the child has been shaped, through reinforcement, to behave in the way they have, in most cases, the child isn't aware that this has happened and doesn't do the behavior with the intention to manipulate but rather simply because their behavior worked in the past.

Another major behaviorism concept is that of *shaping.* This refers to the reinforcement of small steps taken in the desired behavior. So, if an adolescent historically broke his curfew by three hours and was now trying very hard to be on time, the parent might give a partial recognition or reward if the child is only 20 minutes late, as that is heading in the direction of being on time for the curfew and is much better than being three hours late.

Punishment

Punishment, in comparison to reinforcement, applies consequences to an undesired behavior that lead to a *reduction* or *decrease* in the behavior. In DBT, we consider two types of punishment:

WARNING

>> **Effective punishment:** For example, in parenting, punishment can include actions used to decrease behaviors that don't have natural consequences. Examples include losing the car for a week for coming home after curfew, or the loss of dessert or a favorite TV show for having hit a younger sibling. There are, however, punishments that do have natural consequences; for instance, if a person truly cares about her grades, failing a test after not studying would be a natural consequence.

>> **Ineffective punishment:** These are punitive actions used to decrease behaviors that are neither specific, nor time limited, nor appropriate for the unwanted behavior. However, they are consequences that are unlikely to have a long-term benefit or lead to behavioral change because the punishment is so out of proportion to the behavior that instead of teaching anything, it often leads to resentment toward the person applying the punishment. So, if after an adolescent broke his curfew, his parents grounded him for three months and then took every opportunity to point out how irresponsible the child was, this would be an example of ineffective punishment. Ineffective punishment doesn't teach people that what they did was wrong or what they need to do differently next time, and instead leaves people feeling angry and bitter.

Dialectics

REMEMBER

As we explain in Chapter 2, the word *dialectical* describes the notion that two opposing ideas can be true at the same time. In DBT, there is always more than one way to think about a situation, and all people have something unique and different to offer. A life worth living has both positive and negative aspects (happiness, sadness, anger), and all of these aspects are necessary and valuable. It's sometimes hard to accept ourselves and our actions while simultaneously recognizing the need for change. Dialectics allows for a balance between acceptance and change, both of which are necessary for establishing a fulfilling life.

For parents of sensitive children, using the Walking the Middle Path skill is important for effective parenting. This is because parents face what the developers of the skill termed the *dialectical dilemmas* of parenting. DBT focuses on three polarities:

» **Too strict or too loose:** When it comes to household expectations and life rules, parents need to recognize whether their parenting style is too strict with their children on the one hand or too loose on the other. Strong emotions can lead a parent to swing from one pole of the dilemma to the other, and this will cause confusing and challenging parenting. DBT teaches parents that they should have clear rules that should be enforced consistently, while at the same time, parents should be willing to negotiate on certain issues as circumstances change — for instance, if the child starts to consistently follow rules, or become more defiant, or develop a new group of friends, or stick to a commitment to not use a substance — and learn not to overuse consequences.

» **Making light of problem behaviors or too much of typical childhood behaviors:** Another place that parents seek to find balance is by ensuring that they aren't dismissing problematic behavior by saying things like "Oh, that's just normal teen behavior," but on the other hand that they aren't making too much of typical childhood behaviors. For parents, it's important to recognize when their child's behavior crosses the line into behavior that is concerning, and then to ensure that the child gets help, while at the same time knowing which behaviors are typical and developmentally appropriate.

» **Fostering dependence and forcing independence:** Finally, parents want to guard against fostering dependence, meaning that the parent consciously or unconsciously encourages their child to rely on them for all their needs. The problem then is that the child doesn't learn to deal with many of life's challenges. On the other hand, parents want to be careful not to force independence by insisting that their child start to take care of life's responsibilities before they are ready to do so.

Embracing Cooperation and Compromise

Cooperation is consistent with dialectical synthesis in that it strengthens the underlying nature of a relationship through balanced interchange and integration of each person's point of view. But compromise, within the context of relationships, is a double-edged sword that poses a dialectical opportunity. On the one hand, it can mean that each person in the negotiation gets some of what they want, which can be a good thing. On the other hand, inherent in the definition is that it implies that at least one person, and likely both people, in the transaction are giving something up, and in these situations compromise can leave both feeling bitter. Nevertheless, both compromise and cooperation have their place in relationship building.

There's more than one point of view to each situation

There's more than one perspective to look at in a situation, as we explain in Chapter 3. From a purely physical point of view, for example, an elephant looks different if it's being seen from behind, from the front, or from the side. It becomes more complicated when emotional and cognitive perspectives are added. If a person has been bitten by a dog and they see that same dog, that person's experience will be different from that of a person who hasn't been bitten by the dog.

Continuing along this line of thinking, two things that seem like opposites can both be true. From a DBT perspective, this comes into play around the behavior of self-injury. For instance, from the perspective of a parent seeing their child self-injure, they understandably consider this behavior to be a problem. From the point of view of the child engaging in self-injury, the behavior is a solution. For the child, the problem is an inability to deal with emotional intensity in a different way, and so self-injury is both a problem and a solution at the same time. These opposite perspectives are both true and co-exist.

A corollary to this is the understanding that a person with whom someone has disagreements can still have correct opinions. DBT recognizes that other people's behavior and thoughts make sense from their own point of view given their experiences, perspective, and biology. The DBT way to address different points of view is for a person who comes up against a contradictory position to ask themselves, "What am I missing?" or "What is the kernel of truth in the other person's position?" It encourages people to let go of extreme ways of speaking, and so statements like "You always come home late" or "You never help me" become statements that have words like "sometimes" followed by highlighting the impact that the behavior has on the person making the statement. The idea is to further the conversation by being curious, rather than certain, as to why a person is behaving the way they are behaving, and so rather than the statement "What is wrong with that child?" they consider with genuine curiosity, "I wonder what happened to that child that they are acting in that way."

For the patient and the therapist in DBT, there is a way to practice recognizing multiple points of view. When they are triggered and notice a sudden change in emotion or level of anxiety, or when they notice an urge to do something ineffective, they stop and ask themselves whether they can come up with three or four alternative explanations for what could have happened.

Change is the only constant

Nothing is constant. Everything is in motion all the time. Some of this change is visible in real time, like waves in an ocean; some of it happens at a slightly slower pace, like an ice cube melting in a drink; some of it happens even more slowly, like the human body growing; and some of it even occurs over millions of years, like the formation of mountains and canyons. And yet, throughout all of this change, the molecules and atoms in waves, ice cubes, humans, and mountains are vibrating, and electrons are whizzing and spinning. Nothing stays still even if it feels that way. In psychology, every time things feel like they have become "okay," something happens to make it not so, and similarly, when things aren't going well, things change and life becomes easier.

From a DBT perspective, many patients, their families, and therapists feel as if nothing is ever going to change; however, by recognizing that it cannot be that something is not going to change, they can push on and continue the therapeutic work. Many patients and their families struggle to deal with the unfamiliar, and so accepting change can be particularly difficult, especially when it's uncertain how things will turn out or whether it will require a different way of doing things or maybe even a different way of life. What is key here is that change will happen whether a person wants it to happen or not, and so when a person actively participates in more effective choices, the possibility of a healthier future — one brought on by enduring skills practice — will leave that person with greater control of their own life, rather than feeling that their decisions are solely dependent on outside forces.

TIP

For the patient and the therapist in DBT, a way to practice this is to recall every time in the past that they imagined that things would never change. They can then remember just how many times things have in fact changed, and that in this context, not only have they gotten through those moments of being stuck, but have perhaps even succeeded.

Change is transactional

Everything that happens in the universe impacts something else. At a quantum level, the spin of an electron impacts its twin. At a much larger scale, the moon impacts tides and the light of the sun impacts the growth of plants. What people say to one another impacts each of them. DBT gets people to pay attention to the effect that they have on others and their environment.

Another aspect of this recognition is to focus on letting go of blaming others for things that happen, and rather, to consider how both one's actions and those of other people were caused by a life of learning and the interactions that occurred in the past. And so, because things are caused, rather than getting stuck on blame, a person practicing DBT sees that people do things for reasons that make sense given their historical transactions.

TIP

For the patient and the therapist, one way to practice is to examine some transaction that happened during the day and then to consider the ways in which other people and the environment influenced what happened in that transaction, as well as asking in what ways they themselves may have influenced other people. Another way to think about this is for the therapist and the patient to reflect on whether they would have acted in the same way if the transactions they had with the environment and other people hadn't occurred.

4

The Mechanics of DBT Therapy

Discover the benefits of individual therapy.

Reap the rewards of learning skills in group meetings.

Find out how to ask for help when problems arise outside of the therapy hour, through the use of skills coaching.

Realize that your therapist is also receiving help by connecting, and consulting on difficult clinical matters, with other DBT therapists in a consultation team.

Check out a few more important concepts and skills in DBT: dialectical dilemmas and strategies, structuring your environment, tracking your habits, and gaining (and keeping!) motivation.

Chapter **14**

Exploring Therapy Basics

Understanding the components of DBT is the first step in setting up an effective treatment. A comprehensive DBT treatment has four components: individual DBT therapy, a DBT skills group, phone coaching, and a consultation team for the individual therapist. For adolescent DBT, the skills group is typically attended by both the adolescent and the parents and is referred to as a multi-family skills group. If that is unavailable, adolescents will attend a skills group and parents will receive parent-skills training separately.

In this chapter, we review DBT individual therapy, DBT skills groups, and phone coaching. In Chapter 17, we discuss the DBT consultation team.

REMEMBER

Entering into a DBT treatment is a big commitment. You'll be asked to attend individual therapy once or twice a week, as well as a weekly skills group. Most DBT therapists and group leaders have strict attendance policies that will be reviewed when you begin treatments. This often comes in the form of a contract. Multiple unexcused absences aren't tolerated.

One on One: Individual Therapy

When people are referred to DBT, the first step is to identify an individual therapist. Depending on where you live, this can be a challenge. It seems that while there are DBT therapists around the world, there tend to be cities with high concentrations of DBT therapists, and by contrast, DBT deserts where there are no DBT therapists for hundreds of miles. Part of the reason that you find areas with a higher concentration of DBT therapists is because trained DBT therapists work on teams. You learn more about the consultation team in Chapter 17; however, it's important to know that while you may never meet the members of your therapist's consultation team, they, too, are part of your treatment by supporting your therapist. DBT is a team of therapists treating a group of patients. With the increased use of telehealth, some DBT providers are able to work alone because they meet with their teams over video platforms, but this is more the exception than the norm.

The following sections help you find a therapist, set goals, and get the most from individual sessions.

REMEMBER

DBT is a very specialized treatment that requires extensive training. Only a small percentage of therapists elect to get the training to practice DBT because it's a rigorous therapy that involves working with patients who are frequently at high risk for suicidal behavior. DBT also requires the individual therapist to be on call for skills coaching much of the time. As DBT becomes a more popular treatment and is modified to treat different types of symptoms, our hope is that it will become easier to access. Many people say they are doing DBT, but it's important to know how to differentiate a therapist who says they do DBT from therapists practicing the evidence-based form of DBT that you are looking for. Because DBT has become more popular, you may find many therapists who say they do "DBT light." Generally, this means that they have some training in DBT but offer only some of the required components of the full treatment.

Finding an individual therapist

When you begin your search for a DBT therapist, you want to know whether they offer DBT with all of its components. Around 2014, two different groups began offering a DBT certification, so asking whether the therapist is DBT Certified is one way to answer this question. That being said, certification requires a commitment of time and money, and therefore this process is advancing at a low rate. Many excellent DBT therapists have decided to not go ahead with the certification process.

REMEMBER

You don't need a DBT-Certified therapist, but you do need to do some investigating to find out whether the therapist is sufficiently trained and that they have fidelity to the DBT model. These four questions will be your guide to finding a therapist who practices all of the components of DBT:

» **Do you offer individual DBT?** When you ask this question, you can also ask whether they have been either foundationally or intensively trained by Behavioral Tech. Behavioral Tech is a subsidiary of the Linehan Training Institute (Dr. Marsha Linehan is the founder of DBT; see Chapter 1). This is the gold standard training for DBT. While "intensively trained" may sound better, the only difference is that intensively trained therapists went with their consultation teams to learn how to set up a team, and foundationally trained therapists went on their own, but already had established consultation teams to join.

Behavioral Tech has a list of DBT therapists who have completed their training on their website, which you can find at https://behavioraltech.org/resources/find-a-therapist/. Unfortunately, this list only offers a small number of DBT therapists, but it is a good place to start.

» **Do you offer a DBT skills group or skills training?** The skills group doesn't need to be run by the individual therapist or even be in their practice; however, they need to be able to help you find a group or individual skills trainer that has an opening, either when you begin individual therapy or soon after. (Find out more about group therapy later in this chapter.)

» **Do you offer on-call, after-hours skills coaching and intersession contact?** This is a critical component of DBT that offers patients in-the-moment support to use their skills. (We talk about skills coaching in more detail later in this chapter.) This is one of the components of the treatment that can be the hardest for therapists to commit to, as it means you're on call for your patients after work hours, on weekends, and during holidays.

» **Are you on a consultation team?** The consultation team is the last critical component of this treatment, as it supports your therapist, ensures they are practicing fidelity to the treatment, and helps monitor and address their burnout so that they remain helpful and effective when working with you. (Flip to Chapter 17 for more about consultation teams.)

REMEMBER

The individual therapist must answer "yes" to these four questions. Answering "yes" means that they practice the treatment that is evidenced-based. If the answer to even one question is "no," then you will no longer be receiving a DBT treatment because what has been studied is the treatment that includes all four components.

Setting a reachable goal

Changing behavior is not an easy task and can be quite complicated. Many of the behaviors that bring people to DBT are simply defined by others as problematic, but there is almost always a dialectic that is missed. By dialectic, we mean that many of these behaviors are both problems and solutions. That is, the behaviors have both a problematic consequence and at the same time provide some solutions for difficulties with emotion regulation. For example, staying in bed may make you ultimately lose your job or get poor grades in school; however, in the moment, staying in bed may be helping you manage unbearable anxiety.

REMEMBER

One of the most effective ways to change your behavior is to link the change to some long-term goal. This will help you in the moment when you have to decide to use skills and do something different, or succumb to the familiar but problematic behavior. We frequently see patients who tell us that they want to change a behavior for a girlfriend or boyfriend, a friend, or a parent. This is problematic because our feelings for that person or relationship could change, and with that, your motivation to change. When that happens, all of a sudden, changing that behavior doesn't seem to matter anymore. Change needs to happen for yourself, so slow down when you're thinking about changing behavior, and work with your therapist at the outset to link it to some goal that is important to you.

Getting the most from individual sessions

TIP

As therapies go, DBT is a demanding treatment. Like most things, the amount of work, effort, and commitment you put into your therapy has a big impact on what you get out of it. Here are some ways that you can get the most out of your individual sessions:

» **Make a commitment and show up!** For your treatment to be effective, you have to show up consistently. This may sound obvious, but your individual therapy will be hard work. You'll be faced with painful emotions, problems to sort out, and new skills to use. You'll also be with someone who is committed to help you and walk with you through the process. Many people who come to DBT struggle with mood-dependent behaviors. You need to get to your therapy sessions, no matter what your mood is!

» **Complete your diary card consistently.** During your initial sessions, you and your therapist will create a diary card. This is the DBT system that helps you track your behaviors, urges, emotions, and skill use. You'll be asked to complete your diary card daily, typically at night, reflecting on the day. This is one of the single most important tools for your individual therapy.

» **Bring an agenda.** DBT individual therapy is a very active process. To get the most out of your sessions, bring agenda items. Some agenda items will naturally flow from your diary card. Be sure to make notes in the notes section of your diary card to help you remember what agenda items you want to cover in therapy. Don't leave it all to your therapist to ask you questions; this is your time.

>> **Call for skills coaching.** While skills coaching happens outside of your therapy hour, it's critical for both your skills generalization and in many cases your relationship with your therapist, as you learn to effectively ask for help in situations when you would like to be more skillful. We discuss skills coaching in more depth later in this chapter.

>> **Do your skills group homework.** Completing your weekly skills group homework will help you learn and practice the DBT skills and concepts that you learn about each week. As you learn more skills, you and your individual therapist will work on specific ways that you can integrate them into your life, as well as look at what barriers are arising that make skill use challenging. If your individual therapist has to take too much time teaching and reviewing new skills with you, you'll miss out on the opportunity to get help with specific things going on in your life. (We cover group therapy in the next section.)

All Together: Group Therapy

DBT group therapy is very specific. DBT groups are skills group. The goal of these groups is to teach you skills from the DBT modules. Learning the skills in a group allows you and your individual therapist to work on ways that you can generalize the skills to your goals and your life. Unlike many groups, DBT skills groups don't focus on processing things going on in your life or even having you put topics on the agenda; it's completely focused on teaching you the critical skills of DBT. At the end of each group, you'll be assigned homework from your skills workbook.

The following sections discuss joining a group, sharing strategies in a group, and making the most of your group time.

Joining a group

Once you have found an individual therapist (covered earlier in this chapter), they should be able to guide you toward a group. If you're working with a therapist in a large practice, the practice may offer DBT groups. If that isn't the case, because DBT therapists work on teams, your therapist will refer you to a group in your area.

Most DBT groups require their members to be in treatment with a DBT individual therapist. For that reason, that may be one of the first questions they ask you when you call to join the group. The groups are typically divided by age: adolescent or teen groups, young adult groups, adult groups, and multi-family groups. In areas with only a few DBT therapists, you may find only adult and adolescent groups. Some groups offer admission at any time, while other groups have specific points of entry during skills teaching, such as at the beginning of a skills module.

TIP

DBT skills groups require a significant time commitment; six months to one year is common. Some people will elect to stay in the group longer because they find that repeating the modules helps them consolidate their skills.

Sharing strategies

REMEMBER

Most of the sharing that you'll do in group will be related to your homework review, feedback to group members about their homework, or questions you have about the skills. It's generally understood that while many members are working on self-injurious and suicidal behaviors, the details of self-destructive behavior aren't shared between members during or outside of groups. Many groups will ask members to refer to specific self-destructive behaviors as "target behaviors," but this does vary from group to group.

Many groups also have rules about romantic relationships, asking members to refrain from these types of relationships with one another while in group together. Should a romantic relationship develop, when possible, the members are asked to attend separate groups.

Gaining from the group

TIP

Here are some ways that you can gain the most from your group:

>> **Show up.** While it may seem like you can read your skills manual and learn the skills on your own at home, there are many nuances that are not captured in the book, as well as important contributions by your fellow group members that occur only in the group setting. Your group leader will teach the skills and talk about how and in what context you can use them, as well as what may get in the way.

>> **Do your homework and be prepared to share it.** Completing weekly homework is required for the group, but more importantly, it will help you think about and practice skills in your daily life. Be active in group, give feedback, and answer questions.

>> **Fully participate.** Use your "fully participate" mindfulness skills. Be present in group, and don't multi-task. Make the most out of your time in group.

Time to Connect: Phone Coaching

Phone coaching is one of the most unique parts of DBT. It's the only therapy we know of that uses intersession contact as an integral part of the treatment.

REMEMBER

As you find out in the following sections, you can use skills coaching for four things: asking for help, asking for validation, repairing the relationship, and sharing good news. It's critical to understand that skills coaching isn't a therapy session over the phone. Coaching should last 7 to 12 minutes. When you call your therapist, you need to do your best to be clear about what you're asking for. If you're calling for help, the goal of phone coaching is to help you practice a skill in a moment when you are stuck and need help so that you can learn how to do something different in a difficult situation. The idea is that once you get help in the moment with that situation, the next time you find yourself there, you'll have an idea of what skills to try. If you're trying to change how you manage strong emotions and self-destructive behaviors, it isn't as effective to wait until your next therapy session to ask your therapist for help, as you miss the opportunity to do something different in the moment. In-the-moment coaching is a more effective way to learn and practice new skills.

Before you begin: Setting parameters

There are very specific parameters around coaching, which you'll discuss in detail with your therapist. For example, there is some variation in the hours during which your therapist will be on call; this can range from 24 hours a day, seven days a week, to a schedule that could look like 8 a.m. to 9 p.m. daily. When the hours are more restricted, your therapist will give you instructions for alternative places to access help should you need it.

In addition to talking to your therapist about the hours you can call for coaching, you should also review what is expected. One important question to ask is whether you can text for coaching. Therapists have mixed feelings about this, so it's important to clarify. When we meet with our new patients, we orient them to the hours we are available as well as our expectations. For example, we require that before calling for coaching, our patients try at least one skill on their own. Often these skills come from skills plans that you complete in a session.

We also orient patients that once they call, they are making the commitment, to the best of their ability, to refrain from engaging in a problematic behavior until we return the call. This may be one of the more challenging agreements because we'll likely answer the call or text; however, there will be times when it takes your therapist some time to get back to you. You should have a plan for what you can do while you're waiting for your therapist to call you back. Typically, you'll find distress tolerance crisis survival skills (discussed in Chapter 11) to be helpful while you wait.

When your therapist calls you back, they will ask you to give them a brief explanation of the situation and what you need help with. Your therapist will ask you what skills you've tried and then suggest a series of skills to do. Another agreement we ask for is that you be open to the skills suggestions and not say "no" to everything your therapist suggests. Be open minded even if it's hard. If you think one or more of the skills may not work given where you are or what you have access to, you should actively collaborate with your skills coach to make a plan that you feel will be helpful.

It isn't uncommon for your therapist to ask you what has worked in the past. Sometimes when you get emotionally dysregulated, it's hard to remember which skills work. Hearing your therapist ask can, at times, help you regulate you emotions, feel calmer, think more clearly, and remember which skills have been effective in the past. This is very common and is called *co-regulation*. Once you've agreed to the series of skills, you and your therapist will problem-solve any barriers that could get in the way of following your skills plan, and then you'll end the call. A lot of focused work can happen in a short coaching session.

REMEMBER

Take a moment to get clarity on what you're asking for before you call your therapist. Knowing this information will make your coaching call much more effective. The rest of this chapter discusses the four ways in which you can use coaching: asking for help, asking for validation, repairing the relationship, and sharing good news.

Calling for help

Calling for help is the most common use of skills coaching. As therapists, we recognize that you may have mixed feelings about calling, for a couple of reasons. Some common barriers to calling for coaching are thinking that nothing can help, that you don't deserve help, that you don't know what you need help with, that you aren't skilled at asking for help and don't know how, or that you don't want to bother your therapist and interrupt them outside of work. If you see yourself in any of these barriers, you aren't alone. We would ask you to work with your therapist to use skills and tackle these barriers.

TIP

It can be helpful to begin with practice coaching calls. Calling your therapist after hours when you believe it will interrupt them and trusting that your therapist will answer if they can, and if they are busy that they will call you back, is a great first step. This would be using the emotion regulation skill of opposite action (see Chapter 10). You may be surprised, but worrying about bothering or being "too needy" for your therapist is a very common worry, and one that many people overcome.

Before you call for coaching, take a moment to think about what you need help with. Do you know what the problem is? Do you need help managing urges for a certain behavior? Do you need help completing a task? Do you need help with a relationship? Do you need help getting out of bed? When you're stuck, coaching can really help you get unstuck. Sometimes, it isn't that clear and you may call because you're having a hard time even defining the problem or knowing what is wrong; you can ask for help with that as well. Other times, you may know what the problem is and a possible solution, but you need help putting that solution into action.

REMEMBER

If you're someone who struggles to ask for help, skills coaching will initially be a challenge, but if you can master the skill, it will make a huge difference in your life. Asking for help is one of the most important skills we can teach you in DBT.

Asking for validation

Validation is finding the truth or value in your own or someone else's emotional experience. Most people who come to DBT have experienced significant invalidation and really struggle to validate themselves. While ultimately we want you to be able to validate yourself, if you're really struggling, asking your therapist for validation can be an extremely helpful way to stay skillful and get support while learning to self-validate or get validation from trusted people in your life.

REMEMBER

When we are validated, when someone understands our emotional experience and believes it makes sense, we start to feel more regulated, and when that happens, our thinking becomes clearer. As your emotional intensity decreases, you may find that you're able to think about what you should do next and what skills you may want to use. If you're surrounded by people in your life who are invalidating, calling for coaching for validation can bring you much-needed support.

Repairing the relationship

People with borderline personality disorder (BPD), and those who come to DBT, frequently struggle in relationships. Sometimes it is because they don't have the skills (this is why there is an interpersonal effectiveness module in DBT; see Chapter 12), and other times it is because their emotional reactivity and mood-dependent behaviors damage important relationships. The work you do with your DBT therapist will be hard, and as a result, you may develop a strong connection with your therapist.

WARNING

Given this, when there are ruptures in the relationship, it can be quite painful. You'll get angry and frustrated at your therapist. You may feel misunderstood or even hurt by your therapist, and as a result, you may do or say things that you regret. So many people sit in that suffering, feeling angry, hurt, guilty, and shameful. Holding onto these feelings is not effective and leads to a lot of pain. It may be one of the things that brought you to DBT.

The goal is to be able to address a problem in the relationship with your therapist as soon as possible, make a repair, and not have to wait until your next session. Directly addressing a rupture in a relationship takes a lot of skill, and being able to call your therapist for coaching to make a repair is good practice for the many ruptures, large and small, that you'll experience with other important people in your life.

Sharing good news

REMEMBER

The final thing you can use skills coaching — or in this case, more precisely, intersession contact — for is sharing good news. Sometimes it's nice to be able to share your good news or accomplishments in real time with your therapist. In DBT we believe that the relationship with your therapist is a real one between two people, a relationship with multiple dimensions that doesn't always mean talking about problems but also about successes, accomplishments, and just generally good news. For therapists, these are wonderful calls or texts to receive!

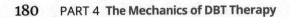

Chapter **15**

Embracing Dialectics

As you know if you read Chapters 1 and 2, the *D* in DBT stands for *dialectic.* In fact, the concept of dialectics is really what defines this treatment and makes it unique. The theory of dialectics is much older than DBT itself, dating back to before the 19th century. According to the *Oxford English Dictionary*, *dialectics* is defined as "the art of investigating or discussing the truths of opinions and the inquiry into metaphysical contradictions and their solutions." So, what do you notice? Dialectics is about two opposing truths existing at the same time. While there are many dialectics in DBT, the foundational dialectic is acceptance and change.

In this chapter, we discuss three areas of dialectics in DBT: the dialectical dilemmas of treatment, the dialectical dilemmas of parenting, and some of the dialectical interventions that your therapist will use. But first, we explain how dialectics came to be a part of DBT and break down the basics of dialectical thinking.

In the Beginning: Stumbling onto Dialectics

When Dr. Marsha Linehan was developing DBT, she stumbled upon the concept of dialectics. Dr. Linehan was determined to find a treatment for women with borderline personality disorder (BPD) who struggled with suicidal and self-destructive behavior. Many years after she had established DBT as the gold standard treatment, we would learn that as a younger woman, she also struggled with these symptoms. A fierce researcher and believer in evidence-based treatments, Dr. Linehan got to work finding an effective treatment for what was then considered an untreatable group of people.

First she tried cognitive behavioral therapy (CBT), but the women she was trying to help became more suicidal. They felt that she was demanding they change and did not understand their pain. So, Dr. Linehan tried the opposite of the heavily change-based CBT and used mindfulness-based therapy, focusing on acceptance. What did she find? The women in her study got worse again, reporting more suicidality and frustration that all her treatment was doing was asking them to essentially accept their misery and suffering, and not helping them change.

Enter dialectics. Dr. Linehan realized that she could create a treatment that used principles of both acceptance (mindfulness) and change (CBT) — two very opposing concepts — as a mechanism that would ultimately support change. She believed that you could help someone change by sometimes pushing change and other times focusing on acceptance.

REMEMBER

Dialectics allows DBT therapists to avoid getting stuck in the way other types of therapy sometimes do by searching for "the answer." For example, a patient may want to give up self-harm and yet *not* want to, or they may want to die and may *not* want to die. Instead of getting caught up in determining which it is, we understand that, in fact, it is both and may fluctuate back and forth based on mood and context. That is not to say that we do not help patients free themselves from these behaviors, but that we understand that when giving up these powerful behaviors, people may be of mixed minds about it, sometimes more committed and other times less so. We have to look at how these behaviors create problems in their lives but also offer an immediate solution to regulating emotion. DBT is a dialectical balance of change-focused, problem-solving (behavioral change), and emotion regulating skills, as well as acceptance skills and interventions that focus on validation and mindfulness. This has proven to be a very effective way to help people, especially emotionally sensitive people, to change problematic or maladaptive behaviors.

Thinking Dialectically

REMEMBER

In DBT, there is always another way to look at something, and always another truth or something we're leaving out. When you're thinking dialectically, you could actually consider the opposite of a truth not to be a lie, but instead another truth. In this treatment, you'll be challenged to not get stuck in the absolute, but when you find yourself at an impasse or polarized, you must look for the synthesis and ask yourself how these two positions can exist together. Dialectics isn't about making a compromise; it's about seeing other positions and working on a synthesis when needed. There are often multiple ways you can solve a problem, but sometimes you may get stuck seeing just one way and miss out on a far more effective way to look at things or to behave.

The skill of dialectical thinking is a powerful one. When you can think dialectically, you can see multiple contradicting positions in front of you, and you can arrive at a position that acknowledges and reconciles these multiple positions. Being able to think dialectically makes you both more effective in relationships and a more holistic problem-solver. It's also a wonderful way to combat the problems of black-and-white thinking and to keep yourself calm in difficult and emotionally charged situations.

Some people's minds work more dialectically than others. In general, strong emotions narrow your thinking and tend to pull you more toward absolutes and certainty. If you struggle with black-and-white thinking, you may observe that it is at its peak when you're dysregulated. During times of strong emotion, it's particularly hard to consider positions other than your own because it's hard to take in new information. Dialectical thinking is quite the opposite.

Like all DBT skills, dialectical thinking is a skill that needs to be practiced. The more you practice dialectal thinking when you're regulated, the easier it will be to think more dialectically when your emotions are intense. Here are some ways to practice dialectical thinking:

>> Observe when you feel absolutely certain about something; you are likely missing some important information about another point of view. Pay attention to what that certainty feels like in your mind and body. Catch it so that you can practice opening your mind.

>> Challenge yourself to find at least two other points of view (that you disagree with or don't value as much as your own), and ask yourself how they make sense and could be valuable.

>> Be mindful of making assumptions about what the other person is thinking. Ask them questions to better understand their perspective.

>> Be wary of using too many "you" statements and lead with "I" statements. Avoid telling people what they did or how they feel, and instead tell them how you feel about what is going on. This opens you both up to being more curious about the other's perspective.

>> Avoid thinking in absolutes. Try to avoid using words like *always* and *never.* Instead, try using words like *sometimes, often,* or *rarely.*

>> Try replacing the word *but* with *and* or *at the same time.* Doing this allows you to give both positions equal weight. For example: "It makes sense to me that self-injury helps you, and it is also true that it is keeping you from doing many of the things that you want to do in your life."

REMEMBER

Dialectical thinking helps you open your mind and synthesize different perspectives so you can make wise decisions. Dialectical thinking is also a powerful way to remain calm and effective in difficult situations.

Looking at the Main Dialectical Dilemmas Tackled in Treatment

There are many dialectical dilemmas in DBT; in fact, we are all often faced with challenging dialectical situations in our lives. However, there are three dilemmas that we highlight for patients in DBT, and they are each defined by their opposite poles. The following sections cover the most common behavioral patterns that people who come to DBT seem to get stuck in. The dilemma is that you get caught at the extremes, sometimes remaining at one extreme but more commonly pinging back and forth.

One of the goals of individual DBT therapy (discussed in Chapter 14) is to reduce the fluctuations between the two extremes and work toward finding more balance, which helps foster awareness and understanding of yourself and your problematic behaviors. Learning and using your DBT skills is critical in this process. In this section, we look more closely at these three dilemmas, and later in this chapter, we review the common dialectical dilemmas for parents of adolescents in DBT. These dilemmas are wonderful tools to help you step back and become aware of both your pattern of behaviors and thinking that is too extreme to be effective.

REMEMBER

The following dilemmas will help you and your DBT therapist better understand both your behaviors and experiences. Although you may not relate to all of these dilemmas, it's very possible that you'll find your experience captured by many of them. BPD and the symptoms that bring you to DBT can be confusing and can feel like opposites. With the help of your individual DBT therapist, DBT skills are designed to help you learn to find ways to live a less emotionally reactive and extreme life.

Emotional vulnerability versus self-invalidation

Emotional vulnerability is extreme sensitivity to emotional situations, where your reactions are strong to even seemingly small circumstances or events. Emotionally vulnerable people often have difficulty hiding their emotional experience and may react very strongly, leaving the people around them surprised or confused by the magnitude of their response.

On the other end of the dialectical pole is self-invalidation. As we discuss throughout this book (particularly in Chapter 23), self-invalidation involves discounting your own emotional experience, telling yourself you shouldn't feel the way you do, judging yourself for your feelings, or rejecting your emotions. You can see how the combination of these characteristics can be extremely painful. Not being able to trust their experience, people who struggle with this dialectic often look to others for how they should feel, oversimplify solutions to their problems, and feel great shame and self-hatred when their goals aren't met.

Active-passivity versus apparent competence

Active-passivity is a helpless approach to problem-solving. You may interact with the environment in a way that results in the people around you solving problems and fixing things for you. This may be overt, but more commonly it is a long-standing behavioral pattern in which people feel the need to take care of or solve problems for you.

On the opposite pole is apparent competence. This is the ability to seem like you can handle all problems with skill and competence. Many people who come to DBT can navigate many of life's problems skillfully; however, this is not consistent. There may be difficulties identifying wants and needs, perfectionism, difficulties saying no to unwanted demands, or an inability to ask for help. For many, competencies are dependent on their mood and the situation, both of which may be frequently fluctuating; for others, these are areas of significant skills deficits. Because these competencies can be inconsistent, the situation can be confusing for everyone. This dialectic can leave people feeling at times helpless to solve problems and lacking confidence that they can do things, and at the same time unable or unwilling to ask for help when they need it, believing they are being left to fail on their own.

Unrelenting crisis versus inhibited grieving

Unrelenting crisis consists of repetitive, impulsive, and self-destructive behaviors like self-injury, suicide attempts, drinking and drug use, excessive spending, dangerous driving, or stormy relationships as a way of coping. This typically occurs when you're unable to return to your emotional baseline before something painful happens again, and you live your life being ruled by your emotion mind.

Inhibited grieving is the extreme avoidance of painful emotions. However, the emotion-minded lifestyle of unrelenting crisis often leads to painful emotions that you desperately try to avoid.

The Dialectical Dilemmas of Parenting: Walking the Middle Path

When DBT was modified for adolescents, Drs. Alec Miller and Jill Rathus created the Walking the Middle Path skill (see Chapter 13) to address common dialectical dilemmas between adolescents and their parents. This skill is also made up of three dialectical dilemmas, as you find out in the following sections.

REMEMBER

The goal is to help parents and adolescents improve communication and nurture their relationship during a very challenging time and in difficult parent-adolescent situations. These dialectics are used as tools to better understand behavior and respect differing opinions and points of view in order to support looking for more effective ways to move forward when they are stuck. Thinking about it this way prevents parents from getting polarized with each other, where both of them land too far on a dialectical poll or swing from one extreme position to the other.

Making light of problem behavior versus making too much of typical behavior

This is the first of the three middle-path dialectics, and it can be more compli-cated than it looks. Parents need to find a balance between not making too much of or pathologizing normal adolescent behaviors when they arise, and under-standing when behaviors and feelings have crossed a line into something that is no longer typical but causing significant problems for their adolescent and his or her ability to function.

Many developmental struggles occur in adolescence as teens grapple with independence, exposure to drugs and alcohol, sex, school achievement and failure, employment, and issues of crime and violence. Strong feelings and reactions accompany these struggles, which are made more complicated by the surge in hormones and general impulsivity and risk taking related to age-appropriate brain development. As you try to sort pathological from normative behavior for your adolescent, it can be helpful to zoom out and consider ways in which their struggles are interfering with their academic, social, and family functioning.

This dialectic becomes more complicated when pathological adolescent behavior becomes paired with normal adolescent behavior. For example, an adolescent may be upset and storm upstairs to their room, slam the door, and the parents don't see them for a few hours. While this is unpleasant behavior, it's typical for adolescents. However, if that behavior of storming upstairs and not coming out of their room when they are upset has been paired with self-injury or suicidal behavior, then it becomes harder to untangle. As parents and teens become more skillful, this needs to be addressed so that as a family, they can figure out how the parents can begin to trust their teen to use skills in these contexts, despite their high levels of fear that their teen is upset and returning to old behaviors.

Fostering dependence versus forcing independence

The next dialectic is striving to find the balance between fostering dependence — doing too much as a parent and thus not allowing your child to learn the skills they need — and on the other side pushing them to be more independent before they have the skills they require to manage effectively. When children are younger, they are very dependent on their parents, and parents solve many of their problems. However, as their children grow up, parents must teach them skills for independent problem-solving. The transition typically goes from doing for children, to doing with them, to them doing it on their own.

When you have a child with deficits, it's easy to fall into a habit of doing for them and unintentionally fostering dependence; although well intentioned, this deprives them of the opportunity to learn how to do the task on their own. Consider a child who has severe attention deficit hyperactivity disorder (ADHD) and struggles to organize their schoolwork and backpack, clean their room, or even remember their medication. This lack of organization causes both the child and the parents a lot of anxiety and conflict. The child lacks these skills, so the parents take care of these tasks to help the child manage, and as a result everyone feels less anxious. There is some conflict, but the feelings of relief that the tasks are complete are very reinforcing, and so the parents' behavior continues.

As the teen gets older and approaches college age, they don't have the needed organizational skills and strategies to be successful. It's easy for parents, exhausted from over-functioning and doing so much for their child, to then swing to the other side and expect that child, who is now 18, to be able to do these tasks because "people your age should know how to do this." Parents then stop doing these tasks, and the teen's reliance on their family to do these tasks for them has left them without the skills to do them on their own, which has dreadful consequences.

TIP

It's also easy for teens who have some deficits to push their parents toward giving them independence because their peers have those freedoms. It isn't easy to find this dialectical balance. It's helpful for parents to ask themselves, when they do tasks for their adolescent, whether there are opportunities to shift to doing those tasks with them to foster some skills that will support them later on.

Being too strict versus being too loose

The final of the three middle-path dialectics is striving to find balance between being too strict and too loose. Another name for the poles of this dialectic is authoritarian control and excessive leniency. It's easy for fear to push parents to either one of these extremes.

When teens are engaging in dangerous or life-interfering behaviors, it's easy for parental fear to drive them toward being too strict, clamping down, and trying to control a situation that is out of their control. At the extreme, they may find emotion-minded consequences — like taking away all items that are important until the adolescent has nothing left to lose, or punishments lasting for excessive periods of time — that are impossible to uphold. When this approach doesn't work, it can be easy to willfully swing over to the other pole, throw their hands up, and get very loose, which is also ineffective. Parents may also find themselves too loose when they are parenting on eggshells and are frightened that limits or contingencies will destabilize their child and cause destructive, dangerous, or relationship-ending behaviors.

This is a challenging parental task, as they will find they may need to be more or less strict or loose, depending on the situation. The best way to find balance in this dialectic is to find their wise mind (the place of inner wisdom) and not be overly driven by fear, which can easily push them to an ineffective extreme.

Understanding Therapist Dialectical Interventions

Your DBT therapist will also be working to find dialectical balance or synthesis in the way they interact with you and work to help you. DBT therapists use many dialectical strategies. If you are new to DBT and have done other types of therapy, you may find this to be a different experience. Some strategies that may be helpful to understand are those of communication. In the following sections, we discuss three different dialectical styles that will help you understand some of the unique ways your therapist will communicate with you during your sessions, as well as how they will approach the problems you need help with. After you understand dialectics with the help of the rest of this chapter, you'll see how your therapist's style is also very dialectically balanced.

Irreverence versus reciprocity

Irreverence versus reciprocity is a dialectically balanced type of communication. Reciprocal communication fosters the relationship between patient and therapist while holding the patient's concerns as the highest priority. This type of communication avoids the more common power differential of expert and patient and instead provides more of a balance in which the therapist relates as both the expert and an authentic person with thoughts and feelings. This type of communication allows for some thoughtful self-disclosure by the therapist to support the patient's therapeutic process and goals. DBT supports a much more egalitarian relationship between therapist and patient.

The counter pole is the use of irreverent communication, in which the therapist is more offbeat or gently pokes fun when communicating. The function of this type of communication is to help shift thoughts, feelings, and behaviors when the patient is stuck. Often unexpected, it helps shift how someone is looking at things. Irreverence is not teasing or making light, but it is a way to help pivot and sometimes foster seeing different options or perspectives. The effective use of irreverence has a lot to do with timing; when therapists use irreverence in a way that doesn't work, they are quick to acknowledge their fallibility and apologize.

Environmental intervention versus consultation to the patient

This dialectic is used to handle the case management part of DBT as well as the patient's interactions with people in their lives. It isn't uncommon for patients in DBT to have multiple providers during their care, as well as family, friends, work, and school to juggle. The therapist works along this dialectic when other providers request or ask information about the patient, when the patient asks the therapist to speak with other providers, or when the patient asks the therapist to solve a problem for them. Keep in mind that one of the main goals of DBT is to help patients learn and practice skills to be more effective in their lives.

The dialectical balance that a therapist strives to find in order to support skills use and generalization is to intervene by changing the environment as little as possible, but of course, there must be a balance. The general principle in DBT is that if the therapist is to intervene in a way that changes the environment for a patient, then the therapist must determine whether the short-term gain for the patient is worth the long-term loss of learning for the patient.

For example, is the short-term benefit of the therapist talking to another provider on behalf of the patient sufficiently necessary that it is worth the loss of the patient learning how to directly communicate with that provider in a way that deepens their relationship and bolsters direct communication and self-advocacy skills? If the therapist decides that environmental intervention is not worth it, then they take the more common position of consultant to the patient. As a consultant, the therapist supports the patient using skills to navigate these challenging situations. As a result, the patient gains a sense of mastery as they apply skills to real-life situations. The therapist takes the position of consultant when they believe the patient has the skills to manage the situation and needs to practice generalizing them outside of therapy.

Problem-solving versus validation

This dialectic is emblematic of DBT. Keep in mind that the foundational dialectic in DBT is acceptance and change. The therapist is constantly balancing the problem-solving skills of CBT with the acceptance skills of mindfulness and validation. You'll find this happening throughout all your sessions. Your therapist will use problem-solving skills of behavioral, chain, missing links, and solution analysis (see Chapter 18), and approaches to problems, skills teaching, and cope-ahead plans, to name a few, when you're working on problem-solving. If you pay close attention, you'll find that your therapist is frequently validating before they move into problem-solving and then may toggle back and forth as you dive into problem-solving tasks. DBT is a change-based treatment, and we use validation and acceptance to help support and move toward change.

Chapter **16**

Structuring the Environment

One function of DBT, and in fact of any effective treatment, is that of *structuring the environment.* This means structuring the treatment, as well as elements in a patient's life, in a manner that most effectively promotes progress toward the patient's goals. In considering this function, the therapist pays close attention to environmental factors that reinforce effective behaviors and don't reinforce problematic behaviors.

In this chapter, we give you ideas to manage the challenges that the environment throws at you. Then you see that there is a structure to the individual and group DBT sessions that focuses the therapy on the teaching and clinical needs of the moment, different from more traditional talk therapies. We also point out that there are only five ways to address a problem when one arises, and which methods are effective and which are not.

Adding Structure to Two Different Environments

REMEMBER

If the environment continues to reinforce problematic behaviors, and in some way punishes clinical improvement, then it makes no sense to expect improvement. For treatment to come to an end, it must help a person by including an environment that more powerfully reinforces clinical gains. It's just as important that the therapist focus on creating a treatment environment that encourages progress and doesn't lead to a relapse.

One way to do this is through the use of family sessions, particularly in the treatment of children and adolescents (see Chapter 13), the use of case consultation meetings with other therapists (in which the patient is always present), and the use of case management services to help with certain logistics in the patient's life. Other services include providing the family with psychoeducation and consulting with schools to help them to keep a student in school. The addition of these services can help structure the environment so that patients and their families can have the greatest likelihood of a favorable outcome.

Structuring the environment can include ways to help patients modify their own environments. For example, say that a person tends to use drugs when they are in a certain social circle or in a particular area of town, or that when a person has had a particularly hard day at work, they are more likely to self-harm. In the first example, the person would structure their life in a way that limits their contact with the social circle, and in the second example, they may perhaps elicit help from their partner or family on the days that they have difficulty at work. Then, if the person relapses or self-injures, they need to understand for themselves and then teach their significant others to be careful not to reinforce the lapse or self-harm by, for example, being overly soothing or supportive.

This may seem like a contradiction, and DBT is full of these seeming contradictions. How can a family member be helpful in one context and not supportive in another? The point is that we want family members to be helpful and supportive when a person is struggling and using skillful means to get through difficult moments, and then less so when the person has used harmful behaviors to deal with these problems. This is with the idea of reinforcing DBT skill-based solutions.

REMEMBER

Ideally, the therapist helps the patient structure their environment; however, and especially early in the treatment, the therapist can take a more active role in doing the structuring. This is because the changes demanded by DBT may be too difficult for the patient to manage on their own, and so the therapist needs to help the patient. For example, say that a patient has just learned about validation (see

Chapter 12) and wants to get their partner or family members to be more validating; they try to explain validation to their significant others, but the explanation is dismissed or rejected. The therapist can step in and do a joint session with the significant others to underscore the importance of validation in the recovery process.

Addressing a Problem in Five Ways

REMEMBER

All types of environmental interventions can be applied to different situations, but environmental interventions aren't the only solution to life's problems. DBT teaches that there are five different ways to address a problem when it arises. Say that the problem is that a person is feeling lonely. What can they do? There are five solutions to solve any problem, regardless of what the problem is, in this case loneliness. Think of the acronym SCREW:

>> **Solve.** Ideally, the best way to address a problem is to solve it. If you can solve it, do so. It's not always easy or possible. In the example of feeling lonely, you could solve the problem by changing your situation to meet new people and form friendships by, for instance, joining a social club or volunteer group, or you could initiate a conversation with some of your co-workers, classmates, or neighbors. You could also try to reconnect with old friends by looking them up on social media.

>> **Change the relationship.** Solving the problem isn't always possible. Another healthy alternative is to try to change your relationship to the problem. For instance, you could recognize that being lonely doesn't mean you're unlikable or unlovable. You could find ways to discover enjoyment out of the time you spend on your own by making sure that you do things you want to do even if you're alone. For instance, you might want to go see a movie, check out a new restaurant, or find a new hiking trail, and not be dependent on the availability of other people. Another way to change your relationship to the problem of being alone is to see how wonderful it can be to be alone. For example, you can recognize that being alone will help you learn how to be more self-reliant or confident.

>> **Radically accept.** You can practice radical acceptance (see more in Chapter 11) and accept that in this moment you are lonely, and that there are times when this is going to happen. You don't have to fight this reality, nor do you have to try to solve it. You're simply accepting this moment as it is.

>> **Entertain misery.** You could choose to stay miserable. This doesn't require any skill and typically involves not doing anything but sitting on your bed and ruminating as to how lonely you are.

>> **Worsen.** Then, of course, you could choose to make things even worse. You could delete all your contacts on your phone, you could call your friends and yell at them that they aren't doing enough to connect with you, or you could decide to avoid all calls and spend time isolating in your room.

The DBT therapist can help you with the first three options, but you don't need help to do the latter two.

Building a Framework

Many therapies aren't exactly clear as to what they are going to do in each session. It's hard to make an informed decision about treatment without knowing what is going to happen in therapy, so the early discussions with the therapist are your opportunity to become an informed consumer. In the following sections, we guide you through the structure of a typical DBT therapy.

REMEMBER

If you're looking into a DBT program, make sure it has all the components of DBT (as we describe in Chapter 14). Many therapy groups and mental health clinics say that they offer DBT, but then only offer groups and not individual therapy. Others have individual therapy, but then only offer it twice per month, or they don't offer phone skills coaching. The entire framework should be clear.

Making commitments

In DBT, commitment to do the therapy is a key concept of the treatment, and the commitment is often a target of the therapist, one that is reinforced throughout the treatment. The commitment to the treatment needs to be covered both before beginning treatment and consistently after treatment starts.

When a person does their initial intake, the therapist uses specific commitment strategies to not only extract a commitment from the patient, but also to increase the likelihood that the patient will use all of the treatment components. While these strategies are sometimes seen as manipulative — and certainly if they are, they are effective forms of manipulation — they are based on the cultural reality that most of us expect to do some negotiating in our social interactions. Typically, when we try to go directly for the commitment we're hoping for, the result is that the patient won't agree and might even refuse outright.

The commitment strategies used in DBT are as follows:

>> **Pros and cons:** Here, the DBT therapist elicits from the potential patient the pros and cons of doing the treatment as well as those of not doing the treatment.

>> **Foot-in-the-door, door-in-the-face:** The foot-in-the-door is the approach of making an initial easy request (such as "Can you commit to not self-injure for four weeks?"), followed by a more difficult request ("How about six months, can you commit for six months?"). This is based on the finding that people who agree to a smaller ask are more likely to agree to subsequent asks.

The door-in-the-face approach begins by asking the patient for a much larger commitment than what the therapist realistically imagines they can get, and then "settling" for something less. The idea here is that people who say no to one thing often feel more obliged to say yes to a different request if that request is reasonable.

>> **Linking the current commitment to past commitments:** If a person who has previously expressed a desire to change is now wavering or expressing doubt, the therapist can review times when the patient has made a commitment to something, and stuck to the task from start to finish, and then link the current commitment to that one.

>> **Cheerleading:** Here the therapist provides encouraging statements and support for the positive changes that a person wants to make in their life.

>> **Freedom to choose in the absence of viable or desirable alternatives:** Social psychology demonstrates that people are more likely to make commitments when they believe that they are free to make a choice, or when they believe there are no other options that are consistent with, or will help them attain, their goals. By combining these two conditions, the DBT therapist will highlight a person's freedom to choose and, at the same time, the lack of viable alternatives.

This is also a dialectical perspective, for how are these seemingly contradictory positions possible? It's because there are always other choices; however, there might not be an alternative that would allow the person to attain the goals they have set, and yet they are also free to choose a different goal if they are unwilling to do what is being asked. However, if the person chooses a different goal and does different behaviors, then this will have its own consequences, and the therapist will highlight this fact as well.

>> **Devil's advocate:** This is a technique where a therapist gets a commitment from a patient but then questions the commitment and considers whether in fact the patient's former approach doesn't have merit. It means arguing the other side of the dialectic, meaning the patient's perspective, or creating a counterargument relative to the patient's position in order to get them to more fully examine the decision they are making.

Devil's advocate can also be used *prior* to getting the commitment. In other words, it can be used as a strategy to get the commitment — for instance, by taking the position that maybe therapy doesn't make sense when a person says they want therapy but they are wavering. By suggesting that they might not need it, this typically gets the person to focus on the consequences of not getting help.

Holding true to your plan

When the therapist has attained a commitment, it's important to set achievable goals for therapy. The therapist/patient team considers and anticipates barriers to fully participating in therapy and to attaining the goals. The task here is to know what the patient hopes to accomplish in therapy, or to imagine what their life would look like if they could overcome the challenges they are facing in their life. The therapist then shows the patient how specific skills can be used to attain their goals.

REMEMBER

Once you have a goal and a plan, the next step is to start the plan and stick to it. Here are the steps:

1. **Visualize yourself achieving your goal.**

   Long-term goals can feel overwhelming and too far off, especially if they require the use of brand-new behaviors. Know this: You're aware of how your life feels the way you're currently living it. When you live differently, your life will change. Whenever your motivation wanes, keep the image of a more capable self in your mind.

2. **Create an accountability procedure.**

   What is going to keep you on track? Is there a friend or relative, or a religious minister or teacher, who can help keep you accountable? Do you need to check in with your therapist on a more regular basis in the first few weeks of therapy? Typically, most people feel responsible for completing their goals if they are accountable to other important people in their life.

3. **Break the goal into smaller steps.**

   No matter what you want to achieve, there are smaller steps between now and then. Rather than insisting that you either complete the goal in one instance or give up, think about smaller steps. For instance, if you want to run a marathon, simply going out and trying to run 26 miles without ever having run before is a daunting task, and it would be easy to give up. Rather than trying the entire marathon or giving up, try one mile, and then two, and slowly build up to the entire distance by setting smaller, more manageable goals along the way. You're much more likely to attain your goal this way.

4. Give yourself a day off.

It may seem counterintuitive, but it's okay to give yourself a day off from practicing new behaviors. Change can be draining. The important thing here is to recognize that you're taking a day off, that you remain committed to your end goal, that it's a day of rest and not a day when you'll return to earlier, maladaptive behaviors.

5. Stop thinking and "just do it!"

Sometimes we think too much, and thinking gets in the way of completing our task. Rather than sitting around and considering your goal as some obligation in your life, consider the steps to attain your goal to be an integral part of your lifestyle and completely non-optional. The more you do something daily, even if it is new, the more quickly it will become a habit.

6. Look back.

If you're climbing a steep mountain, it can feel like an impossible task to get to the top. It's easy to become demoralized by the slog of the effort. Take some time whenever you're feeling down or defeated to look back and see just how far you've come. Perhaps you can track your journey by journaling and then going back to read about older versions of yourself. You'll be grateful when you can notice the changes that have taken place from where you started.

7. Cope ahead for difficult moments.

Research shows that our brains can become impatient or that we can lose self-control and become impulsive. It's important to anticipate and potentially eliminate possible obstacles. Instead of simply trusting your future self to do the right thing, make these potential barriers more manageable by preparing for them, and do so when you're feeling motivated, so that when you're feeling less motivated, you don't have to suddenly start making plans.

8. Know that you can do it.

You wouldn't be setting the goals that you did with your therapist if they were unattainable. While self-control can be depleted, we also know that by simply believing, you have the ability to accomplish your goals.

Structuring Individual Sessions

The individual sessions are where you work toward your specific goals. Different from the skills group, where all the skills are taught to all the participants (see Chapter 14), in the individual session, only the skills that are pertinent to your target behaviors and life aspirations are reviewed, considered, and applied. The following sections take you through a typical session.

Reviewing your diary card

At the start of every therapy session, your therapist will ask to review your diary card, which we cover in Chapter 18. A diary card is a tool that was initially unique to DBT, although more therapies now use it. It is a grid-like form that helps you keep track of your target symptoms, your progress toward your goals, and the skills that you have used in different situations. The diary card is completed every day and is tailored to address the specific targets that you and your therapist have agreed need attention.

REMEMBER

The therapist will carefully review your card at the beginning of each session and will then discuss any situation of concern, such as the risk of suicide or self-injury and patterns of substance misuse. These are the so-called life-threatening or quality-of-life-interfering behaviors that have to be addressed before you discuss other concerns in therapy.

Paying attention to target hierarchy

REMEMBER

Because people who come to DBT typically have multiple problems that require treatment, DBT uses a hierarchy of treatment targets to help the therapist determine the order in which the problems will be addressed. The treatment targets, in order of priority, are as follows:

>> **Life-threatening behaviors:** These behaviors could lead to the person's death and include suicidal behavior and thoughts, as well as all forms of non-suicidal self-injury. These behaviors also include being violent toward others or being a victim of violence. People who are violent often use violence as way to get what they want. Like other destructive behaviors, violence might work in the immediate term but ends up leaving the perpetrator isolated and mistrusted. Similarly, being a victim of violence can lead the victim to avoid life altogether to the point of wanting to escape living.

>> **Therapy-interfering behaviors:** A person can't get better if they don't fully participate in therapy, and so behaviors that interfere with effective treatment are targeted next. These behaviors aren't only the ones that the patient is doing, but they can also be those that the therapist is doing. Such behaviors include coming late to therapy sessions; cancelling appointments; being non-collaborative in working toward treatment goals; or refusing to complete homework, diary cards, or chain analysis.

>> **Quality-of-life-interfering behaviors:** Here the therapist and patient review behaviors that interfere with the patient having a reasonable quality of life, such as relationship problems, substance misuse, and other mental health concerns.

Doing a chain analysis on the highest target

The central point of a chain analysis (described in Chapter 18) is that by analyzing your behavior, you're able to know the cause of the behavior and what maintains it. Knowing this is an important step in changing behavior. Any behavior can be understood as a series of linked moments and components. These moments are linked together in a temporal chain in that they follow in succession, one after the other. One link in the chain leads to the next. Behaviors that are repeated are like well-rehearsed habits, and at first glance, it may appear that episodes of behavior can't be broken down because they seem to just happen at one moment. The therapist conducts the chain, and ultimately the patient is able to do so on their own, by asking a series of questions that effectively unlock the links — links that at times can feel as if they have forever been, and will forever be, fused.

REMEMBER

The purpose of a chain analysis is to precisely define what the problem is, what prompted it, what its function is, what is interfering with using other behaviors than the ones used, and what the ensuing consequences are. Although performing a precise chain analysis requires time and effort, it's worth it in that it provides essential information and clues for understanding the events that led up to specific problem behaviors. Attempts at solving a problem often fail because the problem hasn't been fully understood and assessed. If the behavior occurs frequently, by conducting repeated chain analyses, the therapist helps clarify the problem and better understand the way that the links are connected.

Figuring out the links is the first step in finding solutions to stopping or changing the problem behavior, and this happens by breaking the chain in places where the links can be broken. For instance, if every time a person has three drinks after 10 p.m. they tend to have a fight with their significant other, they may decide to stop drinking by 9 p.m., to not drink at all, or to minimize the drinks to one or two.

TIP

Here is an example of a completed chain analysis:

1. **What exactly is the problem behavior that I am analyzing?**

   Drinking too much and fighting with my partner.

2. **What was the prompting event?**

   I had planned to make a special dinner for my partner, only to have them not return from work on time. My partner arrived late from work and told me that they had gone to a work party and spoken to a co-worker that they know I don't like.

3. **Describe what things within you and in your environment made you vulnerable.**

   I was looking forward to dinner with my partner. I also wanted to let my mother, who is my biggest supporter, know what I was planning to cook for dinner, but when I called her, she was rushed and told me that she was going to a movie with a friend, and that annoyed me.

4. **List the chain of events (specific behaviors and environmental events that actually occurred).**

   A. I felt hurt and started sobbing on the phone with my partner, and I felt angry with them.

   B. I called my mother and she said she was going out to a movie.

   C. I thought, "I can't stand it. I am never anyone's most important. No one loves me."

   D. I felt hopeless after speaking to my partner and my mother.

   E. I thought, "My life is worthless; no one will ever be here for me."

   F. When I looked at my social media, I noticed that everyone seemed to have someone.

   G. I started feeling anxious and thought, "I can't live like this."

   H. I decided to drink a shot of vodka so that I would feel better, but I ended up drinking the whole bottle.

   I. I did everything I could to stay awake, and when my partner arrived at home, I started yelling at them.

5. **What exactly were the consequences in the environment. . .**

   - Short-term: I slept alone, which I haven't done in over nine months.

   - Long-term: My partner is now questioning whether they made the right choice in being with me.

   . . .and in myself?

   - Short-term: I am ashamed that I lost control.

   - Long-term: I will have to face the prospect of being alone.

6. **What harm did my problem behavior cause?**

   It hurt me because I lost control and it broke trust in my relationship.

7. **List new, more skillful behaviors to replace ineffective behaviors.**

    A. Use the GIVE skill with my partner (see Chapter 12).

    B. Check the facts around the idea that my partner is going to reject me.

    C. Call my therapist, explain what is going on, and ask for help.

    D. Use my distress tolerance skills (see Chapter 11) and watch an uplifting movie, or call a friend and go for a walk.

    E. Practice loving compassion meditation (see Chapter 9).

    F. Pour the vodka down the sink so that it will not be a risk.

8. **Come up with prevention plans.**

- Ways to reduce my vulnerability in the future: Make a cope-ahead plan for the next time my partner needs to go to a work party.

- Ways to prevent the precipitating event from happening again: It is nearly impossible to stop something from happening in the future, so I can practice coping ahead and having various plans for how to manage being alone.

9. **Make plans to repair, correct, and overcorrect any harm done to others.**

The focus on overcorrection is one of working to restore the situation to better than its original condition or of going above and beyond what might have been expected in the apology.

Apologize to my partner, reassure them that the behavior is not consistent with my values, and make a commitment for a different outcome next time. Also, commit to working on the issue in therapy so that I can be better prepared and understand and attend to my emotional triggers in a more effective way.

Weaving in solution analysis

Once the therapist and the patient have completed the chain analysis, DBT therapists then conduct *solution analyses* (see Chapter 18) to identify and implement the most effective possible skills or solutions that could have been implemented in the chain. The aim in DBT isn't just to stop the maladaptive behaviors that leave the person suffering, but also to resolve the issues that contribute to the problematic behavior and to relieve the person's suffering as well.

Therapists divide a solution analysis into three basic components: the generation, the evaluation, and the implementation of various solutions:

1. The therapist and patient select a specific link in the chain and then generate various possible solutions that could have been implemented. Ideally, multiple possible solutions are generated, and not immediately discarded.

2. The solutions are evaluated for the possibility of implementation based on how realistic the solutions are, and what the barriers to implementation might be.

3. The solution is implemented.

You can consider the following factors when selecting a link for solution analysis:

>> How strongly does the link control the target behavior?

>> How frequently does the link show up across various chain analyses?

>> How easy will it be to change or modify the link?

>> How closely is the link tied to a patient's goals?

>> How willing is the patient to address the link?

After this questioning is completed, the therapist and the patient move onto the next significant link by repeating the preceding steps.

Interweaving the chain analysis with solution analysis has several advantages:

>> It decreases the likelihood that your therapist only spends time analyzing the causes of your problematic behavior, which prevents them from spending any time on solutions.

>> This approach helps patients become more autonomous in the process of identifying problematic links.

>> The process creates a more automatic connection between problematic behaviors and possible solutions. To decide when to interweave solutions, therapists generally consider how well the link has been understood.

Moving down the hierarchy to discuss skills related to current life situations

Once the more life-threatening targets have been addressed, the therapy then moves down the hierarchy to lower-level targets. This does not mean that these targets are less important; often they are more important. For instance, if a person is wondering how to improve their relationships, this is clearly a very important issue, and yet if they are engaging in dangerous or life-threatening behavior, their life is at risk, and so dealing with life-threatening behavior must come before dealing with the relationship issues, even though to the patient, the relationship issues are more fundamental.

Putting Structure in Different Contexts

One important aspect to structuring the environment is the consideration of the use of DBT in specific settings. Keep in mind that DBT was developed to be used as an outpatient treatment for suicidal people; however, given the power of the treatment, it isn't surprising that it has moved into different settings and with particular populations, as you find out in the following sections.

Prison settings

In most circumstances, prison models are almost the opposite of DBT in that prisons subscribe to a primarily punishment-based model. This system is broken, and in recent years criminal justice systems worldwide have called for prison reform. This makes sense because there is unequivocal evidence that punishment-based systems don't deter or prevent crime. Also, they are financially unsustainable, and they fail to reduce repeat offenders. One of the problems, however, was that there was no empirically based alternative to punishment. This is where DBT comes in.

Forensic settings recognized the utility of DBT as an intensive, well-structured, skills-based cognitive-behavioral program that enhances many of the problems that inmates present with: emotion dysregulation, substance misuse, the inability to tolerate distress, and deficits in effective interpersonal functioning. Further, because DBT has been shown to be effective in difficult-to-treat populations, it's a complete package for prison settings. Also, personality disorders and substance use disorders are important to treat in prison settings because these two conditions are significantly associated with repeat offenses.

The skills taught in DBT address many of the most significant risk factors for criminal activity. Interpersonal effectiveness skills can help people address many of the maladaptive interpersonal styles that are vulnerability factors in the development of relationships with people already involved in crime. Emotion regulation skills can help people manage their anger and aggression.

Clearly some elements of standard DBT can't translate to the prison setting — for instance, phone-skills coaching — and so the structure had to change. One change was to make the language simpler. For example, rather than *emotional dysregulation*, "difficulties in controlling emotions" is used, or instead of *interpersonal effectiveness*, "relationship skills." Then, because of restrictions in prison settings — a prisoner cannot go for a long walk in the woods, take a bubble bath, go to bed when they want, or do an ice dive to regulate emotions rapidly (see Chapter 21) at will — there is instead the use of activities that apply to a custodial environment.

School settings

A significant number of young people engage in risky behaviors. These include marijuana and alcohol use; sexual encounters with multiple, and at times unknown other, sexual partners; and physical fights. These high-risk behaviors are associated with the leading causes of death among young people. Two factors associated with engagement in these behaviors are emotion dysregulation and impulsivity, clear targets for DBT.

There are also stressors that are particular to school settings. Every year there is the need to re-acclimate to the social structure of the new school year. Then, simply transitioning to a new school year with new classrooms, academic material, and teachers is its own stressor.

The modifications for school settings offer ways to structure the treatment for specific needs. For instance, one adaptation of DBT for school is known as DBT Skills Training for Emotional Problem Solving for Adolescents (DBT STEPS-A), which is a social emotional learning (SEL) curriculum adapted by Dr. James Mazza and colleagues for middle and high schools in order to teach all adolescents effective emotion regulation, decision-making, and problem-solving skills. Then there is Teen Talk, which is a program of adapted DBT skills that serve as a disciplinary alternative in education. It's a four-week skills curriculum designed to enhance student coping skills — specifically, awareness and radical acceptance. The program focuses on managing disruptive behavior such as impulsivity, emotional reactivity, and aggression. Whereas a DBT skills group focuses on reviewing skills homework, in Teen Talk, the group is paired with individualized monitoring of academic schoolwork as well as mindfulness exercises, feelings, and responses; the use of interpersonal effectiveness; and distress tolerance and emotion regulation. The Teen Talk lessons are aimed at reducing social isolation, aggression, hyperactivity, and distractibility, as well as depression and anxiety.

TECHNICAL STUFF

Because many students don't want to be seen as needing mental health treatment, to appeal to the students, the skills were renamed to sound more interesting and include names such as *Riding the wave, At the movie theater,* and *Try to bother me.*

Another problem specific to schools is youth school refusal. DBT makes sense because a significant percentage of school refusal cases present with significant emotion regulation problems, and in this context, DBT conceptualizes these cases of school refusal as resulting from these problems, and so the DBT emotion regulation skills make sense. A change from standard DBT is the addition of web-based coaching between the adolescent, their parents, and the primary therapist. This takes place every morning on school days.

These and other ways of structuring the school environment have been found to improve student functioning and to enhance their self-worth and social relatedness.

Hospital settings

Because inpatient hospitalization is unpredictable when it comes to the length of a patient's stay, to structure DBT for inpatient settings, it has to work within the time frame allotted, which can be between 3 and 14 days. One way to structure this is to offer individual therapy, skills training, and medication management during the clinical day, which is typically from 9 a.m. to 5 p.m. at least 5 days a week. Patients with emotion regulation problems are usually selected; however, because all patients can learn from groups that focus on emotion vulnerability factors as they pertain to stress, even patients not typically served by DBT can attend. It also means that the majority of staff have to be familiar with the DBT skills so that they can provide real-time skills coaching.

The entire therapeutic day and all of the groups are dedicated to covering as much of the DBT curriculum as possible, given that the length of the stay is likely to be short. For many patients, it won't be possible to cover the entire curriculum, and so rather than comprehensively going through every single practice or skill within each module, only a few are chosen and reviewed. Another element is that every person who attends should be given psychoeducation as well as an understanding of the biosocial theory (see Chapter 2) and, in particular, the impact of invalidation and the benefits of self-validation.

If the patient finds the groups and the treatment to be useful or of interest, then the hospital case manager can help to find them an outpatient DBT therapist, or at least provide the names of local therapists so that the patient can follow up on discharge.

Therapy for people with developmental disabilities

Despite the logic that all people who might benefit from DBT should be provided with the treatment, it can be difficult to provide the therapy for people with intellectual and developmental disabilities. For instance, one problem is that there are significant cognitive elements to the treatment. In addition, the standard model is full of metaphors and acronyms. Certain concepts are also very abstract, such as the ideas of dialectical synthesis and radical acceptance. Finally, some people with these disabilities also have poor or no reading skills, or they have a poor memory that will make standard DBT difficult for therapists to teach and patients to grasp.

One adaptation of DBT is known as the Skills System, which was developed by Julie F. Brown, Ph.D. It is a developmentally friendly set of emotion regulation skills, designed to help people of various ages and abilities manage emotions.

TECHNICAL STUFF

With regard to dialectics, one of the standard teaching techniques for working with people with intellectual disabilities is to keep things simple by asking questions that have single answers such as right or wrong, or that have a choice such as this or that. This teaching seems to violate the principle of the duality of nature because it portrays the world as black and white without encouraging the search for various perspectives. On the other hand, it's consistent with the principle of doing what is effective and that best meets the needs of the patient.

Many therapists are constantly working on maintaining and learning the therapy, and it can be challenging for therapists to stay abreast of all the nuances, and so it's clear that the treatment can be particularly difficult for people with cognitive challenges. Complicated treatments should be taken on only if there is a strong commitment to the use of the model for the long haul, and this means that the teams working with the developmentally disabled are committed to doing so. For this population, it's very likely that if DBT is used, it will likely be a longer-term treatment and will require multiple and persistent repetitions, with shorter, more narrowly focused sessions, and it will be embedded in a culture where the central assumptions of DBT are core to the milieu.

Another seeming violation of DBT practice is that some people with developmental disabilities have individual service plans, and these often have built into them goals that require consistency of treatment and support by providers. This goes against the DBT approach of *consultation to patient* in which people are taught that they must learn to negotiate the system and generalize their skills to their environment so that they can fend for themselves.

Many people with disabilities live with families, in supervised care, and in some cases independently with case management. The therapist works with the person's non-DBT team and is a consultant to the broader team, supporting them with psychoeducation and clinical leadership in order to strengthen the patient's and the broader team's motivation with the goal of gradual and increasing generalization of skills in the person's community. The therapist also offers training to the broader team — in particular, the practice of validation. This training is also offered to family members. The staff and family then become the coaches for the person, to help as needed.

The therapist may also need to intervene and collaborate with state non-DBT service providers to explain the DBT process. The focus should be on creating a person-centered, user-friendly environment that adheres to the DBT assumptions and principles. Finally, there is often more frequent consultation with the various service elements than would typically be provided in standard DBT.

Chapter **17**

The Therapist Consultation Team

DBT is very effective, and yet the demands of working with a group of people who at times struggle with active suicidal and other self-destructive thoughts and behaviors can take its toll on those delivering the therapy. To address this challenge, and to keep fidelity to the model of the treatment, a therapist delivering DBT therapy has to agree to be on a *consultation team.* They also agree to provide the treatment — its tools, protocols, and principles — consistent with the evidence of efficacy. This means that they don't deviate and use a little bit of DBT, a little bit of psychoanalysis, a little bit of schema therapy, and so on. They are agreeing to do only DBT.

In this chapter, you find out what a therapist does to make sure that they are keeping to the principles and protocols of DBT treatment. You also discover how the treatment team that the therapists belong to is an essential part of the treatment in that they help each other through difficult moments and give each other new ideas and options as to what they might do in the event that they get stuck in your treatment.

Joining a Consultation Team

The consultation team is made up of therapists providing DBT treatment to patients. The founder of DBT, Dr. Marsha Linehan, described the team as "a community of therapists treating a community of clients." Ideally, a team has 3 to 8 people who may come from different disciplines and who may have different roles or professional degrees, but who are all using DBT in the treatment of certain patients. In other words, there can be social workers, psychologists, psychiatrists, nurses, interns, and mental health counselors. In some contexts, especially when there are many trainees, such as in academic centers or larger counseling centers, teams might be bigger, but we have found that if we have more than 12 people in the team, it can be hard to meet everyone's needs. Most consultation team meetings last an hour to an hour and a half.

REMEMBER

Before they join a team, the therapist must be completely aware of the commitment they are making. Just as patients make a commitment to DBT, so therapists must make a commitment to the team. New therapists commit to continuing to actively work on increasing their own effectiveness and adherence to the application of DBT, and commit to being responsible for the care of all patients being treated by the members of the team. Putting this more bluntly, members of the team are agreeing that if a patient being treated by any member of the team were to die by suicide, then all members would say "yes" when asked if they have ever had a patient die by suicide.

The following sections discuss the purpose of a consultation team and agreements that the team members make.

Therapy for the therapists

DBT assumes that effective treatment of self-endangering patients includes as much focus on the therapist's behavior, and their experience of therapy, as it does on the patient's behavior. Treating patients who display chronic suicidal and self-destructive behavior is enormously stressful, and so staying within the DBT therapeutic framework can, at times, seem nearly impossible. Because of this, a core part of the therapy includes the "treatment" of the therapist.

REMEMBER

There are three main purposes of consultation to the therapist in DBT:

>> **The team helps keep each therapist in the therapeutic relationship with their patient.** The role of the team is to help the therapist with any burnout they may be feeling and to cheerlead and support the therapist.

>> **Consistent with dialectics, the team helps provide a balance in the therapist's interactions with their patient.** In providing this balance, the team members might move closer to the therapist's perspective in order for them to hold a strong position, or they might move further from the therapist in order for the therapist to move closer to the patient's perspective and maintain balance.

>> **In the context of programs that are embedded within a non-DBT setting, the team provides the context for the treatment.** For example, in a general psychiatric unit that isn't a DBT unit, if DBT skills are being taught and some of the clinicians are using the therapy, having those clinicians in a team helps support the team members keep fidelity and stay motivated to the model even if they are in the non-DBT setting.

The following sections describe methods used to provide therapy to therapists on a team.

Targeting burnout

WARNING

Therapist burnout is associated with many negative impacts. When therapists feel burned out, this can lead to therapist absenteeism. Burnout can lead to greater staff turnover, increased negative attitudes toward patients, and poorer patient outcomes. Burnout can also take a toll on the therapists themselves, with poorer overall well-being characterized by higher levels of depression, anxiety, insomnia, and substance use.

In some contexts and agencies, one of the problems that DBT therapists face is that of large caseloads and a limited amount of time to review the cases. For very large DBT teams, too many therapists means that some of the therapists might not get a chance to review their cases, and it's possible that some therapists working with very complicated patients will spend a lot of time reviewing their cases. This can also lead to burnout for other team members, and at times, the better option is to divide the large team into two smaller teams.

Within the DBT context, we consider burnout to have three components:

>> Feeling emotionally exhausted

>> Losing compassion for patients

>> Feeling ineffective or incompetent

The team helps reduce team member burnout by providing a listening ear and validation, encouragement, humor, and irreverence, as well as a sense of community and shared purpose. Experienced teams are effective in that they are consistently dialectical; they use radical genuineness with each other; they are direct in addressing problems and honest in the mistakes they make; and they are willing to make repairs. When the team drifts off course, they work on strategies using the DBT framework that help them get back on course. Feeling that the team has the therapist's back is the key to reducing burnout.

Enhancing therapist capabilities

As we mention throughout this book, working with patients who are emotionally dysregulated — often displaying anger, fear, shame, and guilt; threatening or making suicide attempts; and engaging in self-injurious behaviors — is stressful. To become more skilled, as well as to remain motivated to continue to do DBT in these situations, therapists need to acquire, integrate, and generalize the cognitive, emotional, behavioral, and verbal approaches necessary for the effective application of the treatment. In many ways, this isn't different from what therapists need to do with their patients — that is, therapists need to teach their patients so that they can acquire, integrate, and generalize the skills necessary to be able to function effectively in their lives. This enhancement can take place within the team, in individual supervision, through dedicated in-house staff training, and by sending staff to dedicated off-site DBT training sessions.

TIP

Here are some other strategies that can help therapists:

>> **Session recordings:** The therapist records their individual session with a patient to have it reviewed by the therapist's supervisor or other DBT colleague. In this context, colleagues and supervisors can give feedback as to the accuracy of the therapist's application of DBT and their use of DBT treatment strategies. Reviewing session videos during team meetings can be one of the most effective ways to improve DBT adherence for individual therapy.

>> **Didactic teaching:** New ideas in the application of DBT are being developed all the time, and members who have gone to training sessions might return to share with their team any new ideas they have learned or explain new ways of applying DBT techniques. This, in turn, can increase therapist competence and reduce ineffectiveness.

>> **Dedicated use of DBT strategies:** This is the application of the very same DBT techniques that are used with patients, including the use of chain analysis, missing links analysis, and solution analysis with each other (see Chapter 18). There are many benefits to this approach: it can model the use of techniques in the group; the role-play of skills use can be instructive; and it can highlight the difficulty that patients sometimes experience in using the skills.

Consultation team agreements

For a therapist to join a consultation team, they must commit to certain agreements. These make sense in the way that, for instance, a British driver coming to the United States must agree to drive on the right side of the road or else the consequences will be significant. Similarly, without adhering to the treatment that has been developed for suicidal people, the consequence could be serious. The following sections describe agreements that allow for more effective functioning of the team and delivery of the treatment.

Acceptance of a dialectical philosophy

REMEMBER

This agreement is about the stance that a therapist takes in agreeing to deliver DBT. The dialectical philosophy is one that recognizes the subjectivity of experiences, and that therefore there is no absolute truth. This is important because like all humans, therapists can get caught in conflicting opinions. The idea with this agreement is that when this happens, they will agree to look for the elements of truth in each opinion and then search for a synthesis of the positions. They do this by asking questions like "What are we missing?" or "What is the truth in the other person's position?" or "What am I leaving out or not considering?"

Consultation to the patient

With this agreement, the therapists agree that the primary goal of the team is to improve their own abilities as therapists and to help patients develop agency. So, rather than serve as go-betweens for patients and other therapists, or other people in the patient's life, they agree not to treat each other or their patients as fragile in the belief that patients and therapists can speak on their own behalf and that if they cannot, then the compassionate thing to do is to teach them how to advocate for themselves.

Diversity and change

Because change is not only a natural but also a constant life occurrence, the therapists agree to accept diversity and change as they occur. What this means is that therapists don't have to agree with each other's positions about how to respond to specific patients' behaviors, nor do they have to tailor their behavior to be consistent with everyone else's. For instance, one therapist might decide to reinforce wanted behavior by a patient, whereas another therapist might decide to ignore or punish unwanted behavior.

The exception to this rule is one that typically occurs in residential and hospital settings, and that is when a patient is on a behavior plan. If a behavior is being extinguished, then all therapists and members of the treatment team observe the behavior plan.

Observing limits

This agreement holds that each therapist is to observe their own limits and theirs alone. Then, in so doing, they agree to not judge or criticize other members for having different limits from their own. For instance, one therapist might say that it is okay for an adolescent patient to curse during the therapy session, but another therapist might say that this crosses their own personal line. Each therapist is responsible to set their own limits. This does not, however, mean that a therapist can violate the code of ethical behavior set by their professional licensing board.

Stretching limits

Here, therapists agree that although they will observe their own limits, there may be situations when they need to stretch their limits in order to meet the legitimate and justified needs of their patients. For instance, if a therapist has a limit of staying on the phone for only ten minutes when they are doing skills coaching by phone, and a patient who has historically been avoidant of reaching out for coaching does reach out for the first time in a moment of distress, the therapist might decide to go beyond their ten-minute limit in order to reinforce the patient's asking-for-help behavior in that instance.

Phenomenological empathy

REMEMBER

With this agreement, the therapists agree that, all things being equal, they will search for non-judgmental and empathic interpretations of their own, their patients', and their team colleagues' behavior. They agree to assume that their patients, they themselves, and their fellow team members are trying the best they can, and that they want to improve. They strive to see the world through their patients' and colleagues' eyes, considering who they are and the circumstances that could have caused them to be who they are and to behave in the way they do. They recognize that because all behavior is caused, rather than judge a person for the behavior they are displaying, they will instead consider the causes and contexts of this behavior.

Fallibility

Finally, the therapists agree to recognize that they are fallible human beings who, like all other human beings, are prone to make mistakes. They agree that they have likely done at least some part of whatever problematic behavior they're being accused of doing. By accepting this agreement, they can let go of assuming a defensive stance, a stance that can come across as aloof, while hoping to display virtuosity or competence. With therapists assuming this stance, there is also an explicit request and reliance on other team members that they will help point out when the therapist is being defensive, and that the team will help the therapist be more skillful in the future.

Sticking to the Agenda

A key function of the consultation team is to hold the therapist accountable to using the DBT therapeutic framework and to address problems that arise in the course of delivering the treatment. To do this, the group members help each other focus on applying DBT strategies to increase DBT-adherent behaviors and reduce non-DBT approaches. With this in mind, the team agenda focuses on what the individual team members need to deliver the treatment effectively.

The following sections cover the structure of a team meeting and the roles that members play.

Structuring a meeting

There are multiple ways to run a DBT consultation team meeting, and each team can modify the overall structure to reflect their needs. The typical structure includes an identified team leader; this would be the clinician who is generally recognized as the most experienced DBT therapist. Then an observer is agreed upon, and that person has the role of noticing when the team is straying from DBT principles. There are other roles and tasks, and we review the specifics in the next section.

Most teams typically begin with mindfulness practice. Doing this helps team members transition from whatever they were doing previously into the team meeting. Mindfulness practice enhances team members participating fully in the practice and then focusing only on the task of the moment. (Chapter 9 introduces the topic of mindfulness.)

Next is the establishing of the actual agenda. This is set by the team following the DBT hierarchy of targets, with the specific focus on what the therapist needs to effectively deliver the therapy, rather than the problems that any patient is presenting. On our team, the idea is that the therapists themselves have to ask for help. Generally, after considering their burnout, we ask them to consider whether they need help with the following:

>> Getting validation with the situation they are in

>> Defining the problem they are facing if they can't exactly articulate what it is

- Or if they know what the problem is, then considering various solutions

- Or if they know what the solution is, then helping with applying the solution

These questions are considered within the format of the team. Following is one format; however, you can change the format depending on the needs of your team:

>> Therapists assess their own burnout and whether they need help with the burnout.

>> Therapists request help, if they need it, when their clients are exhibiting suicidal or other life-threatening behaviors.

>> Therapists focus on treatment-interfering behaviors such as when their patients don't show up, as well as their own treatment-interfering behaviors.

>> Some teams will add reports of good news and successful interventions.

>> A final agenda item might be administrative tasks or other business matters such as discussing upcoming training sessions.

REMEMBER

Because many therapists in the team might need help, it's important that one therapist's issues not dominate the entire session. In our team, we get individual therapists to estimate the amount of time that they will need, and then hold themselves accountable to keeping to that time. Going over time with any one discussion can mean that other therapists aren't getting their needs met. This is where the observer can take note of members not sticking to the specifics of what they need.

Understanding team roles

The team meets regularly — often weekly — as they support each other in the work of delivering effective DBT. Some teams are very small, and so it may be difficult to fill all the roles. The most important aspect of the team is to conduct regular team meetings. If there are enough members, these are some of the defined roles and tasks:

>> **Team leader:** This person is tasked with monitoring and managing how the team is doing overall:

  • They are the most senior person with the most training.

  • They focus on ensuring fidelity.

  • This role does not rotate.

- » **Meeting leader:** This is the person who leads mindfulness as well as the following:
  - They develop the agenda with team members.
  - They review at least one of the consultation team agreements (as mentioned previously).
  - They determine the order of agenda items.
- » **Observer:** This person observes the proceedings of the meeting and uses a bell that they ring to call attention to when the following situations occur:
  - Team members are polarized, and the polarization remains unresolved.
  - Team members are being treated as fragile.
  - Therapists are being judgmental or non-compassionate of each other or their patients.
  - Therapists are being defensive.
  - Members are not being mindful by doing two things at once such as checking their phones.
  - Members start offering solutions before a problem has been accurately assessed.
  - Members start straying into non-DBT treatments.
- » **Note taker:** This person takes notes that can serve as minutes of the meeting. This does create the risk of the note-taker getting caught up in doing two things at once.
- » **Time keeper:** Some teams notice that the team leader can, at times, get into the weeds of any specific discussion and forget that they are keeping time. As a result, some teams have a dedicated time keeper.

REMEMBER

Whether or not the team leader and observer are sticking to their tasks, it's the responsibility of the entire team to ensure that all team members participate fully to the extent that they have something relevant to say pertaining to the request being made of the team. Also, team members may notice polarization and judgments that the observer hasn't noticed, and it's consistent with team functioning that they bring up these issues.

Chapter **18**

Tracking Your Experience

I n this chapter, you discover the benefit of tracking your experiences on a daily diary card, along with your emotions, and your behaviors, on your journey toward your goal. You find out how to track and see how by doing so, you're also helping your therapist know what your day-to-day observations, struggles, and successes were.

Keeping a Daily Diary Card

One of the problems of traditional weekly therapy is that when you go into a therapy session, you have to rely on your memory as to what happened in the week before. Memory is malleable, which means that it can be stretched or bent into different stories. It can convince you that something is or isn't true, that you heard something that wasn't actually said, or that what you heard was a version of what was said.

REMEMBER

Our memories aren't trying to harm us; rather, the problem is that emotions are powerful forces that are inextricably intertwined with memories. The reason our brain changes what we perceive or how we appraise situations is that the present moment is often seen through the lens of past memories and the emotions associated with those memories. On seeing a dog, a person who has been bitten by a dog will have a different emotional experience compared to a person who has not been bitten by a dog. We call this phenomenon *mood congruency.* Mood congruent memory stores not only the facts of the events but also the memory of the mood. This explains why when you feel happy, you recall other happy memories, but when you feel depressed, you remember other depressing events.

DBT addresses the problem of mood congruency by using diary cards. A diary card is a daily tracker of various aspects of the treatment. It tracks moods, urges, and the target symptoms that the patient and therapist have agreed are the treatment's most important aspects. It is also a way of tracking the use of DBT skills, or the lack thereof.

Figure 18-1 shows an example of the type of card we typically use. It can be modified to focus on each patient's treatment needs.

In the following sections, we explain what you track every day on a diary card, including your emotions, reactions, and skills.

Recording your emotions

One of the most common questions that one person asks another is "How are you?" You're likely to hear this question many times a day. Very few of us answer it in an accurate way that describes our exact emotions. Most of the time, we just say "fine."

It can be hard to focus on emotions for three reasons:

>> You don't know what you're actually feeling.

>> Even if you do know how you're feeling, focusing on your emotions can be painful.

>> You don't want to feel a certain way, so you try to numb or avoid your emotions.

REMEMBER

One of the qualities of good mental health is the ability to know and deal with all emotions, and so emotional tracking is one of the components of the DBT diary card. By focusing on specific emotional experiences, not only do you get a chance to become better at accurately knowing what you're feeling, but you also get a better idea as to what is causing the emotions, and what you might be able to do about strong or unwanted emotions. Tracking emotions on a daily basis also allows you to not have to rely on memory to determine what your mood was like last Wednesday, for example.

DBT Diary Card

NAME: _____ DATE: _____

Date	Self-Injury		Urge to isolate	Exercise	Substance Use		Meals		Excessive calls to boyfriend		Hour you went to sleep	SELF-JUDG MENT	Emotions							
	Urge	Action	0-5	0-5	Urge	Action	Balanced ?	Action	Desire to call	Action	Time		Anxiety	Joy	Anger	Guilt	Shame	Sadness	Fear
													0-5	0-5	0-5	0-5	0-5	0-5	0-5

Behavioral Targets

Suicidal Ideation Scale: **0** = No thoughts **1** = Fleeting thoughts **2** = More intense **3** = Very intense **4** = Developing specific plan **5** = Acting on plan

Urge/Emotion Intensity Scale: 0 = Not noticeable 1 = Barely 2 = Slight 3 = Moderate 4 = Strong 5 = Manageable/powerful 6 = Powerful 7 = Intense
8 = Very intense 9 = Unbearable/overpowering

Notes for the Week:

Mon.	
Tues.	
Wed.	
Thurs.	
Fri.	
Sat.	
Sun.	

Agenda Items:

FIGURE 18-1: A typical diary card.

But what is emotional tracking and how does it work? In its most basic form, tracking your emotions is the ability to measure your emotional state over a period of time. The standard diary card does this over a one-week period, which typically covers the time between individual sessions, and it requires you to describe and measure your experience of various emotions each day. By doing this, you provide information for you and your therapist to analyze. In Figure 18-1, you track these emotions under the section labeled "Emotions."

By carefully analyzing the flow of your emotions, the contexts, conditions, and vulnerability factors, you can get a better sense of the situations that make you happy and those that bring or intensify unwanted emotions. By recognizing just how emotionally volatile you might be in certain situations and the factors that lead to these emotions, you take an important step toward improving your mental health.

REMEMBER

Mood tends to be a more enduring state, whereas emotions tend to be triggered by specific incidents in the course of a day. For instance, you might be in a fine mood, but then your friend posts a photo of herself on social media at a party you weren't invited to, which might spark an angry or sad emotion. When tracking emotions, you're assessing your experience of specific emotions over the course of the day. How was my happiness? How was my sadness? Did I feel shame or guilt? By taking a daily, real-time snapshot of your emotions, you're able to build a bigger picture of your emotional makeup, and so get a more accurate sense of yourself, by further identifying the influences that worsen or improve your overall mental health.

Tracking your reactions

Powerful emotions tend to be associated with strong behavioral reactions or responses. When an event occurs, there is a subjective experience, then the body's physiological response, and finally the behavioral response. The following sections look at each of these elements.

The subjective experience

In the same way that we can't exactly know what another person's perception of the color blue is, we can't know what another person's subjective experience of an emotion is. Your own experience of anger might range from mild irritation to uncontrollable rage.

REMEMBER

Also, for most people, an emotional experience might be more complicated than feeling simply one emotion. We don't tend to experience emotions in isolation from each other, such as pure sadness, guilt, joy, or anger. A mixture of emotions over different events is more typical. For instance, you may feel happy that your friend is getting married but also sad that you won't see her as much as you used to. Another friend may feel envious that the friend was able to find a partner. Thus, the emotional experience is subjective in that different people may have different emotions from yours and may experience more than one emotion, as in your case.

Your physiological response

Like most of us, you have probably felt your body react involuntarily in certain situations. For instance, your heart may start fluttering when you see your loved one, your muscles might tense when you get angry, or you might feel faint when looking down from a great height. Many of the physiological responses you experience when you're having an emotional response — for instance, a racing heart, sweaty palms, or a dry mouth — are regulated by a part of the body's nervous system network known as the *sympathetic nervous system.* This system directs the body's rapid involuntary response to certain situations, and it's controlled by hormones that lead to your mind being more alert, and your breathing and heart rate quickening. This is so that more oxygenated blood can get to different parts of your body for when you need it, as in the classic fight-or-flight response. These hormones also signal your body to release stored glucose, a type of sugar, so that you have extra energy should you need it.

For most people, this response happens so quickly that they aren't even aware that it has taken place. This makes sense. If a person were to come across a dangerous snake, they would want their body to react quickly rather than spend time pondering about the nature of snakes.

The sympathetic nervous system is a part of a larger system known as the *autonomic nervous system,* which controls all of the body's involuntary responses, such as blood flow and digestion. However, when someone sees a potentially dangerous snake, it is not only the fight-or-flight response that takes place; an emotional response is also triggered. For fear and anger, this response take place in a part of the brain known as the amygdala. The amygdala has all sorts of important functions beyond being activated by anger and fear. For example, when we're hungry or thirsty, activity in the amygdala motivates us to get food and water.

WARNING

One of the significant concerns about the body's physiological reaction is what happens when someone experiences chronic stress. When this happens, the body doesn't learn to differentiate between what is normal and abnormal, and so the stressful way of being becomes the new normal. With chronic stress, the potentially lifesaving reactions are muted, and people can experience headaches, insomnia, irritability, and weight gain.

The behavioral response

Although a person has a physiological response to a situation, this doesn't mean that a specific behavioral response is inevitable. Nevertheless, when there is a behavioral response, this is the actual expression of the emotion. Some behavioral responses are relatively simple, such as raised eyebrows when you're surprised, a smile or laugh when you experience pleasure or joy, or a grimace of pain or a sigh when you're in despair. Research shows that many facial expressions are universal. For example, a furrowing of the brow and a slight downturn of the mouth tend to indicate sadness. More complex emotions have different behavioral responses, which are affected by our upbringing and culture. For example, the way love is expressed can be different both from person to person and from one culture to the next.

Behavioral responses have various purposes. One is that they are an important way to signal to another person how we feel. But there is arguably a more important purpose, one that is linked to our overall well-being: Research shows that these responses are also vital to our actual well-being. It turns out that if we suppress our emotional response, this adversely impacts our body because suppressing our response leads to more stress.

REMEMBER

Accurately expressing your behavioral responses to situations, whether these responses are positive or negative, is better for your overall health than suppressing them. Thus, it's better to smile, laugh, or cry than to suppress these responses. However, it's important to do this in an effective way, and DBT helps patients recognize unhealthy behavioral responses and replace them with more prosocial, long-term, goal-focused, and effective forms of expression as a path to improved mental health. The other benefit is this: When you're able to accurately and effectively demonstrate your own behavioral responses, you become more accurate and effective in understanding other people's behavior and demeanor.

Identifying the skills you use

Imagine that you have a home project to do. You know you need to make some home repairs, but you're not exactly sure what they are. What tool do you bring to the project? Without knowing exactly what the project is, you have to bring an entire toolbox. If, on the other hand, you know that some floorboards are loose and that you need to nail them back in, you know that all you have to bring is a hammer.

Similarly, if you don't have the right skills to manage emotions, or reactions, or distress, or relationships, then life can be difficult. DBT is all about teaching skills for dealing with difficult or unwanted emotions, for handling difficult moments in relationships, for tolerating difficult moments without making them worse, and for focusing on reality.

Figure 18-2 has a detailed list of the possible skills that you can use to address the areas of concern that brought you into therapy as a patient. For instance, say that you had strong urges to use substances on a Wednesday. You noted this on your diary card (introduced in Figure 18-1). You decided to use Intense exercise and an ice dive, part of the TIPP skill. You would then mark this skill (TIPP) off in the Distress Tolerance section of the skills section of the diary card.

Fill in the number for the degree to which you used skills.

1. Realized later: "I should've used a skill or called for coaching." **2.** Thought about using skills but didn't. **3.** Recognized later that I'd used a skill effectively **4.** Mindfully tried to use a skill but it was not, or was barely, effective. **5.** Mindfully used a skill and it was effective.

Category	M	T	W	F	S	S	Skill
Mindfulness							**Wise Mind:** Accessed truth. I was centered and calm. Balanced emotion mind and reasonable mind.
							Observe: Noticed the experience. Focused my attention. Experienced what is happening.
							Describe: Put observed experiences into words. Used only words, **no judgments.**
							Participate: Enter into the experience. Act intuitively from wise mind. Practice changing the harmful and accepting yourself.
							Nonjudgmental stance: Evaluate but don't judge.
							One-mindfully: Do only one thing at a time. Focus only on the task at hand.
Interpersonal Eff.							**Effectiveness:** Focus on what works. Learn the rules and play by the rules. Act skillfully. Don't act out of spite.
							Objective effectiveness: *DEAR MAN: Describe. Express. Assert. Reinforce. Mindful. Appear confident. Negotiate.*
							Relationship effectiveness: *GIVE: Gentle. Interested. Validation. Easy manner.*
							Self-respect effectiveness: *FAST:* Fair. No Apologies. Stick to values. Be Truthful.
							Prioritize: Rank the importance of your objectives, the relationship, and your self-respect.
							Challenge myths and beliefs: Dispute thoughts and beliefs that are not based on facts and which reduce interpersonal effectiveness.
							Intensity of your ask: Determine how strongly to ask for something or say no to something.
Emotion Regulation							**Identifying primary emotions:** Use the model of emotions to identify your primary emotions SUN WAVE.
							Checking the facts: Identify the facts of a situation (rather than thoughts, assumptions, interpretations, or beliefs).
							Problem-solving: Identify the problem, check the facts, articulate your goal, brainstorm solutions, evaluate solutions, and put a solution into action.
							Opposite-to-emotion action: Change emotions by acting opposite to the current emotion action urge.
							Accumulate positives in the short term: Doing pleasurable things that you can do now.
							Accumulate positives in the long term: Making choices that match morals, values and long-term goals.
							Build mastery: Try to do a new thing you've wanted to master and that makes you feel excited each day, and then build on that every day.
							Cope ahead: Imagine how you would skillfully cope with a difficult situation before you get to it.
							PLEASE: Reduce vulnerabilities to strong emotions: treat Physical illness, Limit screen time, balanced Eating, Avoid drugs, balance Sleep. Exercise daily.
							Letting go of emotional suffering: Attending to emotional experiences without avoiding, clinging or ruminating on them.
							Managing extreme emotions: Crisis survival skills, mindfulness of current emotions, apply emotion regulation skills.
							Troubleshooting emotion regulation: Steps to follow the skills you are using don't help in the moment.
Distress Tolerance							*TIPP: Temperature. Intense exercise. Progressive muscle relaxation. Paced breathing.*
							Distract: Wise Mind *ACCEPTS Activities.* Contributing. Comparisons. Emotions. Pushing away. Thoughts. Sensations.
							Self-soothe with the 5 senses. Enjoy sights, sounds, smells, tastes and touch. Be mindful of soothing sensations.
							IMPROVE the moment: Imagery. Meaning. Prayer. Relaxation. One thing in the moment. Vacation. Encouragement.
							Pros and cons: Consider the pros and cons of tolerating difficult moments and the pros and cons of not tolerating them (engaging in impulsive behavior).
							Observing your breath: Focus on the in and out breath.
							Half-smile: Smile gently, create posture of acceptance, willingness, and openness to experience.
							Awareness exercises: Focus attention on allowing yourself to tolerate distress.
							Radical acceptance: Recognize and accept reality as it is. Freedom from suffering – not adding non-acceptance to pain.
							Turning the mind: Choosing over and over again to accept even though emotion mind wants to reject reality.
							Willingness: Doing what is needed in each situation.
Middle Path							**Validated myself.**
							Validated someone else.
							Recognized need for skill but didn't know which one and recognized the need to reach out.

FIGURE 18-2: A detailed list of skills.

Analyzing Your Behavior

Bringing your diary card (like the one in Figure 18-1) into a session is a key part of your individual therapy. The therapist reviews the diary card at the start of the session and then, if there are concerning behaviors, assesses them with you in a moment-to-moment analysis. The reason for this is that to effectively solve the problems that bring you into therapy, you first have to understand the factors that led to the occurrence of the behaviors, recognize the consequences of the behaviors, and then learn and apply new skills and behaviors so that either old behaviors can be replaced or the sequence of events leading to those behaviors can be disrupted.

In the following sections, we describe three types of behavior analysis: chain analysis, solution analysis, and missing links analysis.

Chain analysis

To understand a specific behavior, a thorough assessment of the problem must be conducted. Working through the analysis, the therapist and the patient identify key points in the chain when the patient could have done something different or could have used a skill that led to a different and more effective outcome. In DBT, this assessment is known as a *chain analysis*.

The following sections explain when and how to use chain analysis and offer an example of a chain analysis.

Understanding when and how to perform a chain analysis

The chain analysis takes place in an individual DBT session. The actual chain analysis is typically done in visual form, written either on paper or on a whiteboard. Note that DBT sessions are organized based on target behaviors that a person wants to and needs to address.

REMEMBER

In DBT there is a treatment hierarchy, and the behaviors that a patient brings into therapy are based on this hierarchy:

1. The reduction of life-threatening behaviors such as suicidal behavior and self-harm

2. The reduction of therapy-interfering behaviors such as non-compliance with therapy or not showing up to sessions

3. The reduction of quality-of-life-interfering behaviors such as the treatment of other psychiatric disorders, substance misuse, and unhealthy relationships

4. An increase in the use of more adaptive and effective behavioral skills — emotion regulation, interpersonal effectiveness, distress tolerance, and mindfulness (as we describe in Part 3)

For patients in the early stages of DBT treatment who are engaging in the preceding behaviors, chain analysis is a common part of the individual therapy session. Very early on in therapy, the patient is oriented to the importance and use of chain analysis. After reviewing the diary card, the therapist picks a specific behavior on the card, if one is present. This could be a self-harm behavior, the patient arriving late for therapy, or getting drunk on the weekend.

The chain analysis is a deep dive into the problem behavior. The goal is that in working together, there is an attempt to understand all of the factors that led to the behavior, including the ones known as the *controlling variables*, meaning the factors that influenced the behavior. Some people feel that doing a chain analysis is a punishment — that is, they would rather talk about something else, but the therapist is "punishing" them by having them do the chain analysis.

For a chain analysis to be effective, the following conditions are essential:

>> The chain analysis is a collaborative exercise between the therapist and the patient.

>> The chain analysis provides a complete picture of the sequence of events, including both the internal (thoughts and emotions) and external cues and triggers.

>> Any conclusions drawn from the chain analysis are considered hypotheses that need to be tested, and if new information shows the hypothesis to be incorrect, the conclusion is then discarded.

The reason this point is important is that consistent with DBT theory, it's more important to test a hypothesis and get accurate information than for a therapist to be insistent that they are right about what happened.

Chain analysis need not only be used for problematic behavior. When patients are suffering and then use a skill to find a moment of being more effective or noticing more joy in their life, it can be useful for the therapist and the patient to carefully analyze those moments as well, to see whether the conditions and behaviors that led to the use of skills and wanted emotions are something that can be repeated. This allows patients to see that some elements of the experience of effectiveness are under their control, rather than believing that they are victims to the forces of life's cruelty.

Earlier, we mention that chain analysis is presented visually, in written form. Later, once the patient becomes more expert with chain analyses, they can do them on their own, and they can present them orally with the therapist, but it's important to do chain analysis in written form at first. Having a visual image, a step-by-step chain of events linking one moment to the next, reminds the patient as well as the therapist that all events are connected and don't happen randomly, even if the patient thinks that they do.

Walking through the steps of a chain analysis example

Harriett, a 23-year-old woman with a history of using alcohol as a way of reducing very intense emotions, particularly fear, presents at therapy with her diary card showing that she drank to the point of blacking out on Saturday night. She was upset that she drank so much, as she had been doing well in therapy.

REMEMBER

The chain analysis conducted with the therapist is the detailed series of events that led to what happened, and contains the following five elements:

1. **Identifying the problem behavior:** In this case it was Harriett's drinking to the point of blacking out as a way to deal with her fear.

2. **Vulnerability factors:** These elements pertain to the person, the environment, or life circumstances that leave the person open to the negative effects of intrapersonal and environmental stressors, such as the prompting events. Common vulnerability factors include being stressed from some life situation, such as conflict at work, lack of sleep, not eating properly, or some physical illness. In Harriett's case, she had just lost her job and was going to be interviewing for a new one. Her anxiety about the upcoming job interview led her to sleep poorly. These vulnerability factors made her less resilient and less motivated to use DBT skills.

3. **Prompting events:** These are the events that happened, either external (meaning something in the environment) or internal (meaning something in the patient's mind or body), such that if the event or events had not occurred, the problem behavior would likely not have occurred. These events could take the form of a memory or flashback. In Harriett's case, her abusive ex-boyfriend called her out of the blue, and on seeing his number show up on her screen, she started to panic and became frightened. Without her ex having called her, she had been managing well in therapy, and it was unlikely that she would have started to drink.

4. **Links in the chain:** Links are the sequential external and internal events that occur between the prompting event and the problem behavior. They include the person's thoughts, emotions, and behaviors as well as environmental factors and the behaviors and actions of other people.

For example, between getting the call from her abusive ex and starting to drink heavily, Harriett thought, "If I don't answer the call, he'll get angry." She didn't answer the call and let it go to voicemail. This then led to increasing feelings of fear, which led to the thought "I am never going to feel good about myself," and this was aggravated by the vulnerability factor of having lost her job. This then led her to feel hopeless, which then led to her thinking that if she had one drink, she would feel better. This led her to feel shame, and to feel that she had let her therapist down, and then to fear that her therapist wouldn't want to work with her, which in turn led her to start drinking more.

5. **Consequences:** Consequences are any specific events, thoughts, and emotions that occur after the problem behavior. In this part of the chain analysis, the therapist looks for factors that might cause the behavior to occur again. There might be positive and negative consequences. On the one hand, drinking took the fear away, which was a positive for Harriett. On the other hand, she felt ashamed that she had gotten so drunk, felt sick the next day, and felt that she had no control over her life, all of which were negative consequences.

By doing these chain analyses over time, the patient has a better sense of the situations that can lead to concerning behavior and then learns what they need to do in order to intervene at a much earlier moment in the chain.

Solution analysis

The aim in DBT is not just to stop the target behaviors. This is because patients will often use these behaviors to stop suffering, and if the therapist gets the patient to stop the behavior, then the patient is left suffering. The aim therefore includes helping the patient resolve the issues that contribute to the behavior and relieve the patient's suffering as well. This requires the generation of problem-solving ideas through the use of a more traditional cognitive behavioral therapy approach. This process is known as *solution analysis.*

There are three components to solution analysis:

1. The generation of solutions

2. The evaluation of those solutions

3. The implementation of those solutions

The way this analysis is performed is to review the patient's analysis chain and to select a specific link in the chain. For instance, in Harriet's case (covered in the preceding section), she received the call from her ex, which was then linked to the thought "If I don't answer the call, he'll get angry." This was linked to her not answering the call and letting it go to voicemail.

After selecting a specific link from the chain analysis, the therapist and patient generate solutions for that link. Ideally, they generate as many solutions as possible before evaluating them, or they can also decide to evaluate the solutions as they arise. For instance, Harriett may have done any of the following (using skills in Part 3):

>> Answered the phone and told him not to call again

>> Used an interpersonal effectiveness skill to be clear that she did not want to hear from him

>> Used the opposite-action-to-fear skill by approaching the feared communication

>> Used a distress tolerance skill

>> Blocked him

>> Called her therapist and asked for advice

>> Called a friend and asked them to come over

>> Took a medication to help her calm down

>> Self-validated that the situation was scary

>> Used cognitive reappraisal to recognize that she didn't actually know why he was calling or if he would be angry

When considering each of these options, the agreed-upon solution (or solutions) from the list is then evaluated to consider how realistic it is. Then, if it seems reasonable, they troubleshoot what might get in the way of implementing the solution if a similar event occurs in the future.

Finally, the solution is implemented. Some solutions, such as blocking the person if that is what was agreed to, can be done immediately. Other solutions, such as calling the therapist and asking for help in the moment, would need to wait until a situation arose. Nevertheless, the patient, in this case Harriett, could practice calling the therapist and asking for help for lesser problems as a way to rehearse asking for help in a similar situation in the future.

Missing links analysis

REMEMBER

The missing links analysis is an assessment of an instance or moment when the patient failed to engage in a behavior or skill that they were trying to practice, or one that would have been beneficial in a situation. Different from a chain analysis, which breaks down and carefully assesses problem behaviors, the missing links analysis is used to identify effective behaviors and skills that are missing or that didn't show up when they should have.

In the example of Harriett from the preceding sections, say that the ex-boyfriend calls again, and her behavior of getting drunk happens again. The missing links analysis is a way of assessing why the behavior explored and agreed upon in the solutions analysis didn't show up. There are many reasons why this might happen:

>> It is possible that very strong emotions led to a forgetting of the plan.

>> In the moment, the patient was unwilling to do what was needed.

>> The patient tried to do what was needed, but other factors got in the way.

>> The thought did not even enter the patient's mind.

The missing links analysis is a useful way to more accurately define a problem. For example, many people know that exercise is good for their overall health but don't do it. If they agree to exercise and then don't follow through, it can be helpful to do a missing links analysis. In doing such an analysis, it can also turn out what was originally considered as the problem was not what was getting in the way. For instance, perhaps the person says that the problem is that they don't belong to a gym. They get a gym membership but still don't go. On assessment, it turns out that the gym's hours of operation are incompatible with the person's work schedule.

Chapter **19**

Gaining and Keeping Motivation

lthough the word *motivation* is easy to define, for most of us, motivation is an elusive notion in practice. In essence, motivation is the desire to want to do something. When it comes to therapy, it can be the desire to want to change our behavior, thoughts, feelings, sense of self, or the dynamics in our relationships. In this chapter, we talk about ways to get, build, and keep your motivation for therapy.

Having Motivation for Therapy

It's very easy to stay motivated for something you really want to do. Imagine a parent telling their 15-year-old child who is addicted to video games to go and play video games for ten hours. That, he would be able to do. Motivation to clean his room, do his homework, and take out the trash may be a different matter altogether.

Another aspect of motivation is that there are things you know are good for you, like healthy eating and exercise, and when it comes to those things, motivation comes and goes, seemingly unpredictably. At times it doesn't even show up. The author Zig Ziglar once quipped, "People often say that motivation doesn't last. Well, neither does bathing — that's why we recommend it daily." Just like other skills in DBT, motivation is something we can practice.

A lack of motivation can result in not engaging in therapy, not working toward short- and long-term goals, and then feeling hopelessness and despair. The problem with motivation is that it's often mood dependent: We feel very inspired when we're feeling happy and optimistic, but we feel very unmotivated when our mood is low.

However, to regain control of your life, you can't wait for your mood to be better and for motivation to show up. For people with a chronically low mood, this might take a long time. That means there is a lot of time wasted waiting for motivation to show up. The more we wait, the more time passes, and the more we feel that what we're doing is of little consequence, which can, in turn, lead to demoralization and depression, which, in turn, impacts motivation. It's a vicious cycle of negativity.

In the following sections, we talk about the difference between the motivation to want to change and having the ability to make the changes when you start DBT, and we explain the importance of acceptance as a part of the motivational process.

Distinguishing motivation and ability

For a lot of people entering therapy, their initial reaction is one of skepticism. Many people who come to DBT have been in other therapies that have not been very useful, and so when DBT promises to be helpful, they raise a doubtful eyebrow.

When the patient has this initial reaction — that is, one of doubt — and then they behave in ineffective and maladaptive ways, the therapist has to consider whether the patient is displaying a lack of ability or a lack of motivation. These two constructs are very different, and in many forms of therapy, patients are blamed for not being motivated when, in fact, they don't have the skills or ability to behave any differently from the way they do.

Most people learn social and regulating abilities by observing others and then doing the things that they do. Over time, this should lead to effective functioning. However, not everyone has enough opportunities to observe, or what they are observing is confusing to them and the behaviors used don't make sense to them. Not having a skill is very different from not having motivation. Most people learn how to regulate their emotions starting in infancy. The constant interchange of emotions between a primary caretaker and their baby is the start of emotion regulation training. Some parents are good at this and have the circumstances to be very present. Some try extremely hard to soothe their child, but because of their own personal difficulties, life circumstances, or inability to regulate their own emotions — and in particular if they have an emotionally sensitive child — the combination of the child's neurobiology and the parent's deficits makes it difficult for the child to learn from the parent.

When a patient shows up to therapy, and they are struggling in their life and not making the changes necessary to feel better, the therapist has to evaluate whether the patient

>> Has the ability to change but isn't motivated to change their behaviors

>> Has the ability to change but something — for instance, strong emotions or other people or life circumstances — is getting in the way of applying the more effective behaviors

>> Does not have the ability or knowledge of what they could do differently to make life easier

Without assessing for ability versus motivation, a therapist may incorrectly decide that a patient is being lazy or unmotivated when they don't in fact have the ability to enact change.

Moving to acceptance

From a DBT perspective, motivation and acceptance are connected. You can't change something without accepting that it's there. If you are overweight, or unfit, or smoking too much, you have to accept that these issues are a problem to the extent that they are. Once a person accepts that some aspect of their life is problematic, if they want to change it, the motivation becomes the person they imagine they will be without the problematic behavior.

The problem, though, is that if you want to do something differently — say, go on a diet, exercise more, or stop smoking — it's often easy to be enthusiastic at the beginning, but then to see that established habits, whether helpful or unhelpful, are hard to change. After the initial burst of energy and health-focused behavior, it's easy to fall back into old and familiar patterns of behavior. This is just normal brain function. If you go with your family on vacation to Mexico, with the intention of speaking Spanish once you're there, when you're back in the hotel room, it's much easier to revert to speaking English than to persist in speaking Spanish.

It's easy to accept that things have to change; however, although you might be in control of your intention and motivation, what you might ignore or forget to take into account is that things in your environment might make change more difficult. When you're trying to make changes, what happens when you start to behave differently? Say, for example, you'd like to go on a diet. You know the long-term benefits of reducing your overall calories and eating a healthier diet. But then, as you decide to start, your favorite binge-worthy TV series becomes free for streaming, and your kids have just ordered your favorite deep-dish pizza with all the toppings. It's easy to decide that you'll start dieting tomorrow. Acceptance includes accepting that things are going to be difficult at times.

To stay motivated, it's critical to pay attention to the thoughts and conditions that show up at the time that you're trying to make changes. If sticking to a diet is paired in your mind with missing your favorite TV show and having to watch your kids eat pizza, then you're much more likely to lose motivation to stick to your diet. On the other hand, if eating more healthily means getting the family's support and them making changes to support you — and then rewarding yourself with a Sunday TV binge after a successful week — then you'll be much more likely to stick with it.

You're more likely to repeat a behavior when something positive or rewarding occurs with it. Sometimes these rewards are external to us — for instance, a bonus at work or a good grade at school — but there are also natural rewards that can help keep you motivated. For example, you may feel a sense of pride that you have stuck to your diet and are beginning to see results.

REMEMBER

To make a change, you have to accept that the problems you're facing are what they are. Then, as you start making changes, you have to accept that there are factors that you won't be in control of, and to anticipate these factors so that you can face them as they arise. Finally, you need to recognize that pairing your change in behavior with a reward can be helpful in keeping you motivated.

Increasing Motivation

When motivation is low, there are things you can do to transform feeling stuck and unwilling into being energized and motivated. For many of us, lack of motivation begins with never actually getting started with the change that we want or that we committed to do. The following sections provide tips taken from cognitive behavioral therapy (CBT) and DBT.

Ideas from CBT

If you recall, DBT is a form of CBT, and many skills are common to both forms of therapy. The following sections cover some CBT methods you can use to increase your motivation for therapy.

Cognitive restructuring

Getting stuck in a cycle of lack of motivation can leave you feeling hopeless. Cognitive restructuring is a way to recognize unhelpful and repetitive thinking patterns and then to learn and apply new, more helpful ways of thinking about difficult thoughts and situations. Cognitive restructuring reverses old cycles of thinking in order to increase your belief in your abilities and sense of self.

For example, imagine that you're struggling with anxiety, and that you notice a pattern of catastrophizing in social situations when you're with people you don't know well. Maybe your pattern goes something like this: "I am such an awkward person. Everyone is aware of that, and no one is ever going to want to talk to me. Because of this, I will always be alone." A key element of cognitive restructuring is gathering evidence and checking the facts. To do this, you can work on chain analysis with your therapist (see Chapter 18) or keep a journal highlighting the situations that trigger this kind of response. You can then challenge each of the statements based on the data you have.

If you state that you're an awkward person, what do you mean by this and what are the aspects of the way you act that you can practice doing differently? If you say that no one is ever going to want to talk to you, you could list all the facts that support this, but if someone does talk to you, then you have to list that as a fact as well. Compare the list of facts that support your assertions, and then the list of facts that show that your assertion is distorted or just plain wrong.

Behavioral chain analysis

We review this skill at great length in Chapter 18. Chain analysis is a tool used by you and your therapist to assess the internal and external factors that are contributing to the behaviors that you want to change. By removing or reducing the influence of the causes of ineffective or maladaptive behavior, and then feeling better about yourself, you become significantly more motivated and likely to make the changes that were previously too difficult to make.

Contingency management procedures

Contingency management works from the principle that we tend to do things that are immediately reinforcing and avoid things that are immediately punishing, irrespective of the long-term consequences. This is what happens, for instance, with addiction. People use dangerous drugs because of the immediate reward they feel, and don't take into account the long-term consequence of using the drugs.

Contingency management is used for motivation by helping patients shift the balance of the consequences of their behavior so that their desired behavior becomes more immediately reinforcing and, because of this, easier to do. For instance, if a person with an addiction has the desired alternative of not using drugs, then the focus is on how to make not using more reinforcing; perhaps there is an important relationship that the patient wants to maintain, and that person would agree to spend more time with the patient if they aren't using.

Systematic exposure

For many people who struggle with doing what they need to do, avoidance prevents them from evaluating doing something different in familiar situations. For instance, they might fear judgment from a co-worker and so not approach them with a request to swap a shift at work. Exposure therapy works on the theory that this type of avoidance keeps us stuck in old patterns. So, by exposing yourself to the situations that you would otherwise avoid, you learn that you aren't as incapable as you imagined, and by repeated exposure, your anxiety decreases. Using this type of exposure helps you master the things that you previously avoided and so increases your motivation to do the very things that you previously found to be aversive.

Mindfulness practice

Mindfulness is the core skill of DBT, and we review it at length in Chapter 9. By noticing mental activity as merely events occurring in your brain, you become increasingly capable of engaging in skillful behavior, even if you feel unmotivated. You notice that "I am not motivated" is simply a thought, and that lack of motivation isn't something you need to act on.

The DBT approach

REMEMBER

DBT addresses motivation by targeting the commitment for treatment. Commitment is a related but distinct concept from motivation. One of the things that we know about any treatment is that people who are committed to do the treatment do better than those who aren't committed. This is true of all treatments, whether physical or psychological. Thus, it's important to work on commitment strategies, as these are tools that are used to improve motivation in patients. The commitment is not only a commitment to target the things the person wants to work on, but is in itself a key therapeutic task and one that needs to be attended to on a regular basis. This is because commitment and motivation are never static; they increase and decrease, depending on many variables. Research has shown that making a commitment or agreement to do something is a strong predictor that you'll actually do the behavior that you committed to.

DBT borrows from the insights garnered from various fields, including social psychology and sales techniques. The following are strategies used by therapists to elicit a commitment from patients in order to improve motivation:

>> **The use of pros and cons:** The therapist elicits from the patient the positives and negatives of doing the therapy and the positives and negatives of not doing the therapy, thereby maintaining the status quo.

>> **Foot-in-the-door, door-in-the-face technique:** This is based on the door-to-door salesman approach. The first part is the *foot in the door:* Here, the therapist makes a request of the patient, such as "Can you refrain from self-injuring for the next four weeks?" The initial request is easy, and if the patient agrees to it, then the therapist asks for more. This is based on research that people who agree to one thing are more likely to agree to subsequent things.

The second part of the approach is the *door in the face.* Here, the therapist asks for much more than what they really want or can realistically expect. Say a person has been self-injuring on a daily basis. The therapist might ask, "Can you commit to not self-injure for a year?" In many cases the patient balks at the request as being too extreme, and the therapist then asks what they are willing to do. Suppose the patient then says, "One month." The therapist then settles for the lesser amount. The idea behind this is that people who say "no" to a request often feel more obligated to say "yes" to the next request if it seems more reasonable.

>> **Reflecting on the success of past commitments:** Here the idea is that if the patient is wavering on the commitment, then the therapist elicits a time when the patient made a commitment and stuck to it. The intention is to highlight that a person has been able to keep their word and stick to what they said they were going to do.

>> **Freedom to choose in the absence of any reasonable alternatives:** Here the therapist gets the patient to reflect on what they will do if they choose not to do the therapy. Sometimes patients are court-mandated to do therapy, or families say that their relative can't live with them if they aren't actively participating in therapy, or an adolescent either chooses to do outpatient therapy or risks being sent to a long-term residential treatment center. The patient has alternatives, but they are much worse than the one being offered.

>> **Devil's advocate:** With this approach, the therapist intentionally argues against the patient's agreement or creates a counterargument relative to the patient's position in order to get them to explore their position even further. The therapist might say something like, "You know, I think that it is great that you're agreeing to therapy. But it is going to be hard to do all the new behaviors that DBT is going to ask of you. Perhaps it will be too hard and it's not worth the effort." The therapist would only use this technique once they were fairly sure the patient was leaning in the direction of agreeing to the treatment.

Maintaining Motivation

REMEMBER

As a patient, being motivated to do DBT allows you to persist through all the challenges and successes of treatment. This can give you the experience of accomplishment as you complete each session and each skills group, and it can be a wonderful feeling when others recognize the efforts you've put in and the changes you've made. Maintaining motivation does the following:

» **Helps you experience improved self-confidence:** Patients who remain motivated know that they can set increasingly higher expectations for themselves and focus on their long-term goals.

» **Gives you a sense of purpose:** When you're motivated, you have a purpose for improving your life and becoming more skillful. This purpose encourages you to persist and complete tasks such as homework, chain analysis, and skills coaching.

» **Helps you overcome challenges as they arise:** By remaining motivated, you're able to overcome challenges as they occur in the workplace, in your relationships, and in your personal objectives, because despite these setbacks, you can keep your eye on your long-term goal and purpose.

» **Encourages you to push on and become more skillful:** Even though your initial goal in DBT may be to reduce self-destructive behavior, as you become more skillful, your therapy objectives will change. Motivated patients are able to continually reevaluate their current situation and work with their therapist to assess the things they need to do to attain their next goal.

In the following sections, we give you tips for keeping your motivation and taking action when your motivation falters.

Your eyes on the prize

REMEMBER

Keeping your focus on your goal is key to maintaining motivation. Here are some ideas for keeping your motivation up during treatment:

1. **Choose your goals using wise mind (which is fully reviewed in Chapter 9).**

Deciding on your goal is a critical first step in achieving a high level of motivation and maintaining the motivation. When you're initially choosing your goals, it's important to consider what you want to accomplish, and to be clear as to why you want to accomplish a particular goal (or goals if you have more than one). You can consider the pros and cons of striving for each goal. Doing this early in therapy will help you choose goals that you are most likely to remain committed to.

2. **Set intermediate goals.**

Setting smaller intermediate goals can help you keep motivated, especially when the long-term goal seems too far off. Imagine you are thinking of climbing Mount Everest. It may seem an impossible task to make it to the top, and so you set your goal of making it to the next camp site on the way up.

3. **Remind yourself of each success.**

If you find yourself struggling to maintain motivation in your therapy, you, or your therapist, can remind yourself of all the achievements you have had so far. Congratulating yourself on reaching small goals along the way can help you stay motivated to continue to work toward your ultimate long-term goal.

4. **Surround yourself with supportive people and stay away from people who bring you down.**

Connections are essential to human well-being. Authentic and supportive relationships can help cheerlead you during difficult times and can help you stay motivated. At the same time, there might be people who you like, but when you think about your relationship with them, you realize that interactions with them get in the way of achieving your goal.

Say that you are trying to stop misusing alcohol. A friend who knows you're in therapy sees that you're struggling and invites you to a party: "Hey, we'll have so much fun, and I'm buying your favorite vodka!" Your friend may want you to have fun and may want you to escape from your struggles, but offering vodka as a solution is inconsistent with your goal of stopping alcohol misuse. You need to be clear with your friend that even though they may be trying to help, they are offering a short-term solution that is inconsistent with your long-term goal.

When motivation fails

When motivation starts to fail, it's easy to focus on the negative and not stick to your goals. You don't feel as confident in yourself because you end up avoiding the bigger picture and just trying to get through the day. This can impact your confidence and your mood. When your confidence takes a hit, your motivation can start to fail. One of the metaphors we use in DBT is that in order to climb out of hell, you need to use a ladder, but when you get to the ladder, you notice that it is hot, and it can seem an impossible task. Pushing onward in therapy, despite the work being hard, is the only way out.

TIP

If this starts to happen, one of the skills you can consider is that of building mastery. You can read more about this skill in Chapter 10. Building mastery is an excellent way to increase your self-confidence. It's the skill of doing things that make you feel accomplished, and it does so either because you're getting better at doing something new or because you feel confident from learning something new.

Here are some other ideas for when you're beginning to feel less motivated. As with all DBT skills, many of these skills are easier written about or said than done, particularly when you're in a low mood or feeling hopeless. Still, continuing to practice when you're in a low mood will ultimately teach you that you can handle the situations you want and those that you don't:

1. Keep your long-term goal in mind.

When motivation fails, people tend to give up because they lose the focus of their goal. Imagine that you're committed to doing your first 5K race. You're jogging along, and when you get to the 4K mark, you feel that you cannot take another step. You can stop and call an Uber to take you back home, or you can remind yourself that you've committed to finish the race. It may be tough if you're feeling tired, but you can slow down and start to walk. Reminding yourself of your goal is one way to address failing motivation.

2. Use your experiences as learning opportunities.

Therapy, like any other endeavor, will have its share of successes and setbacks. If you hit a period of slow progress or what you consider to be a failure, you have the choice of changing your relationship to the challenges you're facing; you can see them as an opportunity to learn something new or to see that adversity need not derail you. By overcoming such moments, you'll learn that you might be more capable than you had previously imagined. Seeing setbacks as a learning opportunity can help you stay motivated in pressing on.

3. Practice being patient.

Be kind to yourself and self-validate. Doing new behavior takes time, and learning new skills and then implementing them takes trial and error. By slowing down, being patient, and being kind to yourself, you can set realistic goals and expectations. There is an old Zen joke that goes like this:

"Master, how long until I reach enlightenment?" asks a student.

The master says, "Five years?"

"Five years?" asks the student. "That's too long! What if I try really, really hard?"

"Ten years," says the master.

The point is that we can't rush what we're trying to achieve. Trying to go faster than we can may cause us to make mistakes and further demoralize us. If the person running the 5K slows down and walks to the end, they will get there, but if they try to force running on untrained legs, they are liable to hurt themselves. By setting realistic and achievable goals, you stay motivated because each success becomes evident.

5

Putting DBT into Action for Specific Conditions

IN THIS PART . . .

Implement DBT to overcome the suffering associated with borderline personality disorder (BPD).

Incorporate DBT into exposure therapy to address post-traumatic stress disorder (PTSD).

Consider DBT as an alternative approach for when standard therapies haven't been effective in conditions like substance use disorders and eating disorders.

Tackle dangerous behaviors and become healthier with the help of DBT.

Chapter **20**

Building Mastery for Mood and Personality Disorders

I n this chapter, you discover how DBT skills can be used to help with the hall-mark symptoms of borderline personality disorder (BPD) as well as the useful-ness of the skills in mood disorders such as depression and mania. You also find ways to apply the skills for dealing with anxiety.

Addressing Borderline Personality Disorder

DBT was originally developed by Dr. Marsha Linehan to treat highly suicidal and self-destructive people. At the time of its development, Dr. Linehan didn't focus on a specific diagnosis; however, over time, it was clear that many of the people who struggled with these symptoms had a condition known as *borderline personality disorder* or *BPD.*

TECHNICAL STUFF

BPD is a common mental health condition. Depending on the research, somewhere between 6 and 15 million people in the United States suffer from BPD. Although the diagnosis is well known to mental health professionals, it isn't well known to the general public. Nevertheless, in outpatient clinics, about 20 percent of patients have BPD, and in inpatient units, nearly 40 percent of the patients have BPD.

So, what exactly is BPD? There are various ways of looking at BPD. In the following sections, we introduce the most widely implemented DBT perspectives using the *Diagnostic and Statistical Manual of Mental Disorders* (DSM), and we share Dr. Linehan's five areas of dysregulation along with tips on how you can use DBT to address those areas.

The nine DSM criteria for BPD

In the mental health profession, both in the United States and many other countries around the world, there is a handbook considered by many to be the authoritative guide to diagnosing mental disorders. Known as the *Diagnostic and Statistical Manual of Mental Disorders* (DSM), it contains descriptions, symptoms, and other criteria for diagnosing all types of mental disorders. The DSM defines BPD as "a pervasive pattern of instability in interpersonal relationships, self-image, and emotion, as well as marked impulsivity beginning by early adulthood and present in a variety of contexts, as indicated by five (or more) of the following [criteria]."

The following sections contain the nine criteria that the DSM uses for BPD.

Frantic efforts to avoid real or imagined abandonment

You might have a strong fear that someone near and dear to you is going to leave you, and because of this fear, you become desperate and then engage in excessive behaviors to prevent abandonment from happening. The fear of abandonment might be triggered by what seems like a minor rejection, such as a friend canceling plans to come for dinner or a therapist not returning your call immediately. This can lead people with BPD to feel uncared for or unimportant. At times, this can lead some people to express the fear as anger. To others, this anger might seem disproportional to the cancellation of dinner plans or the therapist not returning the person's call, but to that person, the fear can be experienced as near intolerable suffering.

When you're feeling abandoned, whether factually or not, you might resort to "reassurance-seeking behaviors," which are behaviors that you use to get reassurance that you won't be left. This might be the excessive calling or texting of your friend or therapist, and at times this might lead your friend or therapist to become annoyed by your behavior. Ironically, these behaviors can ultimately lead to the destruction of relationships and to the very abandonment that you fear.

Unstable and intense interpersonal relationships

Often, because of the fear of abandonment, some people with BPD tend to become rapidly and intensely attached to others. It can be the experience of meeting someone and suddenly falling in love or a similar form of attachment. At first, this can lead to the idealization of the person. However, because the level of attachment is unsustainable, this can lead to the person with BPD feeling let down or disappointed, and the feeling of idealization can lead to one of devaluation. When this happens, it can cause the person with BPD to speak and behave in hurtful ways toward the other person. This in turn can cause the person with BPD to feel ashamed and regretful for what they said, and then to reverse course and begin idealizing the person again.

For the person on the receiving end of the swing of idealization and devaluation, this experience can be confusing and unpredictable, and they can often they feel like it's too much. As you might imagine, these kinds of relationships are stormy and not very stable.

Identity disturbance

Trying to decide who you are, what your values are, and what you're going to do with your life can be difficult, especially if you have strong mood swings. People who struggle with identity disturbance often notice that they have relatively frequent, sudden, and unexpected changes in their life goals, interests, political and religious views, romantic preferences, and values. At times they look to others to see what they should believe in and how they should act. These sudden changes can lead to a confusing sense of self, an erratic employment history, and chaos in their intimate relationships, and also make them unpredictable to not only others but to themselves as well.

Dangerous impulsivity

WARNING

Impulsivity is a common reason for many people with BPD to seek out DBT treatment. Dangerous impulsivity is behaving quickly without evaluating, or even regarding, the consequences of behavior. There are many examples of dangerously impulsive behavior in BPD, but typically the ones that can lead to enduring life problems include disordered eating, unprotected sex with unknown or casually known partners, excessive spending, and reckless driving. Although these behaviors are not dangerous in the same way that suicidal behaviors are, they are very concerning and can have a long-term impact on the person's mental and physical health.

Recurrent suicidal behavior and self-injury

WARNING

Like impulsivity, self-injurious and suicidal behavior is a common reason for wanting DBT treatment. Often, behaviors like self-injury work to calm unbearably intense emotions, and because self-injury works so quickly and is relatively effective in the short run, it can become a frequent go-to behavior. Another reason why patients say they self-injure is to stop the feeling of being numb. People who self-injure say that it helps in the moment, and yet the solution of self-injury is often seen as a problem by other people. This is another dialectic. What one person sees as a problem, the person who self-injures sees as a solution to the problem of how they feel. Most people with BPD ultimately realize that self-injury is not a long-term solution.

Emotional instability

Many mental health experts consider emotional instability to be at the core of BPD. In fact, in some countries BPD is known as Emotionally Unstable Personality Disorder (EUPD). Instability of mood, together with difficulty controlling up and down emotions, is a defining problem for people with BPD.

The hallmark of the mood shifts is that they are often triggered by frustration and interpersonal conflict, and they typically last from a few minutes to a few hours to perhaps a day, although not weeks or months. It is the intensity of the emotions and how uncontrollable they are that makes them different from mood shifts in mood disorders like depression and bipolar disorder. Another aspect is that when powerful, miserable emotions show up, it can feel to the person with BPD as if they have always felt that way.

Chronic feelings of emptiness

People with BPD often feel that they are empty inside. This experience is often the feeling of aloneness. When people feel empty and disconnected, this often leads to their feeling that life is pointless. If you feel this way, you might consider that this sense of emptiness can be alleviated by closeness to others; this certainly makes sense but also leads to the problem that others may find your need for closeness to be more than they can provide or handle.

Expressions of intense, uncontrollable anger

Many early researchers into BPD felt that a person was unlikely to have BPD if they didn't exhibit intense and uncontrollable anger, often triggered by seemingly trivial situations. Today, this criterion isn't essential, although many people with BPD find that they do become extremely angry. Often, the anger is a secondary emotion to sadness, as they are sad that others have seemed, or been, insensitive toward them, and yet rather than experiencing sadness, they rage against the other person. To others, the anger may seem excessive, as if the person with BPD is making a big deal out of nothing. When people with BPD are told that they are making a big deal out of nothing, this in turn can make them feel misunderstood, and even angrier.

Dissociative and paranoid symptoms

If a person with BPD has experienced trauma, and many people with BPD do, they can present with dissociative symptoms and paranoid thoughts. Also, people who are under a lot of stress can experience these symptoms:

» *Dissociative symptoms* are the experience that a person has when they don't feel real or the world doesn't feel real. Typically these symptoms happen during times of high stress.

» *Paranoia* can manifest with the temporary belief that other people are intentionally trying to hurt them or make their life miserable.

Dr. Linehan's five areas of dysregulation

Other than the DSM, another approach is that taken by Dr. Marsha Linehan, who reorganized BPD symptoms into five areas of difficulties or dysregulation. Her approach is a more practical way of considering the disorder. In reconfiguring the disorder in this way, the DBT approach is easily tailored to the treatment plan.

REMEMBER

The word *dysregulation* essentially means "difficulty in managing." DBT considers the following five areas of dysregulation in BPD:

1. **Emotion dysregulation** is characterized by difficulty in effectively managing emotions. It's the experience of being thrown around or driven by strong and rapidly changing emotions. The behavior that ensues is often mood dependent and inconsistent with the person's long-term goals.

2. **Interpersonal dysregulation** is the experience of chaos in close relationships. Frequently there is difficulty managing and maintaining relationships, coupled with the fear of being abandoned by the important people in their life.

3. **Self-dysregulation** is the experience of not seeing oneself as a whole, integrated person and instead struggling to define a sense of self. It's

characterized by an instability in core values, identity, self-image, goals, and ideologies. It can lead to a feeling of loneliness, boredom, and emptiness.

4. **Behavioral dysregulation** is the inability to effectively control the behaviors that are driven by strong moods. It's characterized by the use of behaviors like self-injury, suicidality, exposure to dangerous sexual situations, misuse of drugs and alcohol, disordered eating, dangerous driving, and other potentially life-threatening behaviors to regulate emotions.

5. **Cognitive dysregulation** is the experience of problems in thinking. These include cognitive distortions such as black-and-white or all-or-nothing thinking, or the cognitive experience that either they or the world around them aren't real. The person might also experience episodes of paranoia, such as believing that others are intentionally trying to make their life miserable.

So, how does DBT address the symptoms and difficulties of BPD? Find out in the following sections.

Regulating your emotions

Given that emotional dysregulation is one of the areas of disorder in BPD, and that the characteristics of BPD either are a direct result of emotion dysregulation (such as extreme anger) or function to reduce emotional intensity, DBT is based on the idea that people with BPD don't have the skills to manage these emotions. The idea is that if a person did have the ability to regulate their emotions, they would. Why wouldn't they?

REMEMBER

Given that people with BPD struggle with emotions and their regulation, the goal of teaching the emotion regulation skills (which are fully reviewed in Chapter 10) is to

» Help people with BPD have a better understanding of their emotions. DBT does this by teaching what the function of the emotions are and then what the basic building blocks of a healthy emotional life are.

» Reduce the person with BPD's emotional vulnerability to intense emotions by focusing on factors that intensify and enhance emotions, as well as factors that reduce their intensity.

» Decrease emotional suffering by teaching ways to reduce the level, duration, and impact of intense emotions.

Improving your relationships

Interpersonal dysregulation is another area of disorder in BPD. There are two main ways in which BPD impacts relationships:

>> A person with BPD tends to have relationships that are characterized by sudden attachment, filled with intensity, with extremes of over-idealization and devaluation of the other person. Then, because these relationships can initially feel so good, the person with BPD fears that the other person will leave them. At times this fear is justified, and at other times not. Sadly, the untreated, at times destructive, behaviors of someone with BPD can leave their friends and partners confused and bewildered, and then not wanting to remain in the relationship. When the fear of abandonment is experienced, the person with BPD can become terrified and then display frantic, persistent, and ultimately ineffective behaviors to prevent the real, or imagined, abandonment from happening.

>> Another aspect is that given the emotion dysregulation, which involves all emotions, self-judgments, and the unstable sense of self, someone with BPD has many barriers to effectively addressing conflict, advocating for themselves, tolerating minor empathic failures, and so on. By addressing these symptoms, the person is not then plagued by the insecurities that these symptoms can cause.

REMEMBER

Given that people with BPD struggle with relationships, the goal of teaching the interpersonal effectiveness skills (which are fully reviewed in Chapter 12) is to achieve the following three objectives:

>> **Objective effectiveness** is focused on a person getting what they want when it's their legitimate right, when they want to get another person to do something for them, or in order to refuse an unwanted or unreasonable request. The interpersonal effectiveness skills are also used to resolve an interpersonal conflict or to get one's opinion to be taken more seriously.

>> **Relationship effectiveness** is focused on establishing and maintaining healthy relationships. Thus, the interpersonal effectiveness skills teach the person with BPD ways to keep people in a relationship with them, as well as liking and respecting them. These skills also focus on balancing the immediate goals of the person with BPD with the goals of a long-term relationship, and then remind the person with BPD why the relationship is important to them now and why it will be in the future.

>> **Self-respect effectiveness** is focused on a person with BPD feeling good about themselves. To do this, the person is taught to know and respect their own values and beliefs, and to act in a way that feels moral and also makes them feel capable and effective.

Reassessing your self-image

An unstable sense of self is another core symptom of BPD. This is often tied to not being clear about one's own values, and years of invalidation. As you can imagine, having been told year after year that the way you think, feel, and behave is not right can leave you feeling very uncertain about yourself and your values. The skills of DBT covered in Part 3 focus on getting the person with BPD to ask themselves the following questions:

>> What are my values?

>> Does my behavior reflect these values?

>> What are my goals?

>> Is what I am doing getting me closer to my goals?

>> Will I feel better or worse after I do this?

>> What does my gut tell me to do?

Adjusting your behavior

In DBT theory, one of the problems that an inability to regulate emotions causes for a person with BPD is that instead of adaptive emotion regulation strategies, maladaptive and dangerous behavior might sometimes arise. The idea is that if unwanted emotions become sufficiently intense, people with BPD tend to turn to maladaptive behaviors instead of healthier adaptive ones. The reason this happens is because people with BPD typically find that maladaptive behaviors such as self-injury often have a more immediate effect or are simpler to employ than more adaptive ones.

Unfortunately, although maladaptive behaviors can be effective in reducing unwanted mood states in the short run, they are ultimately problematic, either because of negative consequences such as loss of trust, relationships, self-respect, or hospitalization, or because the behaviors aren't effective over the long term. All of the DBT skills in Part 3 target behavioral dysregulation.

Taming your thinking

People with BPD tend to have *cognitive dysregulation*, which is faulty and inaccurate thinking. People with BPD, and particularly those who have experienced trauma like abuse, can respond to stress with hyper-vigilance or by dissociation:

>> *Hyper-vigilance* is a state of extreme alertness, one that impacts the person's quality of life. This is because they are always on the lookout for hidden

dangers, whether they are real or imagined. There can also be a feeling of paranoia, which can leave the person with BPD feeling picked on or mistrustful of others, or feeling that people are deliberately being mean to them or out to get them.

>> **Dissociation** is a sense that the person doesn't feel real or that the world around them isn't real. They can experience a disconnection between their emotions and their physical self.

REMEMBER

DBT uses mindfulness (see Chapter 9), checking the facts, and grounding skills to address cognitive dysregulation. Grounding skills are techniques that can help the patient pull away from flashbacks, unwanted memories, and negative, challenging, and disconnecting emotions. The goal of these practices is to help move the person from flashbacks of what happened in the past and then, by initially distracting them from whatever they are experiencing, to change the point of focus to the present moment.

Managing Your Moods

DBT has expanded beyond the treatment of borderline personality disorder and is now also used in the treatment of mood disorders, either by itself or as an adjunct to medications. In the following sections, we explain how DBT can be used for depression and mania.

Dealing with depression

Depression is a common mental illness that leads to feelings of sadness, a loss of interest in activities that the person previously enjoyed, low energy, hopelessness, difficulty in concentrating, and at times self-destructive thoughts, including those of suicide. It can lead to various emotional and physical problems and impact a person's ability to function in their work, family, and personal life.

The treatment considered to be most helpful for depression is a combination of antidepressant medication and cognitive behavioral therapy (CBT). Other types of therapy that have been shown to have some benefit for depression include group therapy, interpersonal psychotherapy, and psychodynamic psychotherapy.

REMEMBER

From a DBT perspective, one of the observations is that if a person is depressed, they tend to give up the things that make them happy and not the things that make them depressed. Say that a person enjoys gardening, going for a walk, and reading a book, and that they dislike not showering, staying in bed all day, and not exercising. If that person becomes depressed, in many cases, they stop doing the things that brought them joy and start doing more of the things that don't make them happy. The DBT perspective is that in order to be happier, you have to live an antidepressant life. Self-validation and behavioral activation are key practices:

>> Self-validation is to say, "I am depressed, and it is hard for me to do things that require energy, while at the same time, staying in bed, not exercising, eating, or showering will make me more depressed."

>> Behavioral activation is one of the most important skills used in treating depression. It works because behaviors and feelings influence each other powerfully. Because depression often keeps people from doing the things that bring them enjoyment and meaning, the depression begins to feel even worse. Here are the practices for behavioral activation:

- Understand the downward spiral of depression.

- Monitor your daily activities.

- Identify your goals and values.

- Focus on overcoming difficult moments by building motivation and energy through pleasure and mastery.

- Intentionally schedule daily activities, and purposefully engage in enjoyable and meaningful activities.

- Problem-solve what may get in the way of your being active and engaged.

- Focus on target avoidance (more about this in the next section).

- Be patient yet persistent. Notice frustration if things don't change immediately, and be kind to yourself.

TIP

Central to using behavioral activation is determining the activities that improve your mood and then focusing your attention on doing those things. Make a list of these activities and keep it with you, especially if you're prone to feeling low and you need a reminder. Some activities work more quickly than others. It's important that you know how each activity affects you. The types of activities that many people list as mood enhancers are exercise, meditation, hobbies, time with friends, walking in nature, eating regularly, mastering something that they have wanted to for some time (knitting, a musical instrument, a new language), maintaining a spiritual practice, volunteering, and many others. Notice what works for you. Write them down. When you're feeling low, do those things over and over again, and if one thing doesn't work, try something else. Don't do nothing. If *nothing* would have helped with the depression, you wouldn't be feeling depressed.

WARNING

Another key to targeting depression is to avoid things that worsen the depression. Certain drugs and alcohol can make depression worse. Some music keeps people feeling low; not eating can lead to depression; not showering can make people feel worse about themselves. Staying alone and disconnected can also worsen the problem.

REMEMBER

When you're depressed, do *less* of what makes you more depressed and *more* of what makes you less depressed. This idea may seem obvious, but when you're depressed, it's hard to remember, so it's important to cope ahead for when this arises.

Handling mania

If depression is a mental health disorder where the person's mood and energy are low, mania is the opposite. It is a period of extreme high energy or elevated moods and is one of the core features of bipolar disorder. So, although everyone's mood and energy levels change throughout the course of a day, people with mania not only have elevated mood and energy for days, weeks, and even months on end, but they also experience behavioral and thinking changes.

The main treatment for the mania associated with bipolar disorder is medication — in particular, a class of medications known as mood stabilizers. Therapy is often added to the treatment plan; however, until recently, DBT hadn't been considered.

Nevertheless, there is growing evidence that because DBT is so useful for emotion regulation, it can be used in people who are at risk of having manic episodes. Current studies have reported that the skill sets of mindfulness (see Chapter 9), distress tolerance (see Chapter 11), and emotion regulation (see Chapter 10) lead to reductions in mania and depression, as well as an improvement in *executive function ability,* which is the ability to think and plan.

One factor that could contribute, at least theoretically, to the use of DBT skills in managing mania is that people who are depressed and then begin to feel manic temporarily enjoy the higher mood and energy level, and it's often at that time that they stop taking their medications in order to continue to feel the high. This is often done without the supervision or agreement of the treating psychiatrist. This makes sense in the short run: If you've been feeling low, why wouldn't you want to feel high? However, in the long run, the consequence of allowing mania to run its course is that it can impact relationships and work.

REMEMBER

DBT would be useful for focusing on vulnerability factors that contribute to mania, such as poor sleep patterns and eating behaviors, and then helping the patient to make decisions related to their treatment. For instance, you could compare the pros and cons of stopping the medication with the pros and cons of continuing the medication, and also review the importance of directly communicating with the psychiatrist. In doing chain analysis of the patient's behavior (see Chapter 18), the therapist would also look at the consequences, in the long and short term, of discontinuing medication without being under medical supervision.

Alleviating Anxiety

Anxiety disorders are states of experience marked by excessive fear that often occurs with avoidance behavior. These states are often in response to specific situations but can also occur in the absence of true danger. In other words, the threats can be either real or imagined. In the following sections, we describe anxiety's components, signs, and chemistry, and we provide tips on tackling anxiety. We also explain how anxiety can be good for you (yes, really).

Understanding anxiety's components

To temper the effects of excessive anxiety, it's important to know how it manifests. There are three components to anxiety: cognitive, physiological, and behavioral.

Cognitive

The cognitive component of anxiety shows up as cognitive distortions in various aspects of brain function, including attention, interpretation of events, and the storage of memories. For example, when anxiety is excessive, it can impact attention in that the focus becomes very narrow. This makes sense to some extent. If you're being threatened by a bear in the woods, you want to keep your eyes on it and not focus on your phone or contemplate what you're going to have for dinner. On the other hand, if you're worried that you're going to encounter a bear in the woods, and there is no evidence that there is one, you can spend so much time focusing on the possibility of a bear sighting that you don't enjoy your hike. This can also manifest as racing thoughts.

Thoughts or cognitions are related to overestimating the actual threat and are paired with the minimizing or underestimating of your ability to cope. Thoughts can include the following:

"I'm in danger."

"Something very terrible is about to happen."

"I'm not going to be able to deal with what is going to happen."

Physiological

The physiological component of anxiety is how it shows up in your nervous system. It can impact body functions, resulting in insomnia, nightmares, loss of appetite, and difficulty in digesting food, as well as physical sensations such as a rapidly beating heart, shortness of breath, nausea, and a tremor in your leg.

Physical sensations, whether or not the danger is real, include

>> **A rapid heartbeat:** The benefit of this sensation is that it takes blood away from the parts of the body that don't need it immediately and sends the blood to the muscles that need it, in case you have to fight or run away. If you feel tingly sensations in your fingers and other body parts, it's often because blood is being redirected from the skin and periphery to the big muscles.

>> **A faster breathing rate:** You breathe faster to get more oxygen into your system, and then the faster-moving blood carries this oxygen to the muscles that need it. After a while, though, you might experience shortness of breath, chest pain, and the feeling that you're choking.

>> **Tense and shaking muscles:** In excess, this can also cause muscle aches and pain.

>> **Sweating:** This stops the body from overheating.

>> **A dilation of your pupils:** This improves your vision in the event of an attack or a need to escape.

Behavioral

The behavioral component of anxiety consists of the actions that a person takes to prevent the exposure to the perceived or real feared threat. Typical behaviors associated with anxiety include avoidance, such as avoiding bridges, certain people, the outdoors, or public speaking. They also include the use of substances such as alcohol and prescribed medications to lessen the feeling of anxiety in situations where there are a lot of people, which can happen in conditions such as social anxiety.

Examples of behaviors include the following:

>> Avoiding certain people, places, or situations

>> Refusing to leave the house

>> Only going to places with someone you trust

>> Having a plan to leave somewhere early the minute anxiety shows up

>> Using drugs (prescribed or not) and alcohol to numb yourself before facing a potentially anxiety-provoking situation

>> Using safety behaviors like playing with a fidget toy, twirling your hair excessively, using compulsions like tapping on wood so that "bad things" don't happen, and not looking someone in the eye

Checking out anxiety's common presentations and chemistry

Commonly experienced types of anxiety presentations include the following:

>> **Panic attacks:** These are characterized by episodes that typically last only a few minutes and have symptoms such as a rapid heart rate, sweating, trembling and shaking of the body, shortness of breath, chest pain, dizziness, and a fear that you are going crazy or are going to die.

>> **Specific phobias:** These are anxiety attacks that are caused by a fear of specific situations or things such as heights, spiders, snakes, or enclosed spaces. A form of this is *social phobia,* which is a marked and persistent fear of social situations.

>> **Generalized anxiety disorder:** This is the broad presentation and experience of anxiety. To be diagnosed with this disorder, the experience of excessive anxiety has to have persisted for more than six months. People who suffer from anxiety disorders recognize that the anxiety affects various aspects of their life and that they have a difficult time controlling their anxiety. Typical symptoms include restlessness, poor sleep, fatigue, difficulty concentrating, irritability, gastrointestinal problems, and muscle tension. All of these can cause significant impairment in a person's day-to-day life obligations.

So what exactly happens to your body when you experience anxiety? When you encounter a perceived threat — say, having to meet your boss for some unknown reason — some neurons deep in your brain send an alarm throughout your body. Through a combination of various signals, the adrenal glands, which are located on top of your kidneys, release a surge of hormones, of which adrenaline and cortisol are the most relevant.

Adrenaline causes your heart rate to increase, your blood pressure to elevate, and your body to release energy stores. Cortisol, which is the primary stress hormone, increases blood sugar levels and enhances the brain's ability to use glucose; it's also a potent anti-inflammatory that prevents tissues from being damaged. Cortisol also stops the body from performing non-essential activities that would be detrimental in a fight-or-flight situation. For instance, it slows the digestive system, which wouldn't be necessary in a fight-or-flight situation.

WARNING

Although cortisol is an essential chemical, when the body continues to produce it beyond the point that it is useful, it can have negative effects. For instance, it can lead to persistently increased blood sugar levels, increased weight gain, a suppression of the immune system, high blood pressure, heart problems, and memory problems.

Tempering excessive anxiety

So, once you understand how anxiety works, what do you do when you experience it? You can identify and address anxiety triggers, as well as apply specific DBT skills.

Steps to identify and address triggers

It would be wonderful if you could just know at any point exactly what led to your anxiety, but this is often not the case. Typically, we suddenly notice that we are anxious and have little idea where it came from. Without identifying triggers, it's difficult to do anything about them. Here are the steps to take in order to do so:

1. **Identify the triggers to your anxiety.**

   Ask yourself, "What are the situations, when are the hours of the day, who are the people I am with, that I am likely to be more or less anxious?" See whether you can establish a pattern. This is like doing your own chain analysis (see Chapter 18). If you do see a pattern, then ask yourself whether there are things that you can do differently in situations where you're facing similar circumstances.

2. **Do things differently than the behaviors that keep you or make you more anxious.**

   People with anxiety often perform what are known as *safety behaviors*. These behaviors make the person feel more comfortable in the situation by providing temporary relief from anxiety created by the situation. Examples of such behaviors include the following:

- Not making eye contact to avoid being noticed by others

- Drinking alcohol or using drugs to feel less anxious before you face a situation

- Tapping on wood if you believe something bad will happen if you don't

- Wearing a turtleneck or scarf so people don't see your neck if it tends to become red when you're anxious

The problem is that safety behaviors lead to the persistence of anxiety and don't allow for the anxiety to improve. And so, if avoiding situations and using safety behaviors leads to the maintenance of anxiety over the long term, then it makes sense that learning to confront anxiety directly will be uncomfortable at first.

You've identified the things that make you anxious, and now the commitment is to make a plan to gradually do the very things that normally make you anxious! For instance, if you normally avoid speaking on the phone or using a video application to connect with your friends, then start by picking someone you're more comfortable with and call them. Don't pick the person you're most anxious to speak to in person. At first it will feel uncomfortable; however, the more you put yourself in the situation of actually speaking by phone and not using safety behaviors, the sooner you'll notice that you have mastered anxiety.

If you have a fear of going to a certain place, perhaps it brings you unwanted memories because something bad happened there, and you're avoiding going to that place. You can start by driving near the place, then driving to the place, and finally getting out of your car at the place and walking around. Of course, we're assuming that the place isn't naturally dangerous. If you were swimming near some rocks during a stormy ocean and got hurt on the rocks, the task isn't to go back to those rocks during a stormy ocean day and try again, but if you're avoiding the beach altogether, then you can go back to the beach and find a safer place to swim.

REMEMBER

It's important to recognize all the safety behaviors you might be engaging in. List them all and make sure you haven't left any out. Then, in anxiety-provoking situations, start by dropping the least important ones.

DBT skills for when you're feeling anxious

Although DBT wasn't developed to treat anxiety disorders, many of the skills can be useful when you're feeling anxious. In addition, people with conditions like BPD are also prone to have anxiety and so they are familiar with the DBT skills;

rather than coming up with other skills, they can use the ones they know. Check out the following steps:

1. Use the STOP skill, which we cover in Chapter 11.

2. To deal with anxious thoughts, check the facts of the situation:

- What precisely am I reacting to?

- What are my fears?

- What is the worst that could happen? Use the Negotiate skill covered in Chapter 12.

- Is my current response proportionate to the threat?

- If the situation happens, do I have the skills to cope?

- Am I suffering ahead of when I need to suffer?

- Do I really have the ability to predict the future?

- What advice would I give a loved one if they were in my situation?

- Can I ask a friend or colleague for help?

- If I react in a certain way, are there negative consequences to that way of reacting?

3. To deal with the physical sensations of anxiety, try these tips:

- Practice paced breathing, with a slow in-breath and a slower out-breath.

- Practice a visualizing breath: Breathe in and picture yourself calm, and then breathe out and picture yourself strong.

- Do some aerobic exercises to burn off any excess energy: Go for a walk, a hike, a jog, or a swim, work in the garden, or do necessary housework.

Experiencing anxiety as a helpful signal

Anxiety is the feeling of worry, nervousness, or being unsettled, and it typically shows up when something threatening might be about to happen or when there is an uncertain outcome to something that is important to you. Anxiety also has an upside. It is the body's way of responding to being in danger or signaling that you're under threat or that you're worried about something. A certain dose of anxiety can help you be more alert, attentive, and focused. For example, just prior to an exam, a little anxiety is what you need. Being too calm and thinking about your beach vacation would be detrimental. Some exam anxiety can have a positive effect and keep you focused on the task of taking the exam.

Like any signal, it's important to pay attention to it and what it's telling you, and so if the exam anxiety were to spill into non-exam life, this would lead to the adverse effects of anxiety. When your body reacts anxiously to real or imagined threats, your brain produces adrenaline and cortisol. Memory loss can occur if the process of cortisol production happens when the fear or anxiety is excessive or persists beyond the duration of the actual threat.

REMEMBER

Some anxiety can be beneficial. It can help you focus, pay attention, and remember things better. When things we need to remember are stored with an emotional tag, they are easier to remember. However, there is a limit to the beneficial effects of anxiety, as too much anxiety for long periods of time can lead to adverse health effects.

Chapter **21**

Taming Trauma

D espite the efficacy of DBT, for many years there was a large gap in our ability to treat trauma for those who came to us with traumatic experiences or post-traumatic stress disorder (PTSD). In fact, the field as a whole struggled to treat trauma when it was co-occurring with self-destructive behaviors.

The dilemma was glaringly clear: There was a subset of patients who experienced trauma and who also struggled with self-destructive and suicidal behaviors. DBT could treat the self-destructive and suicidal behaviors, but would not target the trauma until patients could be free of those behaviors for one year, and clinicians who specialized in trauma would not treat people who struggled with self-destructive and suicidal behaviors because they feared that the treatment would exacerbate these life-threatening symptoms. They tried, but the requirement to be free of high-priority targets such as suicidal behaviors and self-injury for one year proved almost impossible because it was often those very behaviors that were helping patients cope with the unrelenting and untreated trauma symptoms. While patients learned skills, it was too long to wait for the treatment they needed. This was a huge problem. It turns out that about 66 percent of people with PTSD have two or more psychiatric disorders, and up to 30 percent of those people attempt suicide.

In 2005, Dr. Melanie Harned, who worked closely with Dr. Marsha Linehan (DBT's founder), began developing DBT Prolonged Exposure (PE) treatment to address this gap. Her goal was to treat what she called "high-risk multi-problem" patients (adults and adolescents) who were already receiving DBT and were also diagnosed with PTSD or trauma. She took two gold-standard, evidenced-based treatments — PE to treat trauma and DBT to treat self-destructive and suicidal behaviors — and integrated them to create DBT PE. Her goal was to decrease the time that DBT patients had to wait before they could receive trauma treatment. On average, DBT PE treatment starts after 20 weeks of DBT treatment, and the trauma treatment takes an average of 13 sessions. Multiple studies have demonstrated the effectiveness of this treatment, and it was a groundbreaking development in the field of psychology. Not too long after, in 2013 Dr. Martin Bohus of Germany also developed an evidenced-based treatment using DBT to treat trauma. His treatment was called DBT-PTSD.

In this chapter, we look closely at DBT treatment for trauma. We discuss how it works and how you know when you're ready for this treatment, as well as skills you need to develop to be successful.

Understanding the Basics of DBT PE

REMEMBER

Like DBT, DBT PE also uses stages as the foundation to deliver the treatment. DBT PE has three stages:

>> **Stage 1** treatment is standard DBT. You attend weekly individual DBT therapy and a weekly skills group, your therapist participates in a consultation team, and you have access to off-hours skills coaching (all covered in Part 4). The goal of this stage is to help you gain control over your life-threatening behaviors and learn the four skills of DBT: mindfulness, distress tolerance, emotion regulation, and interpersonal effectiveness (see Part 3). You learn the skills you need to effectively work on your trauma without moving back into self-destructive behaviors to cope.

>> **Stage 2** begins your trauma treatment. Once you have achieved behavioral stability and not engaged in life-threatening behaviors for eight weeks, you're eligible to begin. Prior to the development of DBT PE, the waiting period was one year free from life-threatening behaviors. During Stage 2, the structure of your treatment changes from a weekly 60-minute session to weekly 90- to 120-minute sessions. During this stage you'll continue to receive standard DBT as well.

>> **Stage 3** begins after you've completed your PE work. Now you return to standard DBT to work on any remaining problems that are impacting your life. During this time, you may work on increasing skills to use at work or school, or on improving relationships in your life.

In the following sections, we discuss one of the main issues in PTSD — avoidance — and how DBT PE works to treat avoidance. We also give you pointers on determining whether you're ready to try DBT PE.

Breaking down types of avoidance

Many people who struggle with anxiety avoid things. Avoidance can be any behavior, including thoughts or actions that you take to escape from difficult or painful thoughts or emotions. Avoidance is key in PTSD. In fact, avoidant behaviors are one of the symptoms of PTSD that actually perpetuate PTSD and can prevent recovery.

REMEMBER

There are two common types of avoidance that you may engage in when you have PTSD:

>> You avoid thinking about your trauma or feeling emotions around your trauma. People use many strategies to avoid thinking about what happened. Some may be able to just ignore it, numb themselves, or distract themselves when the memories come to mind, but more commonly, people rely on *dissociation* (becoming disconnected from the present moment as a way to avoid coping with painful memories or feelings related to their trauma) as well as self-destructive or other problematic behaviors to shift their attention.

>> You avoid reminders of the trauma. For example, you may stop seeing or talking to certain people, going to certain places, doing certain activities, wearing certain clothing, and so on.

WARNING

The challenge with avoidance is that it works in the short run. That is, you avoid a situation or person or push away a thought or a feeling, which reduces your distress. However, this is only a short-term solution, as this strategy unfortunately makes your symptoms of trauma worse in the long run.

Seeing how DBT PE works

PE works on your avoidance. DBT PE teaches you ways to stop avoiding so that you can effectively process your trauma with your therapist without returning to self-destructive behaviors. The process of doing this is called *exposure*.

REMEMBER

You do two types of exposure work in DBT PE: imaginal exposure and in vivo exposure:

>> *Imaginal exposure* involves sharing, in detail, the events of your trauma with your therapist. You'll describe out loud to your therapist, in as much detail as

possible, what happened to you. Initially you may not remember all of the details, but it's common that the more you engage in imaginal exposure, the more details you'll remember.

During the second part of your exposure session, you and your therapist will talk about your thoughts and feelings during and after the exposure. Your therapist will help you think about what happened to you in ways that will begin to reduce your trauma symptoms and help you find new perspectives about what happened. During your imaginal exposures, your therapist will help you focus on different parts of the trauma and support you as you skillfully navigate the thoughts and feelings that arise.

These imaginal sessions will be recorded, and your therapist will assign you homework to listen to these sessions at home in order to continue working on the imaginal exposure outside of your individual sessions.

>> *In vivo exposures* help you tackle the "real-life" things that you've begun to avoid because they remind you of your trauma, or safe things that you've begun to feel are dangerous as a result of your trauma. For example, part of your trauma may have involved an elevator, and as a result you have begun to avoid all elevators. As a result of your trauma, you feel elevators are dangerous and should be avoided; however, in general, elevators are safe spaces and are of significant convenience, especially if you live or work in an apartment or office building. In this case, learning how to use elevators again without feeling extreme distress could be an in vivo exposure task.

You and your therapist will brainstorm a list of these "real-life" things; they could be places, activities you used to enjoy, people you liked to spend time with, and even foods. Together, you'll create what is called hierarchy and rate your level of distress for each task. You and your therapist will decide where to start. You'll practice in vivo exposures outside of your therapy sessions.

REMEMBER

While challenging to do, both types of exposure have been found to be very effective in reducing avoidance and therefore reducing symptoms of trauma. Before and after each exposure, you'll fill out a special exposure recording form. This form will help you rate the intensity of certain thoughts, feelings, and urges, and it will also help you track the effectiveness of each exposure as well as the entire exposure process throughout the treatment. It isn't uncommon for people with trauma to avoid so many things that it's difficult to feel like they are living at all. These exposures will help them open their life back up so that it feels more meaningful and enjoyable to live.

When you've completed your exposure sessions, you and your therapist will create a relapse prevention plan. By the end of this treatment, you'll be an expert in exposure. You and your therapist will think about ways you can continue to practice exposures on your own and begin living what we call an *exposure lifestyle*. This kind of lifestyle keeps you aware of how your anxiety may lead you to return to old avoidant behaviors and encourages you to practice making decisions using your wise mind rather than letting your fear interfere.

Knowing when you're ready to start

REMEMBER

Doing DBT PE treatment is a big commitment. We would argue that when you're ready to do it, your hard work will really pay off. That being said, there are criteria to help you know when you're ready to begin this treatment. Dr. Harned has identified six readiness criteria that you must meet to begin DBT PE:

1. You are not at imminent risk for suicide.

2. You have not made any suicide attempts or engaged in any non-suicidal self-injury in the past two months (eight weeks).

3. You are sufficiently skillful and committed to managing urges to commit suicide and self-injure when triggered to do so.

4. You do not engage in *therapy-interfering behaviors* (behaviors that get in the way of effective therapy such as cancelling sessions, not completing diary cards as described in Chapter 18, not doing homework, dissociating as covered later in this chapter, avoiding talking about important topics, using "I don't know" as avoidance, or other behaviors that make your therapy less effective).

5. Your PTSD is your highest-priority treatment goal.

6. You are willing to experience intense emotions without engaging in avoidant behaviors.

REMEMBER

Doing this treatment is hard work. Before you embark on this journey, you'll work on these readiness criteria with your therapist. While your PTSD treatment can start as soon as you have been able to avoid suicidal and self-injurious behaviors for eight weeks, it will likely take a few more weeks before you feel confident about meeting all of these other very important readiness criteria.

DBT-PTSD: Exploring an Alternative Model

Dr. Martin Bohus had a particular interest in treating PTSD resulting from childhood sexual abuse (CSA). In Germany, he developed DBT-PTSD for people with the diagnosis of complex PTSD (c-PTSD) with and without the diagnosis of borderline personality disorder (BPD). While there are differences in these two models of treatment (DBT PE and DBT-PTSD), there are also may similarities, including that they both treat symptoms from CSA. DBT-PTSD is completed over 12 weeks in a residential setting (currently in Europe) or 45 therapy sessions in the outpatient model. The treatment is divided into phases, first pre-treatment followed by seven consecutive phases that are identified by theme:

1. Take a full history of your life and trauma.

2. Provide psychoeducation about your trauma and explain how your PTSD functions in your life.

3. Identify your avoidance behaviors and teach you more effective skills to cope with dissociation and your strong emotions.

4. Identify the first trauma you want to work on.

5. Work on guided exposures to your trauma.

6. Focus on learning to practice acceptance of the past.

7. Planning on using skills for a new life that is free of PTSD symptoms.

When you look at the phases, you can see the overlap with DBT PE. While DBT PE focuses on repeated or prolonged exposures to the story of the trauma and then processing using DBT as well as in vivo exposures to things you are avoiding in your life, DBT-PTSD helps you put the story of your trauma together by exposing yourself to the story of your trauma but focusing even more on the very painful emotions, including a sense of powerlessness, body sensations, and thoughts that you experienced during the exact moment that your trauma happened. This treatment uses exposure but focuses less on prolonged or repeated exposures like you learned about in DBT PE. DBT-PTSD relies less on your "thinking system" than DBT PE. That being said, both are very effective evidenced-based treatments that help you work on both your thinking and your feelings about your trauma.

REMEMBER

Many people ask us, "How would I know which treatment is right for me?" This is a great thing to talk with your therapist about. For many, the decision is made by which treatment your therapist or therapists in your area are trained in. Currently, DBT PE is more common in the United States, but there are DBT therapists trained in both models.

Digging into the Dilemma of Dissociation

WARNING

Dissociation is a common symptom of trauma and one that gets in the way of being able to engage effectively in DBT PE. Dissociation is a disconnection in how you experience yourself and the world around you. Many people feel disconnected from reality, and so they may experience perceptual changes, where things look dreamy or distorted. They may feel disoriented or disconnected from their body or emotions, they may lose track of time, or they may not respond to those around them. Dissociation can be scary and can last for some time, but without intervention, it will eventually end on its own. That being said, it will interfere with your life and will get in the way of your progress when you do PE.

The good news about dissociation is that you can learn skills to manage it, catch it early, and prevent it from taking hold. You and your therapist can get a lot of information about your dissociation by doing chain analysis (see Chapter 18) to identify some of the early signs, or red flags that you can look for that will signal you to use your skills to get grounded. Being able to catch dissociation is a critical skill to learn and practice before you start DBT PE.

TIP

The most common set of skills to manage dissociation are called *grounding skills.* Here are a few skills you can try when you feel yourself heading into dissociation:

>> **Use your five senses.** Try naming five things you see, four things you physically feel, three things you hear, two things you smell, and one thing you taste.

>> **Ice dive.** Fill a bowl of ice and water, and submerge your face in the bowl to activate your dive reflex. Find out more about this distress tolerance skill, called TIPP, in Chapter 11.

>> **Use a balance board.** It's physically impossible to dissociate on a balance board. While it isn't a very portable anti-dissociation skill, it can be helpful to have at home or to use in your therapist's office.

>> **Hold an object.** Keep an object nearby or in your bag that you can hold in your hand and focus on. Some people find it helpful to keep a disposable ice pack with them that they can pop and feel the cold sensation in their hand. Others find things like stress balls or putty to focus on.

>> **Feel the floor.** Try lying on the floor. Feel the back of your body pressing against the floor. Sometimes it's helpful to move your arms and legs along the floor or carpet as if you're making a snow angel. This gives you a lot of sensory information to focus on.

>> **Focus on your floating tongue.** Focus your attention on your tongue. Try to let your tongue float in your mouth so it doesn't touch the sides of your mouth or your teeth.

REMEMBER

Dissociation can be a challenge to manage, but with skills and practice, you can learn how to catch it early and focus your attention to ground yourself. It's very common to work with a therapist to learn more about dissociation and how to manage it so that you experience it less and you can effectively engage in trauma treatment.

Chapter **22**

Tempering Addictions

Many people who engage in addictive behaviors and who then develop an actual addiction find that overcoming the addiction can be challenging. In this chapter, we explain how brain chemistry is central to addictive behavior and the role that the chemistry plays in maintaining the addiction. We also review some ideas from DBT as to how to overcome these behaviors and possible disorders.

A Word about Dopamine

Dopamine is a chemical known as a neurotransmitter. It's responsible for transmitting signals between the nerve cells, which are also known as *neurons.* When neurons that contain dopamine are activated, they release the dopamine. When this happens, there is more dopamine in the brain than normal, which causes the person to experience feelings of pleasure. Typically, this happens when a person is doing something that is enjoyable. In many ways, dopamine is essential for survival as the experience of dopamine reinforces survival behaviors such as eating and sexual behaviors for procreating. However, because it's a feel-good chemical, it's also a key player in addiction.

When we're about to eat our favorite meal or when we're waiting for our love interest to show up for a date, dopamine signals our brain that a reward is on its way. Then, when we actually engage in eating our favorite food or experiencing romantic activities, dopamine sends a further chemical message to the brain: The thing you're doing is rewarding. This message then becomes hardwired, a process known as *conditioning*. It makes sense that food and procreation should be connected to feeling good. This stimulus (food and sex) and reward pattern is critical to the viability and survival of our species (and of all species, for that matter).

However, the use of drugs, alcohol, gambling, pornography, and shopping can also lead to dopamine release, and if a person is addicted to any of these things, the dopamine levels in the brain can be as much as five to ten times the normal level, swamping the mood center of the brain. The person's brain then associates the dopamine rush with the activity, and so creates the desire to repeat it. If the person becomes habituated to the level of dopamine, they then need higher levels of the drug or behavior to achieve any feelings of pleasure at all.

WARNING

Most addictive drugs activate the release of dopamine. When this happens, there is a surge in dopamine in the brain. Because the brain can't handle such a high level of dopamine on a sustained basis, it starts to lower the level of dopamine receptors, and so the person no longer experiences the same pleasurable feeling that they did. This why people need increasing amounts of a drug to feel good. The user attempts to achieve feelings of pleasure at any cost, leading them to ramp up the amount of the drug and the frequency of use, thereby cementing the drug dependency. The increased tolerance to the drug and the elevated level of addiction can become life threatening. However, over time, persistent drug use eventually impacts the brain pathways and neurons, and this can cause permanent brain damage.

Working through Substance Dependence

Although DBT is a well-established treatment for people with difficulty in regulating emotions and who are self-destructive and suicidal, it has moved beyond the treatment of mood and personality disorders. Many people who struggle with self-destructive behaviors also have substance use disorders (SUDs) that complicate their condition. DBT has evolved to help people who also deal with substance misuse. Standard DBT, or even DBT for substance abuse, isn't the standard of care for people who have addiction as their primary diagnosis. However, it can be particularly useful for people who have borderline personality disorder (BPD) as well as a SUD, given that people with both of these conditions are susceptible to emotional dysregulation and the observation that the use of substances is sometimes in the service of emotion regulation that goes beyond the addiction.

In standard DBT, the highest-priority target is suicidal and self-injurious behavior. For people who are dependent on substances, the specific drug of misuse is the highest-priority DBT target within the category of behaviors known as quality-of-life-interfering behaviors. Specifically, the goals of therapy are for the patient to

>> Decrease the use of these substances, including illicit drugs, alcohol, and legally prescribed drugs that aren't being taken as prescribed.

>> Alleviate the physical discomfort associated with withdrawing and then being abstinent.

>> Diminish the urges, cravings, and temptations to misuse drugs.

>> Avoid situations that remind the person of the drug use.

>> Delete the phone numbers of drug dealers and casual acquaintances associated with drug use.

>> Consider getting a new phone number.

>> Throw away drug paraphernalia.

>> Reduce behaviors that interfere with giving up drugs, such as giving up on the goal of abstinence.

>> Increase healthy reinforcements such as a community of supportive friends, pursuing charitable social and vocational activities, and even seeking environments that support abstinence and punish drug-abuse-related behaviors.

The following sections discuss substance use versus substance-induced disorders, important DBT skills for people with SUDs, how DBT for people with SUDs differs from standard DBTs and other therapies, and considerations for using DBT with people who have SUDs but don't have emotion dysregulation.

Distinguishing substance use and substance-induced disorders

The reason why people misuse or become addicted to drugs is that they activate the brain's reward system. Some drugs do so in a very powerful way, and this is what causes addiction. Imagine some very happy moment in your life. Now imagine that you could have that feeling whenever you wanted it and also experience it more intensely. That rewarding feeling created by drug use can be so profound, so all-encompassing, and so powerful that the person neglects all other normal activities in favor of getting and then taking the drug.

The *Diagnostic and Statistical Manual of Mental Disorders*, Fifth Edition, known as the DSM-V or DSM-5, is the guide that mental health experts use to name, describe symptoms of, and expand on the diagnostic features of every recognized mental illness — including addictions. The DSM-5 recognizes substance misuse–related disorders resulting from the use of ten separate classes of drugs: alcohol; caffeine; cannabis; hallucinogens (drugs such as LSD and mushrooms); inhalants; opioids (such as heroin or fentanyl); sedatives, hypnotics, or anxiolytics (and these include legally prescribed drugs); stimulants (such as cocaine and other legally prescribed stimulants); tobacco; and substances that have not yet been defined.

REMEMBER

Although each of these drugs works differently, the activation of the reward system is similar in that they produce a wanted state, typically consisting of feelings of pleasure or euphoria, or of numbness. It's also important to note that not everyone will automatically become addicted to all drugs, and different drugs impact people differently. Also, not everyone is genetically or environmentally vulnerable to the effects and availability of drugs. Further, some people are more impulsive and have lower levels of self-control, traits that predispose them to develop an addiction if they're exposed to drugs.

There are two types of substance-related disorders: substance use disorders and substance-induced disorders.

Substance use disorders

Substance use disorders are defined as patterns of symptoms resulting from the use of a substance that a person continues to take despite experiencing problems and negative consequences as a result of taking the substance.

A variety of criteria are necessary to diagnose a substance use disorder:

>> If prescribed, taking the medication in larger amounts or for longer than it is meant to be taken

>> Wanting to reduce or stop using the substance but not being able to do so

>> Spending a lot of time getting, using, or trying to recover from the use of the substance

>> Having persistent cravings and urges to use the substance

>> Being unable to function at work, home, or school because of substance use

>> Continuing to use the substance, even when it causes problems in important relationships

>> Neglecting significant social, family, work-related, or recreational activities and obligations because of substance use

>> Continuing to use substances, even when it puts the person in danger

>> Continuing to use the substance, even when it causes or worsens physical or psychological symptoms

>> Needing to use increasing amounts of the substance to get the desired effects — this is the development of tolerance

>> Developing withdrawal symptoms, which are then relieved by taking more of the substance

Substance-induced disorders

Substance-induced disorders are mental problems that develop in people who didn't previously have a mental health problem before they started using substances. The conditions include substance-induced psychotic disorder, bipolar disorder, depressive disorder, anxiety disorder, obsessive-compulsive disorder, sleep disorder, sexual dysfunction, cognitive disorder, and intoxication.

The category of intoxication has its own subcategories. The types of intoxication include marijuana, alcohol, cocaine, methamphetamine, heroin, and hallucinogen intoxication, as well as substance intoxication delirium. *Delirium* is a sudden change in brain functioning that causes mental confusion.

Looking at DBT skills for substance use disorders

After the patient has learned the basic DBT skills (see Part 3), there are a set of DBT skills that people with SUDs can use, as you find out in the following sections.

Clear mind

REMEMBER

DBT uses the idea of wise mind being the synthesis of emotion mind (where our thinking and behaviors are driven by emotions) and rational mind (where our thoughts and behaviors are driven by logic). In the modification of DBT for SUDs, patients begin treatment in a mental and behavioral state termed *addict mind.* In this state of mind, the person's thoughts, emotions, and actions are under the control of substances. Once the person has achieved an increasingly lengthy period of abstinence, they then develop a perspective that is termed *clean mind.* In this state, they are no longer using substances; however, they also believe that they are immune from being at risk from relapsing. The synthesis of these two states of mind is *clear mind.* In this state, the person experiences the benefits of abstinence while remaining fully aware of the vulnerabilities that can lead to relapse, and the circumstances that will restore addict mind.

Dialectical abstinence

The fundamental dialectic in DBT is acceptance balanced with change. In DBT for substance use, the therapist works on the idea of *accepting* the fact that if a relapse were to occur, it wouldn't mean that the patient or the therapy couldn't achieve the desired result. At the same time, the therapist pushes for *change* by insisting on the immediate and permanent cessation of drug misuse. This is the perspective of *dialectical abstinence.* This approach is the balance of an unrelenting insistence on total abstinence with a non-judgmental, problem-solving response to relapse. It's critical for the therapy to include techniques that reduce the dangers of overdose and other complications of drug use, such as infections in intravenous drug misusers, as well as other significant health effects.

The task of the therapist is to communicate to the patient the expectation that the patient be abstinent from the very first DBT session. They insist that the patient commit to stop using drugs immediately. Because the expectation of committing to a lifetime of abstinence will often be met with an expression of disbelief, the therapist then suggests that the patient commit to a period of abstinence that the patient feels certain is attainable — a day, a month, or just an hour. At the end of this period, the patient renews the commitment, again for a specific time interval. Ultimately, the patient achieves long-term, stable abstinence by piecing together successive episodes of committed abstinence. This is similar to the idea behind the 12 Step slogan "Just for Today," which attempts to achieve, then invokes, the same goal — a lifetime of abstinence achieved by piecing together one moment of abstinence with the next moment.

Another strategy used to target abstinence is the *cope-ahead plan,* which is part of the emotion regulation skill set (see Chapter 10). Here, the person learns how to plan for, and what skills to use, when they anticipate being in a situation where they might be triggered in the next few hours or days. The patient then proactively prepares a response in case they end up in the anticipated situation, one that might risk their abstinence.

Burning bridges and focusing on acceptance

An important part of the cope ahead is to get the person to *burn their bridges* to their drug-abusing past by doing things that remove access and memories — for instance, getting a new phone number, letting drug-using friends know that they are now off drugs, deleting the phone numbers of drug dealers, and throwing out drug paraphernalia. Burning bridges, and building new ones, is a specific set of strategies that help people remove triggers that cue them to use substances. The triggers might be people, places, or specific items.

Also, in the event that the person is unexpectedly triggered, there is also a set of strategies to help them manage any cravings that arise, such as the use of *urge-surfing*, which employs the imagery of a wave as the urge to use substances, where the urge to use is "surfed" until the wave peters out.

REMEMBER

DBT treats a relapse into substance use as a problem that needs to be solved, so that instead of seeing it as evidence that the patient is inadequate or that the treatment has failed, they see it as an opportunity to press on. When the patient does lapse, the therapist moves quickly to help the patient fail as well as they can by using a chain analysis of the events that led to the drug use (see Chapter 18). In doing so, the therapist considers skills that the patient could have used to avoid using the substance, and what they can do should they face a similar situation in the future.

The therapist also helps the patient make a quick recovery from the lapse, with the goal of rapidly reducing the risk of intense negative emotions, because it is often these very negative emotions that lead people to relapse. The therapist wants to minimize the chance that the patient gives up hope and makes statements like "What's the point? I've already screwed up and might as well use."

The idea of reducing the impact of having failed to maintain sobriety includes repairing the harm that the relapse has caused to oneself and to important others. This is very similar to the approach taken by 12 Step programs like Alcoholics Anonymous, which focuses on making amends as a part of their program. The purpose of this approach is for the patient to increase their awareness of the negative personal and relational consequences of having lapsed, and to recognize those consequences without avoiding their emotions, including the experience of justified guilt. The next step is for the therapist and the patient to validate the lapse, while at the same time making sure that the patient does not get so flooded by these unwanted emotions that they use the experience of these emotions as a reason to continue using the substance.

Community reinforcement

Community reinforcement is the process of actively looking for people, places, activities, and situations that will support and reinforce non-addictive behavior. This includes identifying and spending time with friends and family members who are supportive of the person's recovery, going to places not associated with drug misuse, and taking up hobbies such as learning music or painting in a class, or engaging in a group sport like soccer or an exercise class like yoga.

Alternate rebellion

Alternate rebellion helps patients find ways to rebel that are not destructive or as potentially destructive to them or others in their life. An alternative to more destructive rebellion, it's the use of more skillful and non-destructive ways to rebel against society, but ways that don't involve substance misuse. This skill is particularly helpful for people whose identity as a user is in some way tied to rebelling against society.

TIP

Examples of alternate rebellion include getting a controversial tattoo, painting nails in different colors, wearing very alternative clothes, listening to alternative music at high volume, and many other activities. Often patients themselves can come up with some great ideas.

Adaptive denial

Adaptive denial is a cognitive skill that is used when a patient experiences an unhelpful or unwanted urge or impulse to do something ineffective. The idea is to deny that the actual urge is to misuse the substance, and then reframe that urge as a desire to be close to people, to avoid feelings, or to distract. Then, when the problem is denied, the next step is to avoid, or delay, the use.

Another way to use this skill is to replace the denied urge with a healthier behavior — for instance, to say, "I don't want a rum and Coke, I actually just want a Coke."

Seeing how DBT for substance use disorders is different from standard DBT

DBT for SUDs differs in a couple of ways from standard DBT. For instance, an important part of standard DBT is the use of *contingency management* in order to modify a patient's behavior. Because the relationship with the therapist is often important in standard DBT, the therapist uses the relationship to achieve behavioral change. For instance, if a person with BPD continues to engage in self-harm, the therapist might temporarily interrupt the therapy by using a therapy vacation. This often works well in reducing self-harm.

However, people who are dependent on and misuse drugs are often difficult to engage in treatment. Some do attach readily to their therapists, but others engage only episodically. In these cases, there is behavior such as failing to return phone calls or texts, or not showing up to therapy at all. There is often early termination of treatment. If the patient isn't very attached to their therapist, the therapist often has very little leverage to persuade the patient to come back to therapy.

Because of this, contingency management had to be changed and adapted for SUDs, because when a therapist implements a therapy vacation, they may actually reinforce the substance use. This is because the patient might feel guilty about having failed, and so they may turn to substances to address the guilt or because they feel that they now don't have to be accountable or that they now have nothing to lose. Because of this problem, new strategies, called *attachment strategies,* were developed specifically to use with people who misuse substances. An example of this might be that when a patient misses a few sessions, the therapist would send some encouraging texts saying that they miss the patient.

REMEMBER

Because the relationship with a therapist matters, other attachment strategies are used to increase the connection between patient and therapist. The goal is to re-engage the patient and prevent the negative consequences that commonly occur when patients fall out of contact with their therapist, or out of therapy altogether. As a result, until the attachment is solid and the person is out of significant danger of relapse, DBT therapists are more active than in standard DBT or in other therapies in finding lost patients and seeking to re-engage them in treatment.

From the first session, the therapist orients the patient to the concern that therapy may be difficult and that there is a risk that the patient may start to engage less in therapy. They discuss the possibility of it happening and then have a plan for if it does happen. This includes the patient giving the therapist a list of places they should look, and people they should contact, if the patient suddenly drops out of therapy. The therapist also gets the contact information for supportive family members and friends who can be counted on and contacted to help the patient and the therapist re-engage in therapy.

Other strategies include the therapist reaching out to the patient regularly between sessions, especially during the first few months of treatment, through the use of check-in calls, emails, or texts. There is also the idea of bringing the therapy to the patient by being where the patient is willing to do therapy — for instance, at a coffee shop, on a walk in a park, or at their home. The therapist can also introduce the idea of modifying sessions, such as shortening or lengthening them, to keep the patient engaged in therapy.

Knowing how DBT for substance use disorders is different from other therapies

DBT doesn't focus on punishment as a behavioral consequence. A DBT psychiatrist, for instance, would consider prescribing anti-craving medications, and a DBT therapist wouldn't make individual therapy contingent on abstinence. Note that one of the assumptions about patients is that they are doing the best they can and must continue working to achieve the goal of significant reduction or abstinence from the substance, and so it isn't consistent with the philosophy of DBT to punish the patient for the very reason that they are seeking therapy.

As a result, although many 12 Step programs require complete abstinence from all psychoactive substances, whether prescribed or not, in DBT, the therapist determines the degree of abstinence required for each patient in their individual therapy, and develops a treatment plan based on three ruling principles:

1. **Target the primary substance of misuse.**

   The primary substance is the one that causes the most significant problems for the patient, based on their history of misuse and the consequences of that use.

2. **Target other drugs that reliably cause the use of the primary drug.**

   For instance, some people might increase their heroin use (primary substance) if they use marijuana, and so marijuana would then be the next target.

3. **Ensure that the treatment goal of abstinence is realistic and attainable.**

   With regard to this third principle, patients with SUD who also have emotion regulation problems like BPD often have many difficult challenges. For instance, they might also have self-injurious and suicidal behaviors, a lack of relational support, and financial problems, in addition to those associated with drug abuse. Realistically, there is only so much that a severely compromised patient can be expected to target and change at one time.

From a DBT perspective, the substance misuse problem might not be immediately targeted, even if the consumption is excessive, unless

>> The person states explicitly that they want to stop the drug misuse;

>> The substance is the primary drug causing the person's problems; or

>> The substance is reliably associated with use of the primary drug, or if the drug is associated with a higher-order target — for example, if the person only makes a suicide attempt when they use the drug.

Considering DBT for SUD alone, without emotion regulation problems

There is not enough data to answer the question of whether DBT should be used just for SUD without emotion regulation problems. However, a clinician addressing this question should consider the following:

>> If the person does *not* have a condition like BPD, what does the best research show on treating the substance use problem? That should be the first line of treatment.

>> All things being equal, a less complicated and less comprehensive treatment should be used if possible. Certainly, DBT has a lot of features that can be helpful to most people; however, they aren't necessarily essential for the treatment of the substance use problem.

>> It's important to consider the extent to which a difficulty in regulating emotions plays a role in the person's substance misuse. Because DBT was developed specifically for people who have enduring difficulty in regulating their emotions, DBT could be a good fit for someone who is using substances to regulate their emotions.

Overcoming Eating Disorders

As with other mental health conditions, DBT has been adapted for the treatment of eating disorders and combines individual therapy and skills training components. Although it hasn't always been shown to be helpful for all eating disorders, the one it is most helpful with is binge eating disorder (BED). The following sections cover binge eating disorder, other eating disorders, and the DBT model for treating eating disorders.

Binge eating disorder

BED is a severe, at times life-threatening, yet treatable eating disorder. It is the most common eating disorder in the United States and is characterized by the following:

>> **Recurrent episodes of eating large quantities of food:** These binges are often marked by the person eating quickly, and to the point where they feel physically uncomfortable.

>> **A feeling of loss of control during the binge:** This is often accompanied by the emotions of shame and guilt after the binge.

>> **Typically, avoidance of unhealthy compensatory measures like purging to counter the binge eating:** Purging is more common in other eating disorders such as bulimia (covered later in this chapter).

DBT skills used for BED include those in the following sections.

Mindfulness

As we describe in Chapter 9, mindfulness is the skill of focusing on the present moment, without judgment, and acknowledging that the moment is impermanent and ever-changing. The awareness includes everything that happens within a person's body and mind, as well as everything that happens outside of their body and mind.

From a DBT perspective, binge eating is considered a mindless behavior. Mindfulness increases and improves an awareness of thoughts, emotions, and the body sensations that occur before, during, and after normal eating, as well as during the maladaptive binge.

TIP

A practice that can help you is that of mindfully eating a raisin (you can substitute any small piece of food, such as a slice of apple, a piece of chocolate, and so on):

1. **Start by placing a raisin gently into your mouth.**

   Don't chew yet. Hold the raisin in your mouth for at least ten seconds, exploring it with your tongue, feeling the surface of the raisin and the sense of having it there. (The reason a raisin works well for this practice is that it won't melt, like chocolate would, and has ridges on its surface, unlike a smooth grape, for instance; nevertheless, as stated before, any small piece of fruit will work.) For the ten seconds, notice the pause and that you aren't eating.

2. **When you're ready, slowly chew the raisin.**

   Notice where in the mouth the chewing takes place. Then, with intention, take one or two bites into it, and notice what happens after each bite. Notice the waves of taste as they rise and fall. Continue to chew slowly without swallowing. Notice how the sensation of taste and texture change in your mouth over time.

REMEMBER

This practice can then be used during mealtimes when eating any food or food type. Methodically, mindfully, and slowly chewing the food in this way leads to a greater enjoyment of the food and a reduction of the mindlessness that is characteristic of binge eating.

Emotion regulation

Emotion regulation skills are used to control excessive emotions through the practice of identifying and naming the emotions, reducing and managing negative emotions, accepting and increasing the ability to tolerate and manage extreme negative emotions, and increasing the experiences that lead to positive emotions. Because binge eating is often used as a way to manage strong and unwanted emotions, emotion regulation encourages the use of coping strategies other than binge eating.

TIP

One practice you can do is that of loving your emotion. This is based on the principle that by accepting, and even loving, your entire emotion, you can reduce the suffering caused by avoiding the experience of unwanted emotions. By bringing your awareness to the emotion, using mindfulness of current emotion (reviewed in Chapter 10), you then practice acceptance and love of the entirety of the experience. When your mind turns to saying, "I hate this emotion," you remind yourself that hating and avoiding leads to more suffering. Ideally, this practice happens before the binge; however, it can also be used for the emotions that arise after the binge.

Distress tolerance

The skill of distress tolerance is the practice of dealing with a situation that cannot be changed in that moment. Distress tolerance involves practices where you learn to tolerate negative emotions or crisis situations *without* responding in a maladaptive way, such as bingeing.

TIP

One of the distress tolerance skills (many of which are reviewed in Chapter 11) is known as the *half-smile.* The muscles of the face communicate to the emotional part of your brain, and the brain sends signals to your facial muscles that cause you to smile. A change in your facial expression leads to an emotional change. A smile generates one emotion and a grimace a different one. The half-smile practice changes your physiology and leads to a feeling of increasing serenity. This is much easier to do when you're relaxed, but even when you are not, half-smiling will reduce your level of distress and increase your level of acceptance. Doing this will significantly reduce your urge to binge.

Other eating disorders

As a general principle, there is no need to use one therapy if another one is more effective, and as for other complex disorders, there is no single and reliable approach to eating disorders. There are various reasons why DBT was developed for eating disorders (EDs):

>> The current treatments for eating disorders, such as the aforementioned binge eating disorder (BED) and bulimia nervosa (BN), are effective in only 50 percent of cases. For chronic anorexia, the success rate is even lower.

>> BPD and suicidal behavior are common among people with eating disorders. Suicide is a leading cause of death in those suffering from anorexia nervosa.

>> Many people with eating disorders have difficulty in regulating their emotions, and DBT skills can be very helpful for this.

Eating disorders, especially anorexia nervosa, differ from other mental illnesses in the significant degree of ambivalence about symptoms and treatment. Overall, DBT yielded positive outcomes in the treatment of anorexia nervosa, bulimia nervosa, binge eating disorder, and other eating disorders as well.

Anorexia nervosa has the following characteristics:

>> **Amenorrhea,** the loss of at least three menstrual periods in a row

>> **Low weight,** a body weight that is only 85 percent of what is expected due to dieting, vomiting, over-exercise, and the misuse of laxatives, diuretics, or diet pills

Bulimia nervosa has the following characteristics:

>> **A preoccupation with being thin,** despite the person being a healthy weight

>> **Bingeing on large amounts of food, followed by maladaptive compensation** — dieting, vomiting, over-exercise, laxative misuse, or diet pill misuse

Binge eating disorder (BED) is covered in the previous section. We should note that research shows that BED occurs in more than 30 percent of people with obesity.

The DBT model of treatment for eating disorders

The DBT model is based on a theory of emotion regulation in eating disorders. The basic idea of this theory is that people use eating behaviors as a way to regulate painful emotions, and that they use these behaviors because they have no, or few, other adaptive ways of dealing with these emotional states. The thinking is that behaviors such as vomiting, bingeing, and restricting are used to escape, avoid, or block the strong emotions that are triggered by thinking about or seeing food, or by ruminating on body image, or interpersonal situations that rely on an idealized body. Bingeing also sometimes functions as a way to focus on the binge rather than whatever negative thoughts are in the person's mind. Eventually, because bingeing is effective (even though it's maladaptive) as a way of escaping negative feelings, it becomes a reinforced behavior, meaning that it becomes the behavior that the person goes to, especially if they don't have other skills.

The long-term consequences of disordered eating behaviors like bingeing can include feelings of guilt and shame. If the person doesn't have more adaptive ways of dealing with guilt and shame, then they may turn to the very same disordered eating behaviors that led to the guilt and shame in order to deal with these emotions.

Similar to the function of bingeing behavior, DBT argues that the extreme weight loss that is experienced with anorexia serves to escape strong emotions in the absence of having healthier emotion regulation skills.

Because emotions and eating behaviors are intertwined, DBT targets the unhealthy eating behaviors directly, and then, when strong emotions are generated by efforts to regulate eating, the focus is on increasing emotion regulation and distress tolerance skills. Emotion regulation, from an eating disorder (ED) treatment point of view, includes focusing on the vulnerability factors that adversely impact emotion regulation, as well as focusing on the learning and application of emotion regulation skills. You can find out more about the DBT model for treating eating disorders in the following sections.

Treatment targets

REMEMBER

Just as with standard DBT for conditions like BPD, in DBT for eating disorders, there are four treatment stages that focus on four levels of severity. Within each stage, there is a hierarchy of treatment targets:

>> Stage 1 focuses on reducing suicidal and self-destructive behavior, as well as increasing behavioral and emotional control in people who have both an eating disorder and BPD. Specific to the eating disorder, this includes behavior that puts a person at imminent high risk of death or self-injury, such as starvation through misuse of purgative medication — that is, medication that causes a person to vomit — in people with anorexia and who have an extremely low body weight. This is because these behaviors put people at risk of a heart attack or organ failure. This stage then focuses on therapy-interfering behaviors such as when a person falls below an agreed-upon weight range, or a refusal to talk about the maladaptive behavior in therapy. Then they can move on to a discussion of the eating behaviors that are not life-threatening.

>> Stage 2 is the same as in standard DBT, targeting emotional avoidance. It involves reducing any trauma-related symptoms including those of post-traumatic stress disorder and other traumatic emotional experiences not rising to the level of PTSD. In this stage, the invalidating emotional experiences of childhood can be discussed as well.

>> Stage 3 targets ED behavior that interferes with quality of life, such as decreasing mindless eating; noticing cravings, urges, and preoccupation with food; and weighing, if weighing leads to the maintenance of eating behaviors.

>> Stage 4 focuses on the non-ED aspects of a person's life, which include developing relationships, establishing careers, and generating other sources of enjoyment like hobbies and other activities.

Dialectical strategies

The DBT philosophy that informs treatment is one of moving from extreme and rigid eating behavior patterns to a more balanced way of thinking and eating. Similar to DBT for substance addiction (covered earlier in this chapter) is the concept of *dialectical abstinence,* which balances abstinence from ED behavior with acceptance of, and coping ahead for, the possibility that the person will lapse back into ED behavior.

REMEMBER

Another area of focus is working with the person to recognize more moderate achievements than holding on to an extreme and perfectionist goal. The illusion that overeating is a form of control is challenged, while at the same time, the person recognizes that the changes they are making in treatment mean that they are more in control of the elements in their life that they can actually change. This dialectical perspective is important in targeting the person's ambivalent feelings about treatment, together with any frustration that their family, or the therapist for that matter, may experience.

Change strategies

The DBT diary card (see Chapter 18) is modified to focus on ED behaviors, and allows the person to track and rate their urges to engage in binge eating, food restriction, food preoccupation, and maladaptive use of the scale to check their weight. If there has been an eating behavior, a chain analysis of the behavior (see Chapter 18) is completed, with a clear description of the problem, its antecedents — that is, the thoughts and emotions that occurred before that behavior took place — and the context in which it took place, followed by a review of the consequences of the behavior. The chain analysis also looks at what skills the person used and what they plan to use should the situation arise again.

One of the biggest obstacles to successful ED treatment is ambivalence. For instance, if a person stops restricting, they will likely gain weight, or if they stop purging, they will have to experience their emotions. DBT commitment strategies are leaned on heavily to address this ambivalence. For instance, there is *highlighting the freedom to choose* to continue to stay in treatment against the choice of lack of realistic alternatives and the impact that this lack of treatment has on the person's health. They can also complete lists of the *pros and cons* of continuing their eating behaviors. By using the *devil's advocate* strategy, the therapist elicits reasons for not abstaining from bingeing if the person's goal is to have a life worth living. One of the additions to DBT for eating disorders is the focus on recognizing how culture, social media, and the nutritional environment can be invalidating.

Exposure and response prevention include the use of *opposite action*, where the urge to use maladaptive eating behaviors is overcome by doing the action opposite to the urge. This strategy can also be used for behaviors such as the urge to weigh oneself frequently or repeatedly do body checks. Another focus on change is through the use of contingency management, when the therapist uses the relationship by, for instance, making outpatient therapy sessions contingent on the patient maintaining weight limits. Finally, cognitive modification strategies are used to reappraise beliefs and concerns about a person's weight and shape, and to target the concept of perfectionism.

Acceptance strategies

In DBT for eating disorders, change strategies are paired with acceptance-based validation strategies. Validation includes the genuine response to a person's thoughts and feelings as understandable, given their history and eating disorder.

WARNING

It's important that the therapist not involve validating the invalid by, for instance, validating a person as overweight if they state that they "feel fat" and yet are in a normal weight range. The therapist can validate that experiencing thoughts about being fat are simply thoughts and point out that fat isn't a feeling or an emotion. "Feeling fat" can be a habitual thinking pattern occurring after the person has eaten a meal that can lead the person to have the thought that they are fat, a thought established as habit through years of thinking so. The therapist can also point out that there is no evidence that the thought that a person is fat is actually true, given the person's weight. They might also tie the sensation of being full to the thoughts of being fat. You can read more about validation in Chapter 12.

Gaining Ground on Body Dysmorphic Disorder

Body dysmorphic disorder (BDD) is a mental health condition where the person becomes fixated on a perceived flaw, or multiple flaws, in how they look. They often have intrusive worries and obsessions about the part of the body that they need to "fix."

BDD is an extreme form of concerns that many people have. Many of us might think that we would look better with tighter abdominals, a smaller nose, whiter teeth, lighter skin, darker skin, more dimples, and so on. For people with BDD, the preoccupation with how they see these flaws is so significant that it impacts day-to-day functioning, in that a lot of the time, they focus on the part of the body they are trying to fix. In many cases, these perceived flaws aren't evident to other people.

Unfortunately, BDD isn't made any easier by a culture that focuses on attractiveness, and where products that promise to erase wrinkles, remove body fat, and reshape body parts are everywhere on television and social media. To make matters worse, social media is full of selfies by so-called influencers, which are often filtered through photo-editing software, and which often make people who struggle with BDD feel even worse about themselves.

The following sections describe DBT strategies used to address body dysmorphic disorder, as well as tips for handling specific BDD issues.

Addressing perceived flaws

Because people with BDD present with *perceived* flaws, the perception is often difficult to eliminate completely. BDD itself is also difficult to eliminate because it often co-occurs with other disorders, such as eating disorders (covered earlier in this chapter), obsessive-compulsive disorder (OCD), anxiety, and depression. The approach to treatment focuses mostly on the cognitive behavioral therapy (CBT) elements of DBT, as you discover in the following sections.

Cognitive strategies

Cognitive strategies include identifying maladaptive thoughts, and then evaluating them afterwards and asking the patient to generate alternative thoughts. There are common thinking errors in BDD, such as *all-or-nothing thinking*, a type of thinking that is prevalent in conditions like BPD. For instance, the patient might think, "The curve of my nose makes me look totally ugly." Another type of thinking error is *mindreading* — for instance, "I know that my boyfriend wishes that I got plastic surgery on my nose."

Once these thinking errors are identified, the patient is asked to monitor their appearance-based thoughts in the session and then, as a part of their homework outside of the session, to identify these cognitive or thinking errors. For instance, outside of the session they might say, "I know my co-worker is staring at my nose and thinking how ugly it looks," and then identify this as mindreading. The therapist then points out how automatically these thoughts come into the patient's mind.

Next, once the patient has become more expert in identifying this type of cognitive distortion, the therapist starts to evaluate the thoughts with the patient. There are two approaches:

>> To evaluate the validity of the maladaptive thoughts, which is done using the DBT skill of checking the facts: "What evidence do I have that others are judging my nose?"

>> To examine the usefulness of having the thought: "Is it useful for me to think that straightening my nose would make me happy?"

Next, after the patient has become skilled at identifying and then restructuring their automatic, appearance-related thoughts and beliefs, other thoughts about the self are explored. Common to BDD and BPD are thoughts such as "I am unlovable," "No one will ever want to be with me," or "I am an inadequate human being." Without also addressing these core beliefs, it's unlikely that a patient's BDD will improve.

Another way to target the core beliefs is a form of the cope-ahead plan (introduced in Chapter 10). The therapist repeatedly asks the patient the worst possible consequences resulting from their belief; for instance, in the preceding example, if the patient thinks that their nose is crooked and that people are always noticing it and judging it, the therapist may repeatedly ask the patient, "What would it mean if people noticed that your nose was crooked?" The goal is to get at the patient's core belief. Perhaps the patient answers, "Well, then I know that no one will ever love me." These negative core beliefs can be addressed through the skills outlined in Chapter 7, skills such as cognitive reappraisal as well as working on self-compassion in order to focus on qualities that can enhance self-worth and self-love.

Perceptual retraining

People with BDD often have a complicated relationship with mirrors and reflective surfaces. Because of this, a person with BDD might spend hours in front of a mirror grooming or engaged in skin picking behavior, or they may spend a lot of energy actively avoiding any reflective surface in case they see their reflection.

When they do spend time in front of mirrors, usually the only part of the body that they focus on is the one of concern. Sometimes they use a magnifying mirror and then get very close to the mirror, thereby magnifying the particular area. This has the unfortunate consequence of magnifying the perceived imperfections, and leads to the maintenance of the maladaptive BDD beliefs and behaviors. When this happens, it's typically followed by judgmental and emotionally charged self-criticism: "I have the most hideous nose on the planet."

Perceptual retraining focuses on changing the perception by learning to engage in healthier mirror-behaviors — for instance, not getting too close to the mirror, not focusing on just the area of concern, but at the same time not avoiding the mirror altogether. The therapist also guides the patient in an exercise of describing their body from head to toe while standing at a more typical distance from the mirror. Then, instead of judgmental self-talk, during the perceptual retraining, the person learns to describe their perceived flaw in more objective terms. If there is a bump on their nose, then they could say, "There is a small bump on my nose." Part of the retraining is to use cope-ahead plans to get the person to refrain from previous rituals, such as zooming in on disliked body parts.

TIP

Perceptual retraining includes aspects of mindfulness (see Chapter 9) in that people with BDD are encouraged to focus on other things in the environment. For instance, at a dinner, rather than focusing on their body part, they may focus on the taste of their meal or the content of the conversation with their dinner companion.

Exposure and ritual/response prevention

People with BDD often perform rituals that end up perpetuating their struggle — for instance, excessive checking of the mirror — as well as performing avoidance behavior such as not going to the mall, where they believe the crowds will be judging their physical appearance. Exposure is the best way to tackle certain ritual behaviors.

Exposure response prevention (ERP) therapy is used to prevent the typical response or ritual a person normally has, and it's done through getting the patient to focus for an extended period of time on the part of the body that causes them to become anxious; over time, this will lead to a reduction in the level of anxiety. After a course of ERP, the patient will eventually experience very little, and ultimately manageable, anxiety. Prior to beginning ERP, the therapist and the patient identify the patient's rituals — for example, excessively checking their nose in the mirror — and then they review how the rituals actually lead to the persistence of symptoms.

The therapist and the patient then develop a hierarchy of situations that provoke anxiety and that the patient avoids. It's important that the patient identify all rituals and situations that they avoid in the service of not exposing their perceived flaw. For instance, some people will avoid shopping for clothes and changing in a mirror-filled dressing room, or they might avoid intimate sexual encounters, particularly if the lights are on. The hierarchy should include chosen situations that would increase the patient's exposure to a lot of people, such as going to the mall with friends, as opposed to unchosen situations, such as going to work. The first such exposure should be mildly to moderately challenging so that the chance of success is very high. Ultimately, the exposure to these situations should happen when the patient feels that their nose is at its most crooked.

Validation of just how anxiety-provoking the exposure is, is consistent with DBT. The validation is balanced with change strategies, encouraging the exposure and cheerleading the patient as they push on, while also helping the patient block their performance of the ritual. To reduce rituals, the patient is encouraged to monitor the frequency of the rituals and the context in which the rituals arise. The therapist then teaches the patient strategies that they can use to eliminate the rituals by first practicing resisting the rituals (for example, five minutes before checking the mirror) or reducing the rituals (for instance, not wearing a hoodie that hides the perceived flaw, in this case, the perceived crooked nose, when going to the mall).

The patient is then encouraged to use ritual or response prevention strategies during exposure exercises. It can be helpful to set up the exposure exercises as an "experiment." For instance: "If I don't wear a hoodie, someone at the mall will laugh at my crooked nose." The goal of ERP is to help the patient practice distress tolerance skills (see Chapter 11) during these exposures, and in so doing, acquire new information to evaluate their negative beliefs.

Handling particular problems

Not all forms of BDD are the same, and specific treatment strategies are used to address certain symptoms that affect some, but not all, patients. These include skin picking and hair pulling, as well as the desire for surgery to increase muscularity, change shape, and reduce weight, and for cosmetic surgeries including Botox and facial modification.

Skin picking and hair pulling

REMEMBER

For skin picking or hair pulling, the CBT approach of *habit reversal* can be useful if the symptoms are related to BDD. Habit Reversal Training (HRT) is a highly effective behavioral intervention for people who have unwanted repetitive behaviors or habits. HRT is a form of chain analysis of behavior (see Chapter 18), and it has five components:

1. **Awareness training:** The patient focuses their attention on the behavior they want to change in order to gain better awareness. The goal is for the patient to notice the earliest warning that the behavior is about to take place, where the situation occurs, and then what happens when they are performing the actual behavior.

2. **Competing response training:** The therapist helps the patient come up with a different behavior to replace the unwanted behavior, and then practice performing the new behavior.

3. **Motivation and compliance:** The patient makes a list of all the negative consequences caused by doing the behavior. Important people in the patient's life, such as parents, co-workers, and friends, can be asked to help out — for example, by offering praise and encouragement for every success. The idea is that such praise is reinforcing and will be helpful in getting the patient to stay on the path of not performing the unwanted behavior.

4. **Relaxation training:** This part of the treatment is based on the observation that habitual behavior like skin picking and hair pulling increases when a person is under stress, and so it can be helpful to use relaxation skills such as paced breathing, mindfulness, and progressive muscle relaxation.

5. **Generalization training:** This is the practice of using the new skills in many different situations so that the new behavior becomes automatic.

Seeking surgery

Some people with BDD have significant concerns about their shape or weight. One form is known as *muscle dysmorphia*, or MD, where the person is preoccupied by worries that their body is too small or not muscular enough, despite having a normal build, or in some cases, an objectively muscular physique. People with these categories of BDD often seek to correct their perceived deficits by requesting surgery.

Therapists can use the cognitive strategies mentioned earlier in this chapter to address any maladaptive beliefs about the perceived benefits of surgery, while also taking a dialectical stance by which they help the patient non-judgmentally explore the pros and cons of pursuing cosmetic surgery versus the pros and cons of not pursuing the surgery.

Getting a Grip on Behavioral Addictions

Substances are not the only thing that people can become addicted to. By definition, anything a person becomes addicted to can be incredibly hard to overcome. For people who are not addicted, this can be confusing, as they may feel that motivation and willpower should be enough, and yet even though these are important qualities, they are not enough for a person to attain recovery. Beyond substances, people can become addicted to activities like playing video games, gambling, viewing pornography, and more. The following sections list activities that may become addictive and explain how DBT can help.

Activities that may become addictions

The skills that we review in the earlier section "Looking at DBT skills for substance use disorders" are the same ones that are used for these lifestyle addictions, but not all of them work as well for all addictions. For instance, with addictions to dating websites, social media, or pornography, it can even be hard to burn bridges, because laptops, tablets, and smartphones have become necessary in contemporary life, which makes them hard to avoid.

For a person to be considered compromised by these addictions, as with substance addictions, the activity typically causes the following:

>> Impairment of the person's ability to control the frequency, intensity, and duration of the activity

>> Giving the activity a priority over other interests

>> A continuation of, or increase in, the activity despite negative consequences

>> An increase in interpersonal conflict or in social withdrawal

>> An adverse impact on occupational or academic obligations

>> Difficulty in trying to stop the activity on their own

The following sections note the types of activities or behaviors that might be targeted by DBT if other forms of treatment don't work.

Gaming

DBT's approach to any situation is to consider it from multiple points of view. Video games are often maligned by parents, who see them as an unnecessary distraction from what a child "should" be doing — homework, spending time with friends, and so on. Research shows that video gaming does have some important benefits to the gamer, including improved spatial attention, improved ability to track moving objects in a field of distractors, reduced impulsiveness, and an increase in mental flexibility. Nevertheless, built into the code of video games is the function of novelty. Novelty triggers the release of dopamine — the feel-good chemical that we talk about earlier in this chapter — and in fact, during gaming, the level of dopamine can double, which is about the same level of increase that is triggered by sex.

It is because the level of dopamine increases that video games can become addictive, and when a person is addicted, it can be the reason why they get up in the morning — to go and play — and the reason why they don't go to bed at night. As with other addictions, gaming can interfere with the completion of academic requirements and with relationships by increasing social isolation as well as in-person friend and family interactions.

There are more than just psychological consequences to gaming; physical symptoms also often occur. For instance, people can experience dry eyes, severe headaches, insomnia, backaches, and poor self-care — like skipping meals or not taking showers. And then, if they withdraw from gaming, they can experience mood swings, irritability, or significant boredom, because something that used to occupy a lot of their day no longer does.

Pornography

REMEMBER

Even though dopamine is involved in addiction to pornography, just like all other addictions, addiction to pornography is categorized as a *process addiction.* In drug addiction, the end result is to get high or drunk; however, in process addictions, there is the compulsion to participate in the entire process, like watching an entire pornographic movie or video clip. These types of addictions can cause just as much damage to a person's life as drug and alcohol misuse, especially in terms of the impact on the person's mental health.

Pornography addiction can take various forms, including the use of online pornography sites, sexting, receiving and sending explicit photos, and webcam viewing. Because of the sexual nature of addiction to pornography, it's often confused with sex addiction. For instance, some people are addicted to masturbation, which can happen independent of the use of pornography. Pornography addiction doesn't necessarily include incorporating any actual sexual acts, and the viewing of pornography is often done independent of anyone else. So, someone addicted to pornography is not also necessarily addicted to masturbation, even though masturbation commonly accompanies pornography watching.

Problems occur when the pleasure and dopamine release associated with viewing pornography becomes hardwired. When this happens, intimacy and sexual relations don't live up to the fantasy of the portrayed or imagined scenes because the brain has programmed itself to be turned on by the extremes and fantasy of the unrealistic pornographic depiction. Intimate relationships suffer, and the person can begin to feel isolated and ashamed, and then might in turn go deeper into and require even more graphic and intense pornographic experiences. For some people who start paying for webcam viewings and subscriptions, this can lead to them spending a lot of money, which can take a toll on their finances.

Compulsive sexual behavior

Compulsive sexual behavior disorder is characterized by persistent and repetitive sexual urges, or impulses to do something sexual, which the person experiences as irresistible or uncontrollable. These urges then lead to repetitive sexual behaviors, along with these behaviors becoming all-consuming and central to the person's life, to the point that they neglect their personal care and health as well as significant relationships, and are ultimately unsuccessful in their efforts to control or reduce the sexual behaviors. They continue to engage repeatedly in these behaviors despite negative consequences such as loss of relationships and work-related problems. Typically, the person can't control their urges, and they experience increased tension or physical arousal immediately before the sexual activity, followed by relief of the tension after the activity.

Gambling

Gambling is common in almost every culture; however, most people don't develop gambling-related problems. Nevertheless, pathological gambling can become a problem, especially in adolescents. Pathological gambling is characterized by a progressive and maladaptive pattern of gambling behavior that significantly impacts relationships, employment, and educational or career opportunities. It can even lead to legal consequences due to the commission of illegal acts.

Very few people with a pathological gambling addiction seek treatment, and interestingly, about 50 percent of people with a pathological gambling problem appear to recover on their own. As with other forms of addiction described in this section, DBT relies heavily on the skills of CBT to address the problem.

When to use DBT for behavioral addictions

If the person does *not* have conditions like BPD complicating these addictions, then, if there is a less complicated form of evidence-based therapy, that therapy should be used in place of DBT.

REMEMBER

However, it's important to consider the extent to which difficulty in regulating emotions plays a role in the person's addiction and behavior. For the therapist, one clue is when the patient swaps one set of symptoms for another. For instance, a person may use self-injury, but then when they try to stop, they use an eating behavior, and then maybe use substances. Because DBT was developed specifically for people who have enduring difficulty in regulating their emotions, DBT could be a good fit for someone who uses their addictive behavior as a way to regulate their emotions, and in such cases, the same format and protocols as the ones used for substance use disorders should be implemented (as we describe earlier in this chapter).

Chapter **23**

Dealing with Counterproductive Behaviors

The central idea of DBT is that emotion dysregulation is at the core of emotional dysregulation disorders like borderline personality disorder (BPD). However, even when a person has learned to regulate their emotions, the person must deal with some significant problems. Two such issues are self-invalidation and self-hatred.

In this chapter, you discover ways to be kinder to yourself and recognize that your experiences were valid even when others told you they weren't. You also find the power of self-love and self-compassion in healing, and then see that being alone and feeling empty are not inevitable but are experiences that you can change by using DBT skills.

Tackling Self-Invalidation

Self-invalidation is the rejection or invalidation of your own emotions and experiences. It's also the judging or rejecting of yourself for even having the emotions. For instance, say that you break up with a romantic partner and you feel sad and start to cry. Then you start to tell yourself that you're stupid for feeling this way, that there is something wrong with you, and that "normal" people wouldn't react this way.

DBT theory states that people learn to invalidate themselves from having grown up in invalidating environments. In an invalidating environment, you're told — even if the person doesn't mean to hurt you — that the way you express your emotions is wrong, that you're making a big deal of things, or that you should just get over feeling the way you're feeling.

Whatever form the invalidation takes, a child growing up in such an environment learns that their emotions are "incorrect" and even something they should be ashamed of. As the person grows up, this can lead them to mistrust their own experiences and feelings.

In the following sections, you find ways to get out of a cycle of self-invalidation by recognizing when and how you self-invalidate, why you do so, the consequences of self-invalidation, and then what to do about it.

Removing yourself from the cycle with self-validation

How can you get out of the cycle of self-invalidating when you have an emotion? The DBT skills of mindfulness (see Chapter 9) and emotion regulation (see Chapter 10) are central to dealing with self-invalidation. You start by improving your ability to notice, understand, accept, regulate, and even love your emotions. Using the emotion regulation module, you and your therapist look for opportunities to help you understand, experience, and then regulate your emotions.

When you have BPD and strong emotional vulnerability, managing your emotional system can be like trying to drive a race car with a powerful engine. It takes a lot of skill and training to operate such a powerful vehicle. It doesn't happen overnight, and at times things will spin out of control. People without BPD typically operate the emotional equivalent of a mid-range sedan. It's much easier for them to manage low-level emotions, and they will almost certainly never experience the kind of emotional intensity that you do. People who don't have strong emotions need far fewer skills to get from emotional distress to a place of feeling regulated. Once you're skilled in the practice of emotion regulation, you'll get to the point of being able to step back and then mindfully notice, using the observe and describe skills of mindfulness, to get to a point of regulation.

The process of self-invalidation is that of traveling down a familiar path. Because you've been invalidated and then have self-invalidated, it's a pattern you're familiar with. Self-validation is a form of opposite action to self-invalidation, and it's something you need to learn to do. But like anything new, it takes time. Note that the brain learns by repetition, so the more you repeat self-invalidation, the better you get at self-invalidation, and the more you repeat self-validation, the better you get at self-validation.

People who have been invalidated and self-invalidate will often first experience validation, both as a concept and in practice, during therapy. The therapist teaches the patient to self-validate by asking the patient how it makes sense to them that they are feeling the way they are currently feeling. Because every emotion is caused by the circumstances that came before it, the emotion is valid. People who have grown up with invalidation will often say that their emotions are stupid or weak or that they are making a big deal of things, and this makes sense, because the invalidating environment has often reinforced these very ideas to them. When you ask yourself the question "Does my emotion make sense?" you'll see that it does.

Self-validation doesn't take emotions away; however, people who have powerful emotions suffer. Self-invalidation adds suffering to a situation where a person is already suffering, so self-validation is an act of kindness and honesty to yourself, as you don't have to deal with the dual problem of emotional suffering and self-invalidation.

Stepping away from shame

Related to self-invalidation is the experience of self-directed anger and the emotion of shame, and these often precede self-invalidation. For many people, the emotion that most often interferes with problem-solving is shame. This is because with shame comes the sense that you're simply bad, and with this feeling comes the desire to hide while experiencing the painful and persistent rumination of "You are defective, you are worthless, you are an embarrassment."

So when a person is suffering and seeking to escape their emotional pain, how do they develop these skills while at the same time engaging in behaviors that increase their distress, such as self-punishment and judgmental negative self-talk? There is a paradox in that people who are suffering actively avoid situations that cause shame, while at the same time doing behaviors that will end up causing shame. Self-invalidation tells them that they deserve that shame, and so they seek to verify that this belief is true and that they deserve to suffer.

Another element to self-invalidation is that people who do this — especially those who are self-loathing — prefer negative feedback and criticism to praise. This is because such feedback "confirms" their negative self-view.

People who use self-harm as self-punishment in the context of shame say that the self-harm is effective in reducing shame. However, they also state that it's an effective form of self-punishment. So, because the person believes they are bad, they self-punish, and they feel that this is effective, but then they are trying to escape the shame that makes them feel bad, and self-injury is again effective. Further, in the context of therapy, people who self-injure often feel shame because they feel that they have disappointed their therapist.

Because of this, the therapist has a complicated task. On the one hand, they need to help the patient reduce shame by stopping and then reversing shame-inducing behaviors, while on the other hand, they must help the patient face the experience of shame by using maladaptive behaviors so that they can develop healthier and longer-term solutions.

The most effective way to target shame is through the skill of opposite action (see Chapter 10), which is based on the behavioral principle of extinguishing the behavior through exposure and the use of emotional processing. To experience the exposure, the first step is to identify the specific areas of shame. For many people, these are typically sexual behaviors, sexual thoughts, body image, and feelings of attraction or love. Next is to identify the triggering or prompting event, whether this is a thought or a situation.

The next step is (and this is the same as with working with any emotion) to decide the extent to which the shame is justified or unjustified:

>> Shame is justified if there is a real danger of being rejected by others because you've violated some societal norm, or the behavior violates your core values or morals. If your shame is justified, then the violation of societal norms and your values is the problem you need to fix.

>> Shame is unjustified if there is little to no risk of rejection, and you have to have evidence for this, or your behavior doesn't violate your values or morals. Almost all patients begin by stating that their shame is justified, but the reality is that, when examined carefully, most instances of shame for most patients are largely unjustified.

The most powerful way to target shame experiences is through the use of opposite action. However, for many people, using opposite action is the most aversive option they can imagine. This is because it's a form of exposure, and for many people, exposure to the thing they fear most is almost unimaginable. (Keep reading for more on exposure.)

Experiencing exposure

REMEMBER

One of the most essential and important lessons in this book is that exposure is among the most powerful techniques in DBT, and arguably in all of therapy. The more you expose yourself, tolerate, and skillfully deal with the emotionally uncomfortable or painful situation, the sooner it will cease to control your life. We can't emphasize this enough. Therapists in consultation teams often bring up the difficulty they have in getting their patients to experience exposure. They describe how some of their patients sometimes wait weeks, months, or longer before they do, and then how within a few weeks of fully participating in exposure, patients start to feel better and in more complete control of their lives.

Building motivation for exposure

Once the patient is convinced that they have to do exposure therapy, the next step is to enhance their motivation to do so. By using the motivational strategies that we review in Chapter 19, the therapist and the patient examine the ways in which shame interferes with the patient's current experience and life goals, and the rationale behind the opposite action techniques and behavior. The patient can then list the pros and cons of doing the exposure work. Exposure isn't a therapy that can be forced. There is no way for a therapist to get a patient to do the exposure therapy if it isn't their goal to do so; however, in this case, the patient will often continue to suffer, and will often interfere with their goal of a life worth living and one in which they have more control of their emotions.

The therapist's task is to seriously consider a patient's doubts and skepticism. The therapist might even consider using the devil's advocate technique to evaluate the patient's determination to do the exposure work. The treatment for unjustified shame is the repeated exposure to the events and situations that elicit shame, while at the same time blocking maladaptive avoidant or self-destructive behaviors, and also strengthening the opposite-action behaviors.

Practicing exposure therapy

The skill of exposure to unjustified shame is practiced frequently and for prolonged periods of times. This skill consists of the following components:

1. The person discloses the detailed and factual information about the situation, and particularly the behavior that was previously hidden or undisclosed.

2. They then engage in the previously avoided behaviors.

3. They reveal physical characteristics that were previously undisclosed, including talking about the parts of their body or the sexual behaviors that are inducing shame.

4. The person then physically approaches the very specific social situations and interpersonal interactions that were previously avoided.

WARNING

It's very important that the shame emotion be elicited in therapy and in real life. In the therapy session, talking about the events, imagining them, and role-playing will frequently elicit the shame response. The therapist has to be clear that they — the patient and the therapist together — have agreed to do the work to target shame. Because of this, the therapist and the patient must make sure that neither of them are vague, switch or avoid topics, mumble or use a quiet voice, use judgmental or self-blaming language, avoid eye contact, or use dissociation or escape behavior. Exposure therapy will be effective only if the events and behaviors that trigger shame are completely identified and incorporated into exposure tasks.

REMEMBER

Acting opposite to unjustified shame is the practice of actively approaching avoided situations and people, and in so doing, recognizing that you haven't violated societal norms, that you haven't been immoral, and that if you're rejected, it isn't because you are some shameful being.

TIP

An important part of the practice of opposite action to shame and self-invalidation is that it needs to be done with self-confidence, good eye contact, self-assurance, and the recognition that although it's difficult, it's the best approach. To strengthen and generalize the practice, sessions can be audiotaped or videotaped so that they can be listened to or viewed over and over. It's critical that the patient be exposed to the shame-inducing situation. Say that a patient feels shame when they get any feedback from others, or when they look in the mirror or discuss parts of their body, which are concerns in body dysmorphic disorder (BDD). The key is to keep addressing and talking about — without avoidance or escape — whatever brings the patient shame.

Many people who experience shame come to the conclusion that they are bad people and not deserving of love. Another aspect of treatment is to reconceptualize the shame as a strong emotion that is elicited by problematic behaviors leading to justified shame, or elicited by faulty thinking if the shame is unjustified. The therapist's task is to help the patient change the problematic behavior or distorted way of thinking. For instance, say that you tend to apologize for everything that happens in a relationship, whether or not you've done anything wrong. One of the treatment goals would be to get you to stop apologizing for unjustified guilt and shame. However, to do so, you first have to determine whether the emotion is justified or not.

This kind of exposure is the most difficult yet most powerful intervention. You have to be as explicit as you can. You might need to describe a transgression, body flaw, or sexual act in detail, without judging yourself, and at the same time, validate yourself for the emotions you experience, and recognize that the reasons you got into that situation make sense, or at least did so at the time. Some patients believe that it doesn't matter whether an emotion is justified or not, but keep in mind that an emotion can be valid whether it's justified or not. This distinction between justified and unjustified shame is central for treatment because otherwise, a person's shame worsens if they expose themselves to situations that elicit justified shame, as this ends up leaving them feeling humiliated, judged, and maybe even ostracized from the group.

A patient described it this way:

> For a long time, I could not look at anything that brought me shame. It was all the same to me, whether it was my fault or not. All that my avoidance did was make me suffer all the time and use behaviors that ended with me feeling even more shame. So, I finally started to look at whether the shame I felt was justified or not. For me, it was a matter of slowing down; otherwise, I would get caught up in invalidating thoughts and not checking the facts. You have to create the space for validation. If I don't make the space for validation, I get more upset, and then I come to negative conclusions about myself, thoughts such as "They don't like me, I shouldn't be upset by this, and so on." You have to take a first step, do something different, and remind yourself that your old routine has not worked. I took a marker and wrote the letters *SV,* for self-validate, on the back of my hand. It really worked. I think that I will get them tattooed there!

Seeking reassurance

A person tells his partner, "I need to know that you love me and that you won't leave me." The partner reassures the person and the person feels good, but then something happens — perhaps the partner doesn't answer a text or a phone call — and the person then starts to feel badly again and needs reassurance again. "Are you mad at me?" the person asks. The partner responds, "No." However, just to be safe, the person asks one more time, "Are you sure?"

To an outside observer, this text exchange seems harmless. The person is asking their partner whether they are mad at them. However, the answer isn't enough. The problem is that the person is engaging in a never-ending cycle of seeking reassurance. The problem with receiving reassurance is that it doesn't work as a permanent solution, and when it helps, it helps only for a short period of time. If reassurance were a solution, then you would need to be reassured only once, and that would solve the problem.

In the following sections, you read about various types of reassurance-seeking behaviors, why they can be problematic, and what you can do instead of seeking reassurance.

Types of reassurance-seeking

REMEMBER

Reassurance-seeking is the act of continuously trying to gather information that has already been provided to reduce anxiety. There are different types of such behavior:

>> **Self-reassurance:** This can happen in conditions like obsessive-compulsive disorder (OCD):

- Checking things repeatedly, such as ensuring that a door is locked or that an alarm is on

- Constantly checking physical symptoms, such as constantly taking your temperature

- Mentally reviewing an event over and over, such as a text conversation with a friend, to make sure that there isn't any indication that they are upset or that your responses weren't inappropriate

>> **Seeking reassurance from others:** This commonly happens in conditions like BPD:

- Asking others whether they are mad at you

- Asking for a promise that everything is going to be okay

- Asking for a promise that another person isn't going to leave

The problem with reassurance-seeking

WARNING

You might ask yourself, "What's so bad about asking for reassurance if it makes me feel better?" After all, reassurance-seeking decreases your anxiety in the short term. We call this *negative reinforcement*. This means that you take away (subtracting, hence the term *negative*) something that you don't want — in this case, anxiety — by asking for reassurance, and then when this works, you ask for it over and over again. However, in the long term, it creates a cycle that worsens anxiety and increases your need for more reassurance. Even worse, it causes you to lose confidence in your abilities and increases your self-doubt, which can then lead to more self-hatred and self-invalidation.

How to decrease reassurance-seeking

Because reassurance-seeking can be so gratifying in the short term and yet mostly unhelpful in the long term, it's important to know the ways to reduce the behavior. Here are the steps you can take to decrease reassurance-seeking:

1. **Identify when it's happening.**

   There is a difference between *seeking information* (gathering information *once* for the purpose of understanding) and *seeking reassurance* (continuously trying to gather information that has already been given in an attempt to decrease anxiety).

2. **Label the behavior accurately.**

   For example: "I am anxious and I am seeking reassurance."

3. **Take a gradual approach.**

   Slowly decrease how many questions you're asking each day or how many times you're asking the same question.

4. **Delay or postpone seeking reassurance for a specific amount of time.**

   For example: "I will delay asking for reassurance for four hours today, and tomorrow I will increase the amount of time to six hours."

5. **Eliminate asking for reassurance completely.**

   This step is often the hardest. If you do this, you want to tell your family and your loved ones so that they can be aware of the difficult emotions you'll be experiencing. You can ask your therapist to help educate your family members, and to ensure that if you ask them a reassurance-seeking question, they should *not* respond reassuringly, but instead, answer with something like the following:

   - "What do you think?"

   - "We talked about that a few hours ago. Are there things that have changed?"

   - "Did something happen that led you to ask that question?"

   - "You already know the answer to that question. I am not going to answer that."

6. **Track your progress on a diary card.**

   Because you're doing DBT therapy and you're keeping a diary card (see Chapter 18), reassurance should be a target symptom on the diary card, and you should track it on a daily basis.

More particularly, you should keep a note of the types of questions and specific reassurance-seeking behavior that you're doing. You should also keep a log as to what has helped and what has not, and then when you notice the need to seek reassurance, refer back to your diary card to see how you dealt with it at other times.

7. Continue your gradual approach.

If you're asking for reassurance, say, ten times per day, taper down the number of times you're asking. Go down to nine times the next day, then eight the day after, and so on.

Decreasing reassurance-seeking is very difficult if you are an anxious person. However, without decreasing the behavior, it will be almost impossible to effectively take control of your anxiety.

Handling Self-Hatred

As author Sharon Salzberg writes, "The mind thinks thoughts that we don't plan. It's not as if we say, 'At 9:10 I'm going to be filled with self-hatred.'" Many people with conditions like BPD struggle with the experience of intense self-hate, shame, and feelings of being a failure or inadequate. As Sharon Salzberg points out, these thoughts, even if unwanted, take residence in people's minds. Therapists will often hear the following statements:

>> "I'm worthless."

>> "I can't do anything right."

>> "I *hate* myself."

>> "I am so horrible; no one will ever want to be with me."

>> "Everyone would be better off if I wasn't around."

>> "I am a terrible person — a loser."

These are all negative thoughts — they are not facts. And yet, these manifestations of self-loathing represent the most unrelenting and destructive thoughts in BPD. There is a curious irony in that people with BPD who hate themselves also often have the experience of not having a sense of self. If you don't know who you are, who is the person you're hating? One 27-year-old patient captured the experience when she stated, "I just think about how much I hate everything, my body, my disorder, my emotions, my decisions, my life, how I destroy relationships. Even when I feel better and less hateful, I'm still not happy with who I am. It is hard to explain. At times I feel like I deserve nothing; at other times, I don't feel like I am a person at all, as someone so worthless cannot be real."

TECHNICAL STUFF

Looking for negativity in situations has an evolutionary basis. As we sought to survive very difficult circumstances, we had to be on the lookout for predators that might attack us or bad weather that might freeze or overheat us. To take a naïve and blissful attitude and not consider dangers would have meant that as a species, we wouldn't have survived very long; as a result, it's built into our genetics. However, today, few of us are exposed to tigers or unable to find shelter, yet this need persists to be on the lookout for threats.

REMEMBER

For people with conditions like BPD, this looking for negativity is turned inward, and the threat becomes themselves. The fixation is then on their own inadequacy and failings, which leads to them feeling anger and disgust toward themselves. What is hard for people who hate themselves to understand is that their self-perception is often not the way that others perceive them. This is particularly true in people who have been abused and whose trauma is unresolved. The narrative can be one of having deserved the abuse they endured. For people who are certain that they aren't worthy, it can be hard to believe that others do love them, because the recurrent narrative in their mind is so negative. How can it possibly be true that they are worthy and lovable? If you struggle this way, how can you change that? The following sections can help.

Thinking of self-love as opposite action

REMEMBER

As we explain in Chapter 10, the skill of opposite action is to act opposite to what your emotions are telling you to do. Effective use of opposite action can lead to a powerful sense of mastery that helps make the skill self-reinforcing, meaning it helps you the next time you're stuck to be motivated into doing the hard task of acting opposite. Practicing self-love is opposite to engaging in self-hatred thinking.

You get to a point of self-love through the actions of self-care and self-compassion. It's all about implementing change, and this is where the hard, consistent work comes in. Many say they want to heal, yet they fear leaving their "comfort zone," even if that comfort zone is built on self-hatred and shame.

There is a quote attributed to the Buddha that goes like this:

> In this world,
> Hate never yet dispelled hate.
> Only love dispels hate.
> This is the law,
> Ancient and inexhaustible.

This is completely compatible with the focus of behaviorism in DBT. You aren't going to replace self-hatred by continuing to hate yourself. Only self-love, or at a minimum, self-liking, can replace self-hatred.

Looking at the elements needed to practice self-love

REMEMBER

For people who have never truly loved themselves, the idea can seem impossible if not ludicrous. And yet there are steps you can take to start practicing self-love:

>> **You have to be patient.** You've likely spent many years feeling self-hatred. Creating new brain pathways and new ways of thinking takes time and practice. This is just like any other practice, and it's the way the brain works. Being patient with yourself is the first act of self-compassion.

>> **Ask people who love you for help.** Make a list of the people in your life who have expressed their love for you. Think outside the box; don't list only your friends and family, but also teachers, religious people, co-workers, therapists, and anyone else who cares for you. Asking for help from people who care about you is an act of compassion for yourself.

>> **Don't avoid the self-hatred.** Somewhere in your life, you went from being a child who had no concept of self-hatred to hating yourself. You weren't born hating yourself. How did you get to self-hatred? Exploring how self-hatred developed will be painful, and yet it is by paying attention to it that you'll overcome it. By facing it, we mean acknowledging it is there, noticing it without dwelling or ruminating on it. Ultimately, you'll be able to face it without it controlling your life in a destructive way.

>> **Forgive and forgive and forgive.** If you've done things that you're ashamed of, you are like almost every other person on earth. Keep in mind that you did the things that you did because you didn't know how to love yourself. You must forgive yourself for each act that led to justified shame because most likely, you didn't know better, and if you did know better, then you must also ask for forgiveness from the people who you hurt. Of course, if you're dysregulated, it may be very hard to be skillful and to ask for forgiveness. In that moment, your task is to regulate and then to ask yourself whether asking for forgiveness is what is needed in the moment. If you've determined that you crossed your values and ended up hurting someone, then ask them for forgiveness as well. Do this because it's in your value system. As you become more skillful, you'll be less likely to do things that cross your values. Forgiving yourself is a practice in self-compassion.

>> **Be with the people you love, and do the things you love.** Do you love reading? Then read. Do you love playing a musical instrument? Then play.

Do you love dancing? Put your dancing shoes on and dance. Do you love being with a certain group of friends? Set up a weekly dinner or Zoom call. The more you practice doing things you love, the more you will love. This is opposite to punishing yourself for being someone you hate. Not depriving yourself is an act of self-compassion.

TIP

Here is a Zen practice that is another way to tackle the problem of self-hatred. Think about someone you respect who you consider to be a wise, compassionate person. Now, imagine that person living with you in your mind and body during moments of self-loathing, and see how they might handle it and how they would guide you. Again, this is a difficult task, but with practice you'll find greater self-compassion.

Balancing Solitude and Connectedness

Most people identify close relationships as the essential reason for joy and meaning in their life. Relationships provide structure to your days, whether they are relationships at home or at work. It can feel so good to be with the people you care about, and even better when you're in a good mood. It can feel good to be with close people, even when you aren't feeling all that good. Relationships also matter because they can be your source of support, and the people who you, in turn, can support.

The other side of connectedness is social isolation and loneliness. Seeing yourself as disconnected and separate is painful and potentially destructive to your mental health. Many people who want connection also want, and even enjoy, moments of solitude. However, they want these moments to be of their choice and not because they are forced on them because there is no one in their life.

Loneliness isn't something that only impacts certain people. Feelings of loneliness can affect any of us at any time, and for some people, this is made particularly difficult during times of celebration, like national holidays, birthdays, and anniversaries. Too much isolation can pose mental as well as physical health risks.

In the following sections, we review different experiences of aloneness and steps you can take to deal with each, if that is your goal. It can also be your goal to be comfortable sitting with being alone for a period of time.

REMEMBER

Many people with BPD come to DBT on antidepressant medications. It's true that some may also suffer with depression, but more often than not, it isn't clinical depression. Instead, it's a state of discontent and unhappiness. A more accurate term would be *dysphoria*, which is a state of feeling uneasy or dissatisfied with life.

Dysphoria happens when the person experiences moments of stability, and the hope that comes with such stability, and then disappointment when the stability doesn't endure. In this context, they can feel empty and alone.

Aloneness

While loneliness (which you read about in the next section) is about wanting to connect with others when there isn't someone readily available to connect with, *aloneness* is the emptiness or hollowness that you feel when people you love have left or abandoned you.

REMEMBER

When you're feeling alone, it can be easy to forget that we are all fundamentally interconnected and dependent on each other. Even though it may not feel like it, people rely on you. Think for a moment about how the people in your life rely on you. Sometimes you don't feel that essential, but think about your local barista, who depends on you showing up to get coffee; your employer, who depends on you showing up to work; your school, which depends on you to be a student; your place of worship, which needs your voice in the choir; and your neighbor, who asks you to check in on their cats while they are away for the weekend. When you realize just how connected you are, you also realize that you are not alone, and so it is important not to dwell on aloneness, for it is a temporary, though understandably painful, experience.

Loneliness

Loneliness is the uneasy emotional discomfort that arises from either being, or perceiving oneself to be, alone. There are different perspectives as to how the feeling arises and manifests. One is that it occurs because the inherent need that we have for intimacy and companionship isn't met. Another is that when the desired need for a relationship doesn't reflect the reality of a person's relationships, this leads to the unsettled feeling of loneliness. Whatever its manifestation, loneliness can have long-term emotional and physical health consequences.

REMEMBER

Loneliness affects millions of people. Fortunately, you can do many things to overcome it. The key is to realize how you feel and to find the best strategy for you. Here are some DBT ideas for dealing with loneliness:

>> **Acknowledge that you're feeling lonely.** This means acknowledging that it is *loneliness* that you're feeling, as opposed to feeling abandoned or depressed. It also means articulating the impact that loneliness is having on your life. Let your therapist know that you want to target the feeling of loneliness. Another idea is to talk to your friends and family. It can be difficult to let people know that you're struggling with loneliness.

>> **Know your loneliness behaviors.** Some people get stuck in a feeling without doing anything about it. Or they might feel that they can't do anything about it. Do you decide to stay in your house? Do you turn down opportunities to join friends and family at events? Do you neglect to return texts or emails? Do you spend time ruminating about how lonely you feel? These behaviors are important to know so that you can target them directly.

>> **Recognize whether being online is making your loneliness worse.** Being online can be a double-edged sword when it comes to loneliness. Certainly, online communities can offer a convenient way to connect with others. Activities like multi-player gaming and online dating can offer ways to interact and engage with others, and that can be enough for some people. However, some social media apps make loneliness worse because they typically highlight only the wonderful lives that other people seem to be living. The reality of others' lives is often typically not as it is being portrayed; nevertheless, it can feel real and as if you are being left out. The bottom line is that if being online leads to increased feelings of loneliness, it's probably a signal that you should log off.

>> **Volunteer.** Many communities have opportunities for people to volunteer. Contributing your time and talents, and working alongside others for a cause that you find important, can help you connect with other like-minded people and help you fight loneliness. Volunteering has other health benefits: It can help you reduce stress and feelings of depression, and increase happiness and fulfillment.

If you're interested in working with the elderly, you can volunteer as a visitor at a nursing home. If you prefer working with children, you might be able to volunteer at a children's hospital or become a reader at a library. If you're interested in causes like climate change or the environment, you can see whether there are local chapters of some of your favorite causes. If you're more of an animal- rather than people-person, you can volunteer at your neighborhood animal shelter.

>> **Join a support group.** There are times when people feel isolated from family members because those family members struggle with mental health issues or a substance use condition. Joining a support group like Al-Anon (`https://al-anon.org/`) or the National Education Alliance for Borderline Personality Disorder (NEABPD; `www.borderlinepersonalitydisorder.org/`), can connect you with people who are likely to understand a lot of what you're going through.

>> **Join a hobby group.** Are you interested in reading, painting, chess, card games, singing, and so on? Many communities have a local center that displays clubs and special interest groups that can connect you to other people who enjoy similar interests.

Emptiness

A 23-year-old college senior wanted therapy to help her deal with the dissatisfaction in her life. More specifically, she said she felt empty a lot of the time and that this was unbearable: "I feel so empty inside. Nothing takes it away, although I feel less empty when I am with people. Sometimes marijuana, sex, and spending money help, but only for a short while. What can I do?"

Of all the difficulties that people with BPD have, perhaps the most difficult one to explain to others is "chronic feelings of emptiness." Emptiness is a subjective experience and doesn't have an outward manifestation the way that anger and sadness might. The following sections describe emptiness and how to help relieve it.

Trying to describe emptiness

The feeling of emptiness is hard to explain, and so we asked people who experience it to describe it. The question brought many responses. Some say that it feels like an unbearable void. Others say that it is a hopelessness and purposelessness. Others, that it is a feeling that they are of no consequence and that the world would be just the same, if not better, without them. Some people say that emptiness is part of who they are, yet others say that it is a sense of existential meaninglessness.

One 28-year-old bank manager said, "It's like a giant hole inside of me. It feels like nothing I do, and no one I'm with, can fill the hole. It's so hard to explain. It's like something was there and now it's gone. You know how when people who have lost an arm still feel it? A phantom limb, they call it. It feels like something that was a part of me has been ripped away. I used to think that emptiness came from people not understanding me, but even when I meet other people who also feel emptiness, I still feel empty."

The experience of emptiness is complicated because it's so hard to define; for instance, it's also the feeling of being completely alone despite being in a group of people. "Emptiness is like my skin. It goes with me everywhere," explained a 19-year-old. "Here is what it is. It is not knowing who I am or what I feel or need. It is yearning for something that I can't explain. Emptiness is a horrible way to live, and there is very little relief from it."

Understanding reasons to tackle emptiness

REMEMBER

If you find it difficult to explain emptiness, as you can see, you are not alone. Even researchers can't completely explain what it is. Your therapist will want you to explain what it means to you so that they can recommend skills to use to tackle the emptiness. It's important to do so for the following reasons:

>> Emptiness is closely related to feelings of hopelessness, loneliness, and isolation.

>> Hopelessness, in turn, is a strong risk factor for suicide, and so emptiness puts people with BPD at risk for suicide.

>> Emptiness is more strongly related to suicidal thinking than any other BPD criterion (except the suicide/self-injury criterion itself).

>> Emptiness and boredom are not the same thing. Sometimes therapists use the terms interchangeably, but simply getting people to be less bored does not make them less empty.

Watching out for distractions

WARNING

For many people who feel empty, distraction from the feeling can temporarily help. Some ways of distracting are healthier than others. Healthy distractions like hobbies, sports, work, and home projects can reduce emptiness, but when these activities end, the emptiness returns. One less healthy approach that many people feel will help reduce emptiness is to get involved in a relationship as soon as possible. However, all too often, sudden, impulsive, and intense relationships, which can help reduce the feeling of emptiness, can also have negative short- and long-term consequences.

Practicing mindfulness for tackling emptiness

Once you've established exactly how emptiness impacts you, ask yourself what your goal is: It's likely that emptiness is intolerable, and so you want to end that feeling. Do this practice (and check out Chapter 9 for more about mindfulness):

1. **Set your intention.**

Find a quiet place — somewhere in your house, or a park, or your local library. Start with focusing on your breath. Slowly bring your awareness to the feeling of emptiness. Notice your thoughts and any judgments that arise. As you do this, divide the thoughts into one of three categories, which you label "good," "bad," or "neutral." Notice that your mind has all of these thoughts and that they are only taking place in your mind. They do not exist outside of you. Sitting with an experience that you label as "bad" will not kill or destroy you.

2. Pay attention.

Use the observe skill of DBT to address emptiness. Notice whether you have paired the "bad" thoughts with the fear that they will harm you. Notice the desire to avoid the thoughts. Now, here is the magic! Simply observing all of this will allow you to notice and then realize that all bad feelings and thoughts pass along and move through, just like the good and neutral ones.

TIP

Attention to emptiness is most easily done when there isn't much to distract you from the feeling of emptiness. Notice when there are distractions, because they can powerfully lead you to avoidance of the feeling. You aren't going to overcome emptiness by avoiding it.

This practice will allow you to realize that the thought that you are empty may not feel pleasant, but it's also just a thought, and the thought itself doesn't make you empty. You'll realize that you and empty are not the same thing. How can you be empty if you are full of thoughts? With practice, you'll notice that the thoughts and feelings will pass.

REMEMBER

If you want to end the feeling of emptiness, you need more than simply desire or hope. You need to be willing to see yourself as whole and sufficient. Many people who are emotionally sensitive feel responsible for the problems in their lives, and at times they refuse to acknowledge that there is anything redeeming about them — for example, that they are kind, intelligent, loyal, or lovable. You won't get this from the outside. Your greatness is inside of you. Accept all of who you are. Accept that you feel empty in this moment, that the feeling is a part of you, and that you are open to it. Don't push emptiness away! If you want it to change, you have to be willing to give it your full attention. Freedom is living without fear and being able to face and ultimately accept the most painful parts of yourself. Emptiness is not you but is a part of you. Be willing to meet it with love and compassion.

3. Use a practice in willingness.

Sit for eight minutes and focus on the word *emptiness*. In your mind, do the following:

TIP

- **For the first two minutes,** as you breathe in, say, "I am empty." As you breathe out: "I don't like it."

- **The next two minutes,** as you breathe in, say, "I am empty." As you breathe out: "I can't change it."

- **The next two minutes,** as you breathe in, say, "I am empty." As you breathe out: "I can accept it."

- **The final two minutes,** as you breathe in, say, "I am empty." As you breathe out: "I will accept it."

6

The Part of Tens

Chapter **24**

Ten Mindful Practices

M indfulness is the core skill of DBT. It's critical that you practice this skill and strengthen the mindfulness muscle in your brain. Think of this chapter as your guide for ten different mindful workouts for your brain. As we note in Chapter 9, DBT breaks down mindfulness into the three WHAT skills — Observe, Describe, and Participate — and this is what you do to practice mindfulness. In this chapter, we teach you a number of practices from each of the three categories.

REMEMBER

When you *observe* mindfully, you just notice; when you *describe* mindfully, you observe something and label it using only facts; and when you *participate* mindfully, you enter into the experience fully letting go of self-consciousness and the thinking that takes you out of the present moment. You'll notice that embedded in each practice, you'll practice the HOW skills: one-mindfully, non-judgmentally, and effectively.

Observe an Itch

Find a comfortable seated position on a chair or on the floor. Rest your hands gently in your lap, palms either up or down. Set a timer for two minutes. Close your eyes and begin to observe an itch in your body. Simply observe it. Notice the sensation, the intensity, and any changes you may find along the way.

Your practice is to observe the itch and do nothing about it, just notice. You'll find there is a lot to pay attention to. Notice what happens in your mind. If your mind strays from the itch, notice that your mind has wandered, label it "wandering mind," and return to looking for an itch to observe.

Observe the Urge to Swallow

Find a comfortable seated position on a chair or on the floor. Rest your hands gently in your lap, palms either up or down. Set a timer for two minutes. Close your eyes and begin to observe the urge to swallow. Do not swallow; simply observe the sensations in your mouth and your thoughts. Step back and simply notice the experience and all that comes with it.

Observe Your Hands

Find a comfortable seated position on a chair or on the floor. Set a timer for one minute. Place your hands together in a prayer position. Now for one minute, begin rubbing your hands back and forth quickly so you feel friction between your palms. When the timer bell rings, observe the temperature and sensations on your hands. Do this until you feel that the sensation in your hands returns to normal.

If you notice your mind being distracted by thoughts, catch it and mindfully return your attention back to the practice.

REMEMBER

Observe Your Breath by Ladder Breathing

Find a comfortable seated position on a chair or on the floor. Rest your hands gently in your lap, palms either up or down. You can do this practice for as short a time as two minutes or extend it for a longer mindfulness practice.

Try this practice with your eyes open. In DBT we strive to teach skills that you can then generalize to different areas in your life. Because we live much of our life with our eyes open, doing your mindfulness practices in this way can help you practice the skill while navigating the distractions you may find when your eyes are open. To minimize distraction, rest your gaze gently in front of you, perhaps on the floor or your lap.

TIP

During the practice of ladder breathing, you'll observe your breath as you count. As you inhale and exhale, you'll count one; on your next inhale and exhale, you'll say two, and so on up to ten. Don't worry about matching your breath length to your count; let your breath be natural, not controlling the length. Once you get to ten, you'll return to the bottom and start back at one.

REMEMBER

When your mind wanders, which it most likely will many times during the practice, your task is to notice it has wandered and return to the number one. It isn't uncommon to notice that you've counted beyond ten; this is another way in which our attention wanders, and you can lose mindful attention. If that happens, notice it and return to one. Some people find it useful to label their mind "wandering mind" when they catch themselves thinking about something else during the practice. It's quite common during this practice to not get close to ten without your mind wandering. The goal isn't necessarily to reach ten, but to notice when your mind has wandered and bring your attention back to the practice; it is this that strengthens your mindfulness muscle.

Describe a Social Media Post

Find a social media post that you like. Set your timer for two minutes and describe or label what you see. Stick to the facts. Avoid using judgments, shorthand, or editorials. Now find a post that you don't like. Again, set your timer for two minutes and mindfully describe what you see. Stick to the facts!

Describe a Difficult or Painful Emotion

Find a comfortable seated position on a chair or on the floor. Rest your hands gently in your lap, palms either up or down. Take a few moments to connect with a difficult emotion you're experiencing. Begin to identify judgments about this emotion or emotional experience, yourself, or someone else who may be connected to this experience. It may be helpful to write down these descriptions.

Next, replace your judgments with a non-judgmental description of the emotion and your experience. You can write these descriptions next to the judgmental observations you just listed. Pay attention to how the emotion feels in your body when you describe it mindfully versus judgmentally. Try to practice this way of mindfully describing your painful or difficult emotions the next time you experience them.

Describe the Sounds around You

Find a comfortable seated position on a chair or on the floor. Rest your hands gently in your lap, palms either up or down. This practice can also be done outside while walking. You can set a timer for two minutes if you would like a short practice, or extend this practice for a longer period of time.

Focus your attention on the sounds around you. As you hear a sound, label it and then search for the next sound. Notice when your mind labels the sound and then begins thinking about it. For example, perhaps you think, "I hear someone unwrapping a piece of candy," and then you begin thinking about what kind of candy it could be and then remembering when you last had candy, and so on. That is an example of your mind wandering to thinking. When that happens, catch your mind and turn your attention back to your practice.

Participate in Standing on One Foot

Many people judge themselves quite harshly when it comes to their balance. Set a timer for two minutes and stand on one leg. Enter into the exercise without judgment and worry. Notice these thoughts and turn your mind back to your practice as if nothing else matters in the world right now, other than standing on one leg.

Participate in Writing with Your Non-Dominant Hand

Unless they are ambidextrous, most people are self-conscious about writing with their non-dominant hand, which makes this task a wonderful opportunity to practice mindfully participating. Take out a piece of paper and a pen. Using your non-dominant hand, practice writing the alphabet two times, first in all uppercase and then all lowercase. Throw yourself into this experience, notice self-judgments, and let them pass.

Participate in Driving a Car

We often multi-task while driving. For this practice you're going to fully participate in the task of driving. You'll do this one-mindfully. Set the intention to drive mindfully to your destination. Pick a drive that you do frequently, such as your drive to work, to school, to the gym, to pick up your kids, or to a frequent errand like a trip to the supermarket. Turn off the music and put your phone down. All you will do is drive. Notice what this experience is like when you're done.

Chapter **25**

Ten Ways to Live an Antidepressant Life

Many people who feel depressed take an antidepressant medication. However, not all those who take these medications feel a benefit. And certainly, antidepressants are not without risk. It's true that it takes just a second every day to take a pill, but people on these medications recognize that they have side effects, lead to financial costs that aren't always covered by insurance, and are not always fully effective. As you find out in this chapter, there are other ways to target depression and anxiety that don't involve medication or, if medication is used, that can enhance the medication's effectiveness.

Engaging in Exercise

Of all the non-medication ways to combat depression, exercise is perhaps the most effective. People who exercise feel better, and this is independent of an increase in their level of fitness. Importantly, research shows that the focus should be on the frequency of the exercise rather than its duration or intensity. Antidepressant benefits appear when a person exercises more than 150 minutes — that is, 2.5 hours — per week. In other words, 30 minutes of regular exercise five days per week is a side effect–free mood enhancer.

If you haven't engaged in exercise for a long time, or if you're new to exercise, you should first consult with your doctor to make sure that you don't have an underlying health condition that would prevent you from exercising.

Trying Meditation

More and more research on the impact of mindfulness meditation is showing that it's useful in reducing depression and anxiety. There is stronger evidence that one form of mindfulness known as mindfulness-based cognitive therapy (MBCT) helps people at risk of relapsing into depression. MBCT is an eight-week course with once-a-week attendance, with each session lasting two hours, and a full-day class in the fifth week. It has proven so successful that in the United Kingdom, MBCT is becoming the treatment of choice for recurrent depression in the National Health Service (NHS).

While both exercise and meditation alone have been shown to help reduce depression, new research shows that when combined, they lead to a marked reduction in depressive symptoms.

You can find out more about MBCT at https://mbct.com/.

Eating a Less Refined Diet

Particularly in the West, overly refined and processed food means that diet plays a major factor in poor health. Our diets tend to be energy-rich, with high levels of saturated fats and refined sugar. As a result, our bodies don't have to do too much work to break them down. Not unexpectedly, this is leading to extremely high levels of obesity. Yet it is not only the body but also the mind that is adversely impacted. Many studies show that people who are obese have a higher incidence of mental health problems such as depression and anxiety.

On the other hand, people who eat less refined, less processed, and less calorie-rich foods reduce their risk of depression. Given the complexities of measuring the relationship between depression and anxiety and food intake, it's difficult to study cause and effect, but increasing evidence shows that lifestyle changes that include a less refined diet contribute to having a less irritable, less anxious, and less depressed brain.

REMEMBER

Before making any drastic or significant changes in your diet, you should contact your doctor or nutritionist to make sure that the changes you're considering are healthy and balanced.

Being Careful with Alcohol and Various Drugs

Many studies show that people diagnosed with substance use disorders commonly have a mood disorder such as depression. Alcohol specifically, and especially in large quantities, leads to chemical changes in the brain that in turn lead to anxiety and depression. People who drink excessive amounts of alcohol are up to three times more likely than those who don't drink it excessively to develop anxiety and depression. Depressed people who drink are also at a much higher risk for suicide than depressed people who don't drink. In the short run, people who drink excessively and then stop may experience some depressive symptoms; however, in the long run, the stopping of, or marked reduction in, alcohol intake improves various aspects of physical and mental health.

However, whereas many drugs worsen depression, some drugs seem to help. Caffeine is one of them. A widely used psychoactive drug, it can improve attention, alertness, and mood.

REMEMBER

From a DBT perspective, the focus is a little less on the specific substance and more on the impact on the individual. While it's true that some people may experience very concerning effects when they use drugs and alcohol, others may not. The DBT therapist can work closely with their patient and assess whether the substances are impacting the patient's mood. If you're worried that you might have a substance use disorder, or others are worried for you, your doctor can recommend specific treatment options and counseling.

Getting Enough Sleep

For many people, a good night's sleep is the bedrock of their mental and physical health. Depression is associated with major disturbances in the quality of sleep, and many people with depression note significant insomnia. It's a vicious cycle, as people with insomnia are then more prone to depression.

Improving sleep reduces the impact of depression, and a person can do specific things to get better sleep:

>> **Avoid certain chemicals.** These include caffeine, alcohol, nicotine, and stimulant medications that can interfere with sleep.

>> **Turn their bedroom into a sleep-only environment.** This can be achieved by using blackout shades, using white noise machines, wearing an eye mask, removing all monitors and screens, keeping pets out of the room, and keeping the room cool, somewhere between 60 and 70 degrees Fahrenheit.

>> **Establish a relaxing pre-bedtime routine.** Activities such as taking a warm bath, reading an article in a magazine, watching certain television shows, and practicing relaxing breathing exercises can be soothing. On the flip side, people should avoid any interaction or activity that leads to stress. These should be left for the next day. Part of the routine should include going to bed at the same time each night, within a 30-minute window.

>> **Go to bed when tired.** Many people feel they should be able to fall asleep when they go to bed, only to find that they can't and instead stay awake, tossing and turning. If a person isn't asleep in 20 minutes, they should get out of bed, leave their bedroom, and do some relaxing activities before heading back to bed.

>> **Avoid naps.** If a nap is needed, it should be in the early afternoon rather than directly before bedtime.

>> **Eliminate heavy meals before bedtime.** People who eat heavy meals just before getting into bed often experience insomnia. Dinner should be finished several hours before bedtime, and if a snack is needed, it should be a light snack.

>> **Stay well hydrated.** This is particularly important in summer, when people lose more fluid than they imagine. They should drink enough non-alcoholic, non-caffeinated beverages in the evening so as not to wake up thirsty, but not so much that they need to make frequent trips to the bathroom.

>> **Exercise.** Covered earlier in this chapter, exercise often helps promote sleep. However, if it's done too close to bedtime, it can be overly stimulating and have the opposite effect. Because of this, any exercise should be completed no later than three hours before bedtime.

Maintaining Social Interaction and Connection

Another key antidepressant influence is the presence and quality of social interaction. Loneliness — and this is particularly true for older people — is highly correlated with depression and suicide. On the other hand, supportive, connected relationships with friends and family have long been shown to maintain and even improve mental health and psychological well-being.

REMEMBER

The need for social connectedness is deeply ingrained into our human nature. It has evolved together with all the neural, hormonal, and genetic factors that are directly associated with bonding and companionship, and from an evolutionary perspective, it's directly connected to the survival of the human species.

Because of this, overwhelming feelings of isolation and the loss of relationships lead to a decline in cognition and a worsening of mood conditions like depression. Loss of relationships can lead to worsening sleep and to an increase in cortisol, which are both associated with depression, a deterioration of the functioning of the immune system, and weight gain. On the other hand, reconnecting with others and maintaining relationships reverses these negative effects of isolation and leads to a reduction in depression.

Adding Recreation and Relaxation to Your Routine

Another element in the management of depression is ensuring that pleasurable recreational activities are integrated into a daily routine. Engaging in ways of caring for the self, such as a hobby, a sport, gardening, cooking, or another activity not done as a chore, can combat depression. Whether it's an established recreational activity or one that a person is considering taking up by building mastery in a new skill, such moments provide an opportunity for the person to experience pleasure and to direct their mind away from the ruminations and worries that plague people with depression.

TIP

Although this hasn't been used in isolation as a way of enhancing mental well-being, it's a core part of the ABC PLEASE skills of the emotion regulation module and one that DBT therapists encourage their patients to practice. See Chapter 10 for details.

Accessing Green Space and the Environment

Many environmental factors have been implicated in mental health conditions. These include access to green space and factors such as noise, air, and water pollution and climate.

The one environmental factor with the largest evidence base is exposure to green space, including parks, forests, and agricultural land. Such exposure appears to reduce the risk for developing many psychiatric disorders during adolescence and adulthood. In a large Danish study published in 2019, which tracked residential green space using satellite imagery, the researchers surveyed nearly a million Danes and looked at their mental health. They found that citizens who grew up with the least amount of nearby green space had as much as a 55 percent increased risk of developing psychiatric disorders such as depression and anxiety.

Although it's possible that simply being out in nature can improve one's mental health, this improvement may also be a result of being exposed to clean air and sunlight. There is evidence that exposure to sunlight leads to higher levels of vitamin D, which also leads to a reduction in depressive symptoms.

Taking Care of Pets and Other Animals

Although this likely applies to other pets, most studies on the role of pets improving mental health have been done on dogs. Having a dog creates a sense of purpose and responsibility for another life. Dogs provide physical affection and a feeling of unconditional love. Studies show that owning a dog reduces stress, anxiety, and depression. Playing with dogs increases the feel-good chemicals such as oxytocin and dopamine in the brain, and these create an overall sense of positivity. Owning a dog leads to a reduction in one's sense of loneliness, not only by having the dog itself but also because it leads to socialization with other dog owners. Dog ownership encourages exercise because of the need to meet a dog's regular exercise schedule. Finally, having a dog also improves physical health because people with dogs have lower blood pressure and are less likely to develop heart disease.

Beyond dogs, time spent with farm animals by people with mental health conditions has been shown to reduce rates of depression and anxiety.

Making Time for Faith and Prayer

Religion and spirituality are associated with better health, including longer life expectancy and an overall improved quality of life. An interesting finding is that it isn't simply following the rules of institutional religiousness, but rather personal devotion and inner faith that are connected to improved mental health.

Brain imaging studies show that prayer leads to increased activity in the reward centers of the brain, particularly those areas that are associated with *anhedonia*, which is an inability to feel pleasure and is a core symptom of depression; by activating the brain's reward centers, and thereby reducing anhedonia, prayer may lead to a reduction in depression.

Chapter **26**

Ten Myths about DBT

M isconceptions have bedeviled the field of mental health for decades. In our era of information, misinformation abounds, and enduring myths about therapy in general and DBT in particular persist. If you're considering DBT but have reservations, it's worth reviewing the mistruths that might be causing you pause so that you can challenge these with facts.

Myth: DBT Is Used Only with People with Borderline Personality Disorder

Fact: A significant amount of research shows that DBT is helpful for many conditions other than borderline personality disorder (BPD). It has been shown to be effective for eating disorders and depression, and as a co-treatment in conditions such as bipolar disorder, post-traumatic stress disorder, and substance abuse.

TIP

The ever-increasing evidence base can be found at `https://behavioraltech. org/research/evidence/`.

Myth: DBT Therapists Teach Skills from a Manual; It's Not a Real Therapy

Fact: Although it's true that all of the skills taught in DBT are outlined in the workbook manuals, the therapy is a healing engagement that involves a real relationship between two people, each of whom uses skills and a behavioral lens to help change, and in so doing, learn to regulate their emotions and change the behaviors that they find problematic.

Dr. Marsha Linehan, who developed DBT, recognized that the relationship was essential and that a strong therapeutic relationship grew with each authentic interaction between the therapist and the patient. According to Dr. Linehan, the relationship was one where each of them could be honest and vulnerable, and included "the therapeutic relationship and therapist self-disclosure." This approach is in stark contrast to traditional dynamic psychotherapies where analysts argued that the major risk in self-disclosure was the mixing of the analytic process with the real relationship; this would prevent the patient from projecting their own fantasies and so distort the relationship with the therapist, which in turn would compromise the effectiveness of the therapy.

Myth: DBT Takes Years Before You Feel Better

Fact: In the standard DBT treatment, patients commit to six months of therapy, sometimes repeated for another six months. This is because it takes six months to learn all the skills taught in skills training group, the skills being mindfulness, interpersonal effectiveness, distress tolerance, and emotion regulation (see Part 3). Individual therapy happens once or twice per week, and a skills training group once per week. Contrast this with the therapeutic treatment known as psychoanalysis, which generally takes three to five meetings a week, and although the length of treatment varies, in general, psychoanalysis lasts an average of five to six years, and in many cases longer.

Myth: DBT Is a Suicide Prevention Therapy

REMEMBER

Fact: DBT is not a suicide prevention program. Instead, it is a therapy that recognizes that for many people who have considered it, suicide often feels as if it is the only way out of intense suffering. DBT emphasizes that there are many alternatives, and that on the other side of a life of misery is a life worth living. The reasoning behind DBT is that people who are suicidal don't know of other ways to not suffer, and so DBT teaches the skills in Part 3 as a way out of suffering. Certainly, the behaviors of suicide and self-harm are targeted, but DBT doesn't end there. It also teaches skills that help a person who is suffering to take control of their life and build one that is meaningful to them.

Myth: If No Other Therapy Has Helped, DBT Won't Either

Fact: Many people who have failed other therapies find success in DBT. This is typically because the other therapies weren't designed to treat the skills deficits that lead to emotion regulation problems, suicidal behavior, and self-injury. DBT recognizes that simply having insight into problems doesn't change the problems. Many people have the insight that smoking is unhealthy and yet they continue to smoke. DBT combines awareness of skill deficits with the teaching, implementation, and application of new skills. It also includes phone coaching to help generalize the newly acquired skills to all relevant contexts of a person's life.

Myth: Once You Start DBT, You Need to Continue It Forever

Fact: DBT is a recovery-based treatment, meaning that once a person has acquired the skills necessary to function in a life that they can now manage, they can take the newly acquired skills with them and use them as necessary. Most clients graduate from DBT go on to live meaningful lives with far less suffering.

Myth: You Have to Accept Buddhism to Do DBT

Fact: Although Dr. Linehan developed her mindfulness practices from her experiences with Christian and Zen meditation, the mindfulness skill of DBT (see Chapter 9) is common to both secular and religious practice. DBT focuses on mindfulness as a skill of awareness and attention. Devout believers, agnostics, and atheists can practice mindfulness and DBT without the need to change their religious or areligious philosophies or perspectives on life.

Myth: DBT Is a Cult

Fact: If a cult is defined as "a relatively small group of people having religious beliefs or practices regarded by others as strange or sinister" or "a misplaced or excessive admiration for a particular person," then DBT does not meet any of these definitions. DBT has no religious underpinnings, no secret societies, and no levels of ritualistic practice, and instead uses the scientific method to measure decreases in suffering, suicidal ideation, and self-destructive behavior.

TECHNICAL STUFF

Some argue that the reverence of Dr. Linehan makes DBT look like a cult, but this admiration is often from patients who have benefited from the treatment that she developed and from therapists who found DBT to be a system of therapy that made sense and allowed them to help their most troubled patients. Certainly, many people are grateful to scientists who made important discoveries. Patients revered Alexander Fleming, who discovered penicillin, and Frederick Banting, who discovered insulin, and certainly many people are grateful for those who developed the defibrillators that have saved their lives.

Myth: There Is Very Little Evidence That DBT Works

Fact: After many decades of considering conditions like BPD nearly untreatable, the outcomes are becoming far more favorable and there are now multiple evidence-based treatments (EBTs) for BPD, including the following: General Psychiatric Management (GPM), DBT, Mentalization-Based Therapy (MBT), Transference-Focused Psychotherapy (TFP), and Schema-Focused Therapy (SFT).

Of these, DBT is the best-known, best-researched, and most widely available of the evidence-based therapies.

TIP

Moreover, DBT researchers have been willing and open to publish all outcome results, whether favorable or not, and these can be found at

» `https://behavioraltech.org/research/evidence/`

» `https://depts.washington.edu/uwbrtc/about-us/`
  `dialectical-behavior-therapy/`

» `https://blogs.cuit.columbia.edu/dbt/research-studies-on-`
  `dialectical-behavior-therapy/`

Myth: DBT Isn't Interested in "Root Causes" of Mental Illness

Fact: DBT believes that all behaviors are caused, and that all causes have causes. DBT's focus on the present moment and recent behaviors is based on the idea that people are much more likely to remember recent events than past events. Also, the connection between something that happened this morning to something happening now is often far clearer and with fewer variables than something that happened years ago or between childhood and the present moment. To be clear, DBT does, in fact, address more distant causes when they show up in a person's chain analysis. It's often the case that when a patient is no longer struggling with dangerous and self-destructive behaviors, that DBT therapists, like all other therapists, will look at the more distant past if this is a goal of the patient.

Index

A

abandonment, fear of, 246–247

ABC PLEASE skills
  about, 327
  decreasing emotional vulnerability with, 118–121

ability, compared with motivation, 234–235

acceptance
  coexistence with change, 25
  focusing on, 276–277
  moving to, 235–236
  of other perspectives, 90–91
  radical, 139–140
  of reality, 134
  of situations, 138–144
  strategies for eating disorders, 287

Acceptance of a Dialectical Philosophy agreement, 213

ACCEPTS skill, 130–131

Accumulating Positives, as skill in ABC PLEASE, 118, 119

Acknowledge the valid, as a validation method, 155

acknowledging initial emotions, 89–90

acting on urges, 68

action
  awareness of how emotions manifest in, 66
  behavioral, 42
  holding off on taking, 32

active-passivity, apparent competence *versus*, 185

Activities, in ACCEPTS skill, 130

adapting to what is, 90

adaptive denial, 278

addictions
  about, 271, 292
  activities that may become, 293–295
  behavioral, 292–295
  binge eating disorder, 281–283

body dysmorphic disorder, 287–292

compulsive sexual behavior, 294–295

DBT for behavioral, 295

DBT for substance use disorders, 278–281

DBT model for eating disorders, 284–287

DBT skills for substance use disorders, 275–278

dopamine, 271–272

eating disorders, 281–287

gambling, 295

gaming, 293–294

pornography, 294

substance dependence, 272–281

substance use compared with substance-induced disorders, 273–275

adding structure to two different environments, 192–193

addressing
  anxiety triggers, 259–260
  problems, 193–194

ADHD (attention deficit hyperactivity disorder), 187

adolescent behavior, 187

adopting self-soothing practices, 125–126

adrenaline, 258–259

agenda
  for therapist consultation team meetings, 215–216
  using an, 174

agreements
  coming to, 34
  therapist consultation team, 213–214

alcohol
  avoiding antidepressant medication and, 325
  depression and, 255

all-or-nothing thinking, 288

aloneness, 310

alternative rebellion skill, 145, 277–278

ambivalence, 286

Building Mastery, as skill in ABC PLEASE, 118, 119
bulimia nervosa (BN), 283, 284
burning bridges, 276–277
burnout, of therapists, 211–212

C

calling for help, 178–179
calming emotions, 114–115
capabilities, enhancing, 9
case consultation meetings, 192
case management services, 192
causes
  about, 132
  changing perspectives, 133–134
  example of, 132–133
  myths about, 335
CBT (cognitive behavioral therapy)
  about, 182
  for depression, 253
  ideas from, 236–238
chain analysis
  about, 226
  conditions for effective, 227
  steps of, 199–201, 202, 228–229
  when and how to perform, 226–228
challenges, overcoming, as a benefit of
    maintaining motivation, 240
change
  coexistence with acceptance, 25
  as a constant, 167
  increasing motivation to, 9
  of perspectives, 133–134
  strategies for eating disorders, 286–287
  as transactional, 167–168
Change the relationship, in SCREW acronym, 193
Cheat Sheet (website), 4
checking-the-facts skill, 79–80
Cheerleading commitment strategy, 195
cheerleading statements, 124
childhood sexual abuse (CSA), 267
choices, breaking free of rigid, 45–47

choosing
  compared with reacting, 46–47
  mindfulness and, 47
clean mind, 275
clear mind, 275
coaching, phone skills, 9, 23–24, 175, 177–180
cognitive behavioral therapy (CBT)
  about, 182
  for depression, 253
  ideas from, 236–238
cognitive component, of anxiety, 256–257
cognitive defusion, 48–49
cognitive dysregulation, 17, 250, 252–253
cognitive modification strategies
  for body dysmorphic disorder (BDD), 288–289
  for eating disorders, 287
cognitive reappraisal, 78–79
cognitive restructuring, 237
commitment
  making a, 174
  strategies for, 194–195
communication
  enhancing, 91–92
  with GIVE skills, 157
community reinforcement, 277
Comparison, in ACCEPTS skill, 130
competence, increasing for therapists, 10
competing response training, 292
compromise
  compared with dialectical synthesis, 46
  cooperation and, 165–168
compulsive sexual behavior, as a behavioral
    addiction, 294–295
concentrative mindfulness, 107–108
confronting disproportionate reactions, 60–63
connectedness, balancing with solitude, 309–314
conscious feelings, 71–72
consequences
  of behaviors, 11
  in chain analysis, 229
consultation team, 21

distractions
  about, 129–131
  emptiness and, 313–314
distress, causes of, 63–64
distress tolerance
  about, 127–128
  acceptance of situations, 138–144
  alternative rebellion, 145
  building, 127–145
  cause and, 132–134
  changing perspective, 133–134
  crisis management, 138–145
  crisis survival skills, 128–132
  curbing impulsive behavior, 134–138
  as a DBT skill, 12
  distracting yourself, 129–131
  example of, 132–133
  foregoing short-term gratification, 134–135
  improving your situation, 135–137
  skill of using pros and cons, 137–138
  as a skill used for binge eating disorder (BED), 283
  skills for finding emotional balance, 40
  soothing yourself, 131–132
  TIPP skill, 144–145
diverse populations, treatment of, 13
Diversity and Change agreement, 213
Door-in-the-Face commitment strategy, 195
  motivation and, 239
dopamine, 271–272
drugs
  avoiding antidepressant medication and, 325
  depression and, 255
DSM (Diagnostic and Statistical Manual of Mental Disorders), 17, 246–249, 274
dynamics, of relationships, 87–91
dysregulation
  areas of, 249–253
  types of, 16–18

E

Easy manner, in GIVE skill, 157
eating disorders (EDs)
  about, 281
  binge eating disorder (BED), 281–283
  DBT model of treatment for, 284–287
  other, 283–284
effective punishment, 164
Effective skill, 105
effectiveness
  myths about, 333
  when coming to an agreement, 34
either/or, moving to both/and from, 45–46
emotion mind, 30, 99
emotional balance, finding, 40–42
emotional dysregulation, 16, 17, 58, 249, 250
emotional expression, intolerance of, 18
emotional instability, BPD and, 248
emotional regulation
  ABC PLEASE, 118–121
  about, 117–118
  accumulating positives, 119
  adopting healthy self-soothing practices, 125–126
  avoiding mood-altering substances, 121
  balanced eating, 120
  balanced sleep, 121
  being kind to yourself, 123–124
  being your own emotional support, 124–126
  building mastery, 119
  coping ahead of time with difficult situations, 119–120
  as a DBT skill, 12
  exercise, 121
  physical illness, 120
  practicing opposite action, 121–123
  reappraising feelings, 124–125
  as a skill used for binge eating disorder (BED), 282–283
  skills for finding emotional balance, 40

emotional support, being your own, 124–126

emotional triggers, identifying and handling, 67–70

emotional vulnerability

  decreasing with ABC PLEASE, 118–121

  self-invalidation *versus,* 185

emotions

  about, 55–56

  in ACCEPTS skill, 130

  acknowledging initial, 89–90

  awareness of how they manifest in action, 66

  calming, 114–115

  confronting disproportionate reactions, 60–63

  handling problem areas, 63–64

  identifying, 41

  identifying problem areas, 63–64

  justified, 122

  as obstacles, 148

  primary, 44–45, 56–58, 90

  recognizing feelings, 56–60

  recording, 220–222

  reinforcement of strong, 18–19

  secondary, 45, 56–58

  unjustified, 122

  validating, 62

  widening range of, 44–45

emptiness

  about, 312–314

  BPD and feelings of, 248

Encouragement, in IMPROVE skill, 137

Entertain misery, in SCREW acronym, 193

environment

  avoiding antidepressant medication and, 328

  structuring, 10 (*see also* structuring the environment)

environment, invalidating

  about, 10, 18

  dismissal of problems and reactions, 19

  intolerance of emotional expression, 18

  reinforcement of strong emotions, 18–19

  shame, 19

environmental intervention, consultation to the patient *versus,* 189–190

environmental trigger, 67

ERP (exposure response prevention) therapy, or body dysmorphic disorder (BDD), 290

establishing new pathways, 72–73

evaluation phase, in solution analysis, 202, 229

evidence, myths about, 334–335

exaggerated first reactions, 30–31

executive functioning, 91

exercise

  avoiding antidepressant medication with, 323–324

  psyche and, 113

  as a skill in ABC PLEASE, 121

experiences, using as learning opportunities, 242

exposure

  about, 301

  building motivation for, 301

exposure response prevention (ERP) therapy, or body dysmorphic disorder (BDD), 290

exposure therapy

  about, 238

  for body dysmorphic disorder (BDD), 290–291

  for eating disorders, 287

  practicing, 301–303

Express, in DEAR MAN skill, 150

F

fact-checking, 79–80

failure, getting back up after, 141

Fair, in FAST skill, 158

faith, avoiding antidepressant medication and, 329

Fallibility agreement, 214

family sessions, 192

FAST skill, 158, 159

fear, opposite action and, 70

Feel the Floor skill, 269

feelings

  about feelings, 81–82

  conscious, 71–72

  reappraising, 124–125

  recognizing, 56–60

fight-or-flight response, 223, 259
finding
  assumptions, 84
  balance, 161–165
  emotional balance, 40–42
  individual therapists, 172–173
Five Senses skill, 269
Fleming, Alexander (scientist), 334
Focus on your Floating Tongue skill, 269
focused attention training, 112
focusing
  on acceptance, 276–277
  as a benefit of mindfulness, 112
  on goals, 240–241
  on long-term goals, 242
  on your breath, 39–40
Foot-in-the-Door commitment strategy
  about, 195
  motivation and, 239
forcing independence
  about, 165
  fostering dependence *versus,* 187–188
fostering dependence
  about, 165
  forcing independence *versus,* 187–188
frameworks, building, 194–197
Freedom to Choose in the Absence of Viable or
    Desirable Alternatives commitment strategy
  about, 195
  for eating disorders, 286
  motivation and, 239
functions
  of comprehensive treatments, 20–22
  dialectical behavior therapy (DBT), 8–10

G

GAD (generalized anxiety disorder), 258
gambling, as a behavioral addiction, 295
gaming, as a behavioral addiction, 293–294
generalization training, 292

generalized anxiety disorder (GAD), 258
generalizing, 9
generating
  distress tolerance, 127–145
  frameworks, 194–197
  healthy space in your psyche, 113–114
  motivation for exposure, 301
  space, 106
generation phase, in solution analysis, 202, 229
generative mindfulness, 108–111
Gentle, in GIVE skill, 157
"get moving," 42
GIVE skills, 157, 159
goals
  of comprehensive treatments, 20–22
  focusing on, 240–241
  setting, 173–174
  setting for therapy, 196–197
  of therapy, 273
good news, sharing, 180
good practices, enhancing, 94
gratification, foregoing short-term, 134–135
gratitude, practicing, 41
green space, avoiding antidepressant medication
    and, 328
grounding skills, 269
group skills training, 9
group therapy
  about, 175
  benefits of, 176
  joining groups, 175–176
  sharing strategies, 176
guilt
  opposite action and, 70
  as a secondary emotion, 90

H

Habit Reversal Training (HRT), 291–292
hair pulling, 291–292
half-smile, 283

interpersonal dysregulation, 17, 249, 250–251

interpersonal effectiveness
   about, 147, 159–160, 204
   awareness of obstacles, 148–149
   combing GIVE skill and FAST skill, 159
   communicating with GIVE skills, 157
   as a DBT skill, 12
   DEAR MAN skill, 149–153
   FAST skill, 158
   increasing, 147–160
   practicing validation, 153–157

interpersonal relationships, BPD and, 247

Interpretation, in THINK skill, 44

intimidating behavior, 89

intolerance, of emotional expression, 18

invalidating environment
   about, 10, 18
   dismissal of problems and reactions, 19
   intolerance of emotional expression, 18
   reinforcement of strong emotions, 18–19
   shame, 19

invalidation, 18

irreverence, reciprocity *versus*, 189

J

joining
   groups, 175–176
   therapist consultation teams, 210–214

judging
   about, 82
   assumptions, 84
   judgments, 82
   others, 35
   self-judgments, 84–85

justified emotions, 122

K

kindness
   in THINK skill, 44
   to yourself, 123–124

L

ladder breathing, 318–319

learning opportunities, using experiences as, 242

letting go, of hurtful practices, 94

life-threatening behaviors, in target hierarchy, 198

limiting disruption, 67–68

Lincoln, Abraham (US President), 141

Linehan, Marsha (doctor)
   ACCEPTS skill, 130
   biosocial theory, 10
   Buddhism and, 334
   on challenging problems, 23
   on consultation teams, 210
   on crisis survival skills, 128
   DBT Prolonged Exposure (DBT PE), 263–264
   as developer of DBT, 8, 15, 45, 161, 245
   on dialectical synthesis, 26
   on dialectics, 181–182
   on dysregulation, 249–253
   on emotion dysregulation, 16
   on emotional states, 99
   on environmental factors, 18
   IMPROVE skill, 136
   on obstacles, 148
   on suffering and agony, 140
   on therapist relationships, 332
   on validation, 154–156

Linehan Training Institute, 173

Linking the Current Commitment to Past Commitments commitment strategy, 195

links, in chain analysis, 228–229

listening, honest, 92

loneliness, 310–312

long-term goals
   about, 68
   focusing on, 242
   sacrificing for short-term goals, 148–149

loose, being too, 188

lying behavior, 89

M

maintaining motivation, 240–242

making commitments, 194–195

maladaptive behaviors, 11

managing

   depression, 253–255

   emotional triggers, 67–70

   excessive anxiety, 259–261

   mania, 255–256

   problem areas, 63–64

mania, managing, 255–256

matching reactions, 31–32

Mazza, James (doctor), 204

MBCT (mindfulness-based cognitive therapy), 182, 324

MD (muscle dysmorphia), 292

"me time," 123–124

Meaning, in IMPROVE skill, 136

mechanics, of dialectical behavior therapy (DBT), 12–13

meditation, avoiding antidepressant medication with, 324

meeting leader, on therapist consultation teams, 217

meetings, for therapist consultation teams, 215–217

methods of validation, 154–156

Middle Path skill

   about, 161

   behaviorism, 162–164

   change, 167–168

   cooperation and compromise, 165–168

   dialectical dilemmas of parenting, 186–188

   dialectics, 164–165

   finding balance, 161–165

   points of view, 166–167

   validation, 162

Miller, Alec (doctor), 161

mind

   states of, 99–100

   turning your, 141–143

Mindful, in DEAR MAN skill, 151–152

mindful breaths, 31

mindful practices, recommended, 317–321

mindfulness

   about, 97

   benefits of, 112–115

   calming emotions, 114–115

   choosing and, 47

   for cognitive dysregulation, 253

   concentrative, 107–108

   creating healthy space in psyche, 113–114

   of current emotion, 58

   as a DBT skill, 12

   exploring your own mind, 98–107

   focusing the mind, 112

   generative, 108–111

   at its core, 99

   making space, 106

   practicing, 238

   practicing for emptiness, 313–314

   practicing of current thought, 77–78

   practicing with the WHAT skills, 100–103

   receptive, 111

   reflective, 111

   relaxation, 112–113

   setting routines, 106–107

   as a skill used for binge eating disorder (BED), 282

   states of mind, 99–100

   types of, 107–111

   using HOW skills in, 103–105

mindfulness-based cognitive therapy (MBCT), 182, 324

mindreading, 288

minimizing power of emotional triggers, 68–70

missing links analysis, 231

modes, of dialectical behavior therapy (DBT), 8–10

modes of treatment

   about, 22

   individual therapy, 23

   phone/skills coaching, 23–24

   skills training, 22–23

   therapist consultation team, 24

recreation, avoiding antidepressant medication and, 327

Reflect back, as a validation method, 155

Reflecting on the Success of Past Commitments, motivation and, 239

reflective mindfulness, 111

reflective perspectives, 43

reframing triggers with reappraisal, 69

regulating emotions. *see* emotional regulation

regulation, transitioning from recognition to, 61–63

reinforcement, of strong emotions, 18–19

reinforcers
  in DEAR MAN skill, 151
  in Middle Path skill, 163–164

relationships
  about, 87
  accepting other perspectives, 90–91
  defined, 88
  dynamics of, 87–91
  effectiveness of, 251
  enhancing communication, 91–92
  possibilities, 93–94
  repairing, 179–180
  what you bring, 88–90

relaxation
  avoiding antidepressant medication and, 327
  as a benefit of mindfulness, 112–113
  in IMPROVE skill, 136

relaxation training, 292

Remember icon, 3

repairing relationships, 179–180

resources, Internet
  Behavioral Tech, 173
  Cheat Sheet, 4
  evidence, 335
  mindfulness-based cognitive therapy (MBCT), 324

responses
  increasing trust in, 50–51
  physical, 71–72
  reducing sizes of, 68–69

reviewing diary card in individual sessions, 198

ritual/response prevention
  for body dysmorphic disorder (BDD), 290–291
  for eating disorders, 287

roles, in therapist consultation teams, 216–217

root causes, myths about, 335

routines, setting, 106–107

S

sadness, opposite action and, 70

Salzberg, Sharon (author), 306

school settings, use of DBT in, 204–205

SCREW acronym, 193–194

searching for multiple truths, 25–26

secondary emotions
  about, 45
  compared with primary emotions, 56–58

self-care
  about, 124
  practicing for loneliness, 312

self-compassion, 35

self-confidence, as a benefit of maintaining motivation, 240

self-destructive behaviors, switching to healthy behaviors, 49

self-dysregulation, 17, 249–250, 252

self-enhancing lying, 89

self-harm, 192, 300

self-hatred
  about, 306–307
  practicing self-love, 308–309
  self-love as opposite action, 307–308

self-injury
  about, 27, 166
  BPD and, 248

self-invalidation
  about, 298
  emotional vulnerability *versus*, 185
  exposure, 301–303
  reassurance-seeking, 303–306
  self-validation, 298–299
  shame, 299–301

selfish lying, 89

support groups, 311

supporting therapists, 21–22

suppression, 69

surgery, seeking, 292

sweating, 257

switching self-destructive behaviors to healthy behaviors, 49

sympathetic nervous system, 223

systematic exposure, 238

T

Take a step back, in STOP skill, 135

taking a breath, 39–40

target hierarchy, 198–199

taste
  for self-soothing, 132
  self-soothing and, 125

teaching patients new coping mechanisms, 20–21

team leader, on therapist consultation teams, 216

Technical Stuff icon, 3–4

Teen Talk program, 204

Temperature, in TIPP skill, 144

theoretical framework, of dialectical behavior therapy (DBT), 10–11

therapist consultation team
  about, 24, 209
  agenda for, 215–217
  agreements for, 213–214
  joining, 210–214
  meetings, 9
  roles in, 216–217
  structuring meetings, 215–216
  therapy for therapists, 210–212

therapists
  burnout of, 211–212
  dialectical interventions, 189–190
  enhancing capabilities of, 212–213
  finding individual, 172–173
  increasing motivation and competence for, 10, 20

  myths about, 332
  point of view of, 33
  supporting, 21–22
  therapy for, 210–212

therapy
  about, 171
  goals of, 273
  group, 175–176
  having motivation for, 233–236
  individual, 171–175
  modes of, 9
  myths about, 333
  for people with developmental disabilities, 206–207
  phone coaching, 177–180
  for therapists, 24, 210–212

therapy-interfering behaviors, in target hierarchy, 198

thesis, 26, 45

Think, in THINK skill, 43

THINK skill, 43–44

thinking dialectically, 182–184

thinking patterns, setting new, 48–49

thoughts
  about, 75
  in ACCEPTS skill, 131
  accounting for self-judgments, 84–85
  assessing assumptions, 83–84
  checking facts, 79–80
  feelings about feelings, 81–82
  as obstacles, 149
  practicing mindfulness of current thought, 77–78
  reactions, 81–85
  self-talk, 75–80
  using cognitive reappraisal, 78–79

threatening behavior, 89

time delay, 68

time keeper, on therapist consultation teams, 217

Tip icon, 3

TIPP skill, 144–145, 224–225

About the Authors

Gillian Galen, PsyD, is an expert in dialectical behavioral therapy (DBT) for adults, adolescents, and families. She is the program director of the McLean Hospital 3East residential DBT program for girls, which is a unique residential program for young women exhibiting self-endangering behaviors and traits of borderline personality disorder (BPD) and related conditions. Passionate about training DBT therapists, she is the assistant director of training for the 3East continuum and regularly lectures to and trains clinicians in DBT and mindfulness. Dr. Galen has been a staff psychologist at McLean Hospital since 2009, when she completed her post-doctoral fellowship at 3East. She has a particular interest in the use of mindfulness in psychotherapy. Dr. Galen is an instructor in psychology at Harvard Medical School.

Dr. Galen has co-authored two other books with Dr. Blaise Aguirre. *Mindfulness for Borderline Personality Disorder: Relieve Your Suffering Using the Core Skill of Dialectical Behavior Therapy* and *Coping with BPD: DBT and CBT Skills to Soothe the Symptoms of Borderline Personality Disorder* are both published by New Harbinger Publications.

Blaise Aguirre, MD, is an expert in child, adolescent, and adult psychotherapy, and in particular, the clinical application of dialectical behavior therapy (DBT). A trainer in DBT, he is the founding medical director of McLean Hospital 3East, a unique continuum of residential and outpatient DBT programs for young people exhibiting self-endangering behaviors and traits of borderline personality disorder (BPD) and related conditions. Dr. Aguirre has been a staff psychiatrist at McLean Hospital since 2000, and is nationally and internationally recognized for his extensive work and research in the treatment of mood and personality disorders in adolescents. He is an assistant professor in psychiatry at Harvard Medical School and lectures regularly throughout the world on DBT and BPD.

Dr. Aguirre is the author and co-author of multiple books, including *Borderline Personality Disorder in Adolescents: A Complete Guide to Understanding and Coping When Your Adolescent Has BPD* (published by Fair Winds Press); *Mindfulness for Borderline Personality Disorder: Relieve Your Suffering Using the Core Skill of Dialectical Behavior Therapy* (published by New Harbinger Publications); and *Coping with BPD: DBT and CBT Skills to Soothe the Symptoms of Borderline Personality Disorder* (published by New Harbinger Publications).

Dedication

This book is dedicated to the many people who have, through the use of DBT, proven its power to change lives, and to Dr. Marsha Linehan, whose life inspired the development of DBT and who has been a mentor to countless therapists.

Authors' Acknowledgments

We want to recognize five groups of people:

Our families who cheered us on and the ones who we live with who now roll their eyes when we promise them that this is our last book! We love you for all of your support and for giving us the time to do this important work.

To our long-time mentors and colleagues at 3East — particularly, Michael Hollander, Janna Hobbs, Cynthia Kaplan, Judy Mintz, and Alan Fruzzetti — as well as our incredible therapists, psychiatrists, nursing staff, unit counselors, administrative staff, hospital administrators, facilities staff, and our amazing outpatient consultation team. It really does take a village!

To our current and past clients, who have used the treatment to develop the kinds of lives that are meaningful to each of you and reinforced our belief in the DBT model. We also want to thank those of you who reviewed some of our ideas and gave some very helpful feedback.

To our team at Wiley: our senior acquisitions editor Tracy Boggier, our development editor Georgette Beatty, who made sure that we kept to each deadline and was a cheerleader when it seemed like too much, and our copy editor Marylouise Wiack, who caught every missing word, every duplicated sentence, and every superfluous opinion!

To Janna Hobbs, a dear friend and DBT expert, for reviewing our manuscript and making sure that we stayed true to our system.

Publisher's Acknowledgments

Senior Acquisitions Editor: Tracy Boggier

Senior Managing Editor: Kristie Pyles

Project Manager and Development Editor: Georgette Beatty

Copy Editor: Marylouise Wiack

Technical Editor: Janna K. Hobbs, LICSW, Senior Consultant, 3East Continuum, McLean Hospital, and DBT Consultant and Parent Coach, Boston Child Study Center

Production Editor: Mohammed Zafar Ali

Cover Image: © Belitas/iStock/ Getty Images Plus/Getty Images

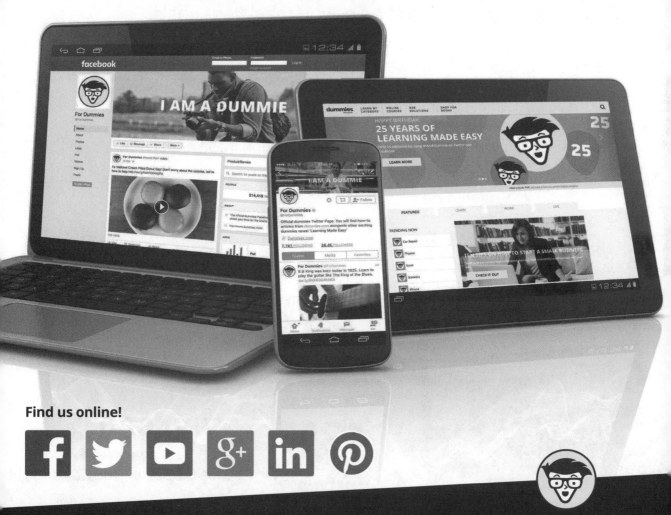
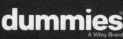

Leverage the power

Dummies is the global leader in the reference category and one of the most trusted and highly regarded brands in the world. No longer just focused on books, customers now have access to the dummies content they need in the format they want. Together we'll craft a solution that engages your customers, stands out from the competition, and helps you meet your goals.

Advertising & Sponsorships

Connect with an engaged audience on a powerful multimedia site, and position your message alongside expert how-to content. Dummies.com is a one-stop shop for free, online information and know-how curated by a team of experts.

- Targeted ads
- Video
- Email Marketing
- Microsites
- Sweepstakes sponsorship

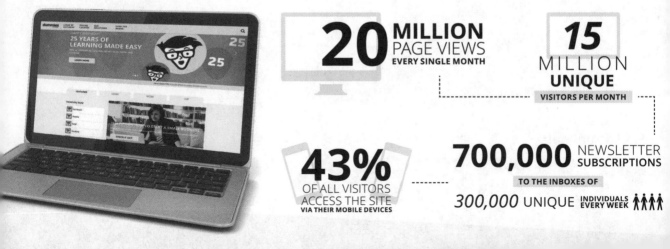

20 MILLION PAGE VIEWS EVERY SINGLE MONTH

15 MILLION UNIQUE VISITORS PER MONTH

43% OF ALL VISITORS ACCESS THE SITE VIA THEIR MOBILE DEVICES

700,000 NEWSLETTER SUBSCRIPTIONS TO THE INBOXES OF

300,000 UNIQUE INDIVIDUALS EVERY WEEK

# of dummies

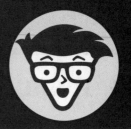

Custom Publishing

Reach a global audience in any language by creating a solution that will differentiate you from competitors, amplify your message, and encourage customers to make a buying decision.

- Apps
- Books
- eBooks
- Video
- Audio
- Webinars

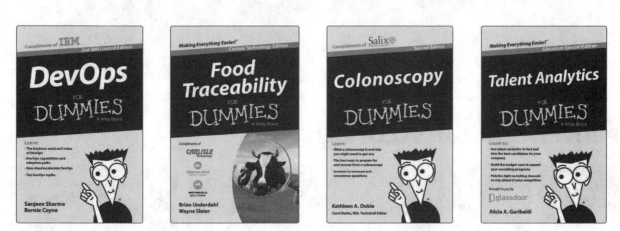

Brand Licensing & Content

Leverage the strength of the world's most popular reference brand to reach new audiences and channels of distribution.

For more information, visit dummies.com/biz

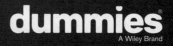

PERSONAL ENRICHMENT

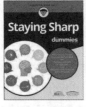 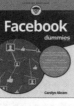 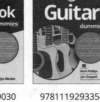 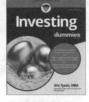 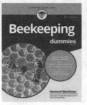

Staying Sharp	**Facebook**	**Guitar**	**Investing**	**Beekeeping**	**Digital Photography**
9781119187790	9781119179030	9781119293354	9781119293347	9781119310068	9781119235606
USA $26.00	USA $21.99	USA $24.99	USA $22.99	USA $22.99	USA $24.99
CAN $31.99	CAN $25.99	CAN $29.99	CAN $27.99	CAN $27.99	CAN $29.99
UK £19.99	UK £16.99	UK £17.99	UK £16.99	UK £16.99	UK £17.99

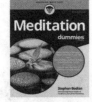 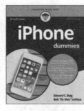 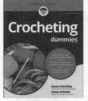

Meditation	**Pregnancy**	**Samsung Galaxy S7**	**iPhone**	**Crocheting**	**Nutrition**
9781119251163	9781119235491	9781119279952	9781119283133	9781119287117	9781119130246
USA $24.99	USA $26.99	USA $24.99	USA $24.99	USA $24.99	USA $22.99
CAN $29.99	CAN $31.99	CAN $29.99	CAN $29.99	CAN $29.99	CAN $27.99
UK £17.99	UK £19.99	UK £17.99	UK £17.99	UK £16.99	UK £16.99

PROFESSIONAL DEVELOPMENT

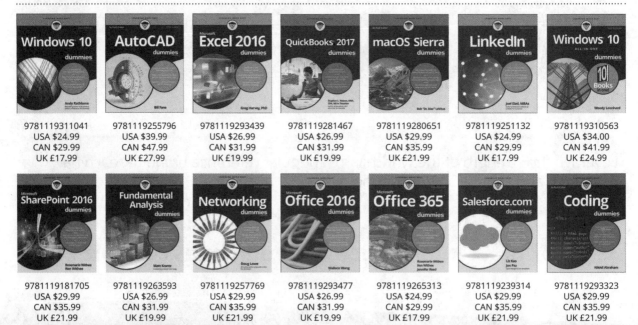

Windows 10	**AutoCAD**	**Excel 2016**	**QuickBooks 2017**	**macOS Sierra**	**LinkedIn**	**Windows 10 All-in-One**
9781119311041	9781119255796	9781119293439	9781119281467	9781119280651	9781119251132	9781119310563
USA $24.99	USA $39.99	USA $26.99	USA $26.99	USA $29.99	USA $24.99	USA $34.00
CAN $29.99	CAN $47.99	CAN $31.99	CAN $31.99	CAN $35.99	CAN $29.99	CAN $41.99
UK £17.99	UK £27.99	UK £19.99	UK £19.99	UK £21.99	UK £17.99	UK £24.99

SharePoint 2016	**Fundamental Analysis**	**Networking**	**Office 2016**	**Office 365**	**Salesforce.com**	**Coding**
9781119181705	9781119263593	9781119257769	9781119293477	9781119265313	9781119239314	9781119293323
USA $29.99	USA $26.99	USA $29.99	USA $26.99	USA $24.99	USA $29.99	USA $29.99
CAN $35.99	CAN $31.99	CAN $35.99	CAN $31.99	CAN $29.99	CAN $35.99	CAN $35.99
UK £21.99	UK £19.99	UK £21.99	UK £19.99	UK £17.99	UK £21.99	UK £21.99

dummies.com

dummies
A Wiley Brand

Learning Made Easy

ACADEMIC

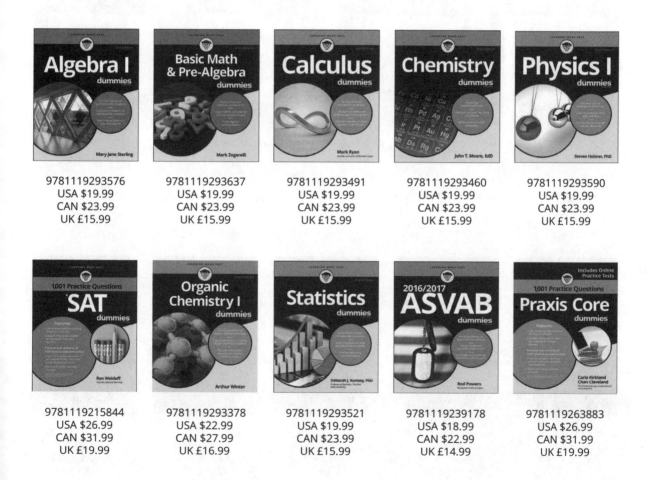

Algebra I dummies
Mary Jane Sterling
9781119293576
USA $19.99
CAN $23.99
UK £15.99

Basic Math & Pre-Algebra dummies
Mark Zegarelli
9781119293637
USA $19.99
CAN $23.99
UK £15.99

Calculus dummies
Mark Ryan
9781119293491
USA $19.99
CAN $23.99
UK £15.99

Chemistry dummies
John T. Moore, EdD
9781119293460
USA $19.99
CAN $23.99
UK £15.99

Physics I dummies
Steven Holzner, PhD
9781119293590
USA $19.99
CAN $23.99
UK £15.99

SAT dummies — 1,001 Practice Questions
Ron Woldoff
9781119215844
USA $26.99
CAN $31.99
UK £19.99

Organic Chemistry I dummies
Arthur Winter
9781119293378
USA $22.99
CAN $27.99
UK £16.99

Statistics dummies
Deborah J. Rumsey, PhD
9781119293521
USA $19.99
CAN $23.99
UK £15.99

2016/2017 ASVAB dummies
Rod Powers
9781119239178
USA $18.99
CAN $22.99
UK £14.99

Praxis Core dummies — 1,001 Practice Questions
Carla Kirkland, Chan Cleveland
9781119263883
USA $26.99
CAN $31.99
UK £19.99

Available Everywhere Books Are Sold

dummies.com

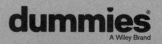

dummies®
A Wiley Brand

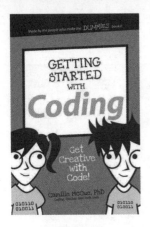
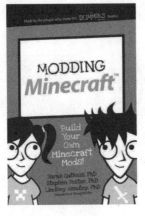
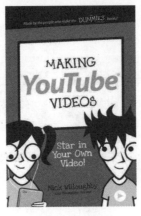
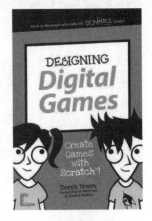
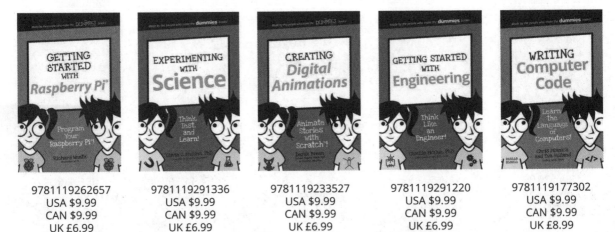
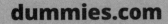
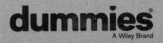